PLAY-BASED INTERVENTIONS
FOR CHILDREN AND ADOLESCENTS WITH
AUTISM SPECTRUM DISORDERS

PLAY-BASED INTERVENTIONS
FOR CHILDREN AND ADOLESCENTS WITH
AUTISM SPECTRUM DISORDERS

EDITED BY Loretta Gallo-Lopez and Lawrence C. Rubin

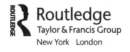

Routledge
Taylor & Francis Group
New York   London

Routledge
Taylor & Francis Group
711 Third Avenue
New York, NY 10017

Routledge
Taylor & Francis Group
2 Park Square
Milton Park, Abingdon
Oxon OX14 4RN

Printed in the United States of America on acid-free paper
Version Date: 2011912

International Standard Book Number: 978-0-415-89075-5 (Hardback)

Library of Congress Cataloging-in-Publication Data

Play-based interventions for children and adolescents with autism spectrum
    disorders / [edited by] Loretta Gallo-Lopez, Lawrence C. Rubin.
       p. ; cm.
    Includes bibliographical references and index.
    ISBN 978-0-415-89075-5 (hardback : alk. paper)
    I. Gallo-Lopez, Loretta. II. Rubin, Lawrence C., 1955-

    [DNLM: 1. Child Development Disorders, Pervasive--therapy. 2. Adolescent. 3.
    Child. 4. Play Therapy--methods. WS 350.8.P4]
    616.85'882--dc23   2011029458

Visit the Taylor & Francis Web site at
http://www.taylorandfrancis.com

and the Routledge Web site at
http://www.routledgementalhealth.com

To my children Emily and Nick, with all my love

LGL

To Randi, Zach, and Becca, my home team

LR

Contents

Foreword

If you enjoy play and strive to bring this important experience to children with autism spectrum disorders and other special needs, you will find *Play-Based Interventions for Children and Adolescents With Autism Spectrum Disorders* compelling. The authors describe the many creative forms of play, play therapy, and the pleasure of play, all of which enable children to interact socially and to learn and grow more successfully. Chapter after chapter validates the significant role of play in the lives of children, from its theoretical and biological foundations to individualized interventions that build on various sensory-motor and symbolic approaches to the creative arts. Each chapter describes common therapeutic elements, such as following the child's interests, encouraging the child's initiative, becoming and remaining connected, and interacting and communicating in the ways children choose or find meaningful for expressing their feelings, ideas, wishes, and desires. Every chapter comes to life through numerous, rich, and engaging case examples that depict play in ways that provoke new ideas, deepen clinical reflection, and provide opportunities for the clinician to integrate new learning into their current practices.

It is important for the reader of this book to put on a "developmental hat" when working through the various chapters, as they each describe very different interventions, theories, and ways to play. The ultimate goal for the reader, as it is for clients, is to climb the developmental ladder—no matter how long it takes. This is because children on the autism spectrum, like all children, will continue to develop if provided with interactive experiences tailored to their individual profiles, and this in turn leads to personal discovery. A developmental lens will further assess the building blocks of the child's developmental foundation and highlight the experiences that are needed to strengthen the capacities to reach higher levels of empathic relationships and abstract thought. In contrast to a deficit view, this approach encourages development, ever moving forward across the lifespan.

The Developmental, Individual Difference, Relationship-Based (DIR®) model, which I developed together with the late Stanley Greenspan, is one of many addressed in this book. It provides a unique integrative lens for viewing the different approaches and for considering how each supports development. First, the clinician asks which developmental capacities are being supported, including shared attention, engagement across a range of emotions, two-way communication, social problem solving, and the creation of representations and abstract and reflective thinking. One follows the child's interests or loves in order to enter his world and help him do what he intends. This helps connect and build the continuous flow of interactions that "deepen the plot" and provide increasing opportunities for problem solving and representation.

Next, the clinician asks how the child's preferences may be part of the solution she has found to express interests, feelings, and ideas in ways that can be successfully executed. If we understand solutions, we can arrive at the problem, i.e., the relative strengths and weaknesses in each child's profile. There may be a reason a child might repetitively push cars back and forth, prefer construction toys that do not fall apart, or dress up rather than use figures, to name just a few examples. These preferences might relate to the child's auditory or visual spatial sequencing and motor-planning abilities. Each child's individual sensory-motor processing and regulatory profile helps us understand how she "takes in," comprehends, and responds to the world, and this allows us to tailor our interventions to promote better comprehension. Informative questions will arise, such as "Can the child use awareness of where he is in space in order to move himself or his objects toward a purposeful destination he desires?" and "Are toys used in simple cause-and-effect, single action ways, e.g., rolled back and forth or up and down, or are they manipulated sequentially to convey an idea?"

Importantly, every author in this book emphasizes how his or her approach encourages and supports the interactions necessary to engage and deepen human involvement. Relationships embrace not only attachments and security but also the mutual regard that leads to empathy and trust. It is within these relationships that children learn to tolerate and symbolize the full range and hierarchy of emotions, from dependency to autonomy, to fears of aggression, as well as anger, jealousy, competition, loss, sadness, compassion, and finally, justice and morality.

Using play to promote symbolic capacities is another significant theme that runs throughout this book. The concept of symbols unites these varied clinical approaches, and as such, deserves some focus. Symbolic development advances as the abilities—to see, hear, and become aware through the senses—evolve into understanding and interpretation of the sensory experiences. What a child sees, hears, and does becomes visualized in her mind, and these mental images are transformed into symbols through the affect that conveys what they mean. Symbols can, then, be manipulated to enable the child to understand feelings, intentions, and ideas. Perception, in turn, becomes separated from actions and represents experience through symbols. One no longer has to have the "real thing" in order to explore ideas, think, and work through experiences: the child begins to manipulate ideas in her mind using symbols that have taken on meaning through emotional interactions.

No longer needing to see the actions to understand what they mean, how they feel, or how they might affect others allows for the development of anticipation, social judgment, and empathy. Development of both emotions and symbols expands as further interactions—which can involve movement as well as affect cues conveyed through looks and gestures—convey further meanings and feelings. Play provides the opportunity to develop symbolic capacities for all children, but it is especially important for children on the autism spectrum since they are compromised in their capacity to comprehend and internalize experiences in the form of symbols. They may find themselves imitating the actions and relying on memory, routine, and rituals to function. As their reality testing remains episodic, they have difficulty putting themselves in someone else's shoes, seeing two sides of the coin, or abstracting what is right or wrong.

Another way to consider symbolic development is from the perspective of how symbols parallel the development of emotions. From infancy, parents offer symbols to their infants at the same time that they offer themselves as agents of love and security. The cuddly blanket, sheep toy, or teddy bear becomes deeply linked to parents' smiles, which are in turn connected with the child's own smiles and feelings of being safe. These emotions eventually become associated with the attachment object when the parent is not present. As development unfolds, emotions play a greater role in developing higher levels of cognitive functioning, as seen in the creation and use of symbols. The earliest symbolic play of the year-old infant—feeding a baby doll or talking on the phone—is derived from her experience of being fed or watching Mommy or Daddy stop everything to answer a ringing phone. Trying again and again to make real use of her toys as symbolic objects, she discovers which ones are pretend and can begin moving into the symbolic world, where the pleasure is as genuine as it was with "real" things. Now she can explore space visually without needing to move through it; she is also able to understand when a toy phone is not a real phone without needing to use it. The more often her perceptions occur independently from her actions—as the process of distinguishing or testing what is real and not real develops—the faster the child will move from the real world to the symbolic world and begin to climb the symbolic ladder of emotion and cognition. Telling a child that a scary sound or idea (monster, ghost, or witch) is not real will not be helpful when emotions still dominate her perceptions and symbolic thinking has not yet evolved.

Symbols take the place of real things as children play; as they learn words, use gestures to represent objects and actions, identify pictures that tell a story, and create stories of their own using words, gestures, and toys. First, real-life experiences are enacted as children visualize what they saw, heard, did, and felt in their minds; how these experiences are enacted reflect the children's emotional and cognitive understanding. As children play different roles, we observe their internalized experience of different characters: how far and wide they venture with their imaginations; what they can find, how careful, controlling, or impulsive they are; and where their adventures lead them.

The symbols a young child chooses reflect the emotional experiences that evolve as the child moves from dependency to autonomy and develops greater mastery over her body, her environment and her thoughts. The child's choice of symbols reflects her level of emotional development and provides a window into the child's inner experience. Symbols—whether expressed with toys and words, dramatic play, or creative movement and art—may reflect positive feelings, longings, and wishes about being loved and cared for, and about security; or negative feelings of jealousy, retaliation, fears, and aggression. Symbols represent the child's ever-widening range of emotional themes—including the unpleasant, the frightening, the opposition, and the power—and follow a predictable hierarchy related to the emotional and psychological development of the child. With development, the child will abstract what is right and wrong, will understand shades of gray and the multiple causes of experience, and will develop a reflective sense of self and of how others experience her. All aspects of sensory-based knowledge, cognition, and interactive relationships combine for the child to know herself and others.

Most clearly, then, development occurs within the dynamic context of personal discovery, interpersonal relationship, and the strengthening of symbolic capacity. Each chapter in *Play-Based Interventions for Children and Adolescents With Autism Spectrum Disorders* will, in its own way, describe how these processes unfold and can be nurtured, as well as provide you with powerful opportunities to discover playful, creative, and effective means of interacting, engaging, and helping your clients. In reading this book, you will be able to better assist your clients in discovering new knowledge and interactive experiences that will form and strengthen their developmental foundation and propel them onward and upward, cognitively, emotionally, and socially.

Serena Wieder, PhD
Clinical Director, Profectum Foundation

Preface

The last two decades have seen a proliferation in the number of children and adolescents being diagnosed with autism spectrum disorders (ASD). Pervasive by definition, and affecting by some estimates 1 in 110 young people, these disorders affect social, emotional, and behavioral functioning in multiple settings including home, school, and community. Parents, teachers, and clinicians struggle to equip those with Asperger's syndrome and autism with the tools necessary to live connected, satisfying, and productive lives. To date, interventions have tended to be either medical or behavioral, with the latter emphasis focusing on interventions based on some variant of applied behavioral analysis.

Increasing attention has recently been paid to the ways play-based interventions can be effectively used to improve social, cognitive, and behavioral functioning with children and adolescents "along the spectrum." While empirical and qualitative research has begun to appear in the literature in the form of journal articles and book chapters, there is as of yet no singular or definitive volume that brings together the voices of researchers and practicing clinicians who are successfully using play and play-based interventions with this most challenging population.

The purpose of this book, therefore, is to provide counseling and psychotherapy trainees as well as practicing clinicians at all levels of experience with a resource that provides a useful integration of theory and practice with regard to the use of play and play-based interventions with children and adolescents diagnosed with ASD. Each chapter will integrate theory with real-world clinical case applications and demonstrate applicability across the wide range of settings in which mental health counselors, marriage and family therapists, school counselors, psychologists, pediatric psychiatrists, social workers, expressive arts therapists (dance/movement, music, art, drama, and play), home-based counselors, and child-care workers provide services.

The book is divided into four parts. Part I, titled "Foundations," provides a discussion of the neurobiology of play, particularly as it manifests in young clients diagnosed with ASD (Bonnie Badenoch and Nicole Bogden), an overview of the role and nature of play in "typical" and "atypical" development (Lawrence Rubin), followed by Part II, titled "Individualized Play-Based Interventions," provides a comprehensive discussion of the many ways play therapy and play-based interventions have been successfully applied to the treatment of ASD, with an emphasis, when applicable, on empirically supported treatments (EST) and evidence-based practice (EBP). Written by practicing clinicians and researchers, the chapters in this part include discussions of canine-assisted play therapy (Risë VanFleet and Cosmin Colțea), Family Theraplay (Sue Bundy-Myrow), dramatic play therapy (Loretta Gallo-Lopez), LEGO-based therapy (Daniel LeGoff, G. W. Krauss, and Sarah Allen), developmental play therapy (Janet Courtney), child-centered play therapy (Dee Ray, Jeffrey Sullivan, and Sarah Carlson), Jungian play therapy (Eric Green), filial play therapy (Risë VanFleet), and sand tray-centered play therapy (Jane Ferris Richardson). Part III, titled "Programmatic Play-Based Interventions," describes larger-scale, evidenced-based, play-centered interventions including Developmental, Individual Difference, Relationship-Based (DIR®) Floortime (Esther Hess), The PLAY Project (Richard Solomon), and the drama therapy–based ACT Project (Lisa Powers-Tricomi and Loretta Gallo-Lopez). The final part, titled "Expressive/Creative Interventions," describes the effective implementation of nonplay yet highly playful, creative, and expressive therapeutic modalities in the treatment of autism spectrum disorders. These include art therapy (Cathy Goucher), music therapy (Darcy Walworth), and dance/movement therapy (Christina Devereaux).

As you will see as you read this book, the clinicians who have shared their knowledge and experiences with us demonstrate how flexibility of thought and practice, creativity, a desire for connection, and, most importantly, playfulness can shine light into the shadows of uncertainty, rigidity, and isolation that often burden children and adolescents diagnosed with autism spectrum disorders.

Loretta Gallo-Lopez
Lawrence C. Rubin

Acknowledgments

I would like to express my respect and deep gratitude to the many children, teens, and adults with autism spectrum disorders with whom I have had the privilege of working over the past 30 years and to their dedicated, brave, and loving parents. I have learned so much from all of you about determination, perseverance, and true commitment. I also want to thank my children, Nick and Emily—my cheerleaders, my inspiration. You fill my heart with pride and joy, and you are truly the greatest treasures of my life. I am eternally grateful to my parents, Kay and Gus Gallo, who instilled in me a love of learning, a sense of compassion for others, and an appreciation of the family ties that keep us forever connected. I would like to offer many thanks to my coeditor, Larry Rubin, who patiently and tenaciously guided me through the left-brain world of book editing and was always there to support and encourage when the going got tough. And finally, a sincere thank you to my dear friend and mentor Dr. Holly Steele, who through her wisdom and good humor taught me most of what I know about connecting with and helping individuals with special needs.

Loretta Gallo-Lopez

First, I would like to acknowledge my coeditor, Loretta Gallo-Lopez, whose clinical passion and insights into the lives of children and teens on the autism spectrum have been a steady source of motivation and inspiration for me. Next, I would like to thank my wife, Randi, for her unwavering support of my scholarly and literary efforts, and my children, Zachary and Rebecca, who believe that "Dr. Daddy" has something to offer. I am deeply appreciative of all the clinicians and researchers who shared their experiences in this book, many of whom were performing cutting-edge clinical work, even during the final round of edits. My parents, Esther and Herb, ages 93 and 95, respectively, have always been in my corner, believing in me for as far back as I can remember. I am honored to contribute yet another volume to the shelves of their private Larry Rubin library. And finally, I would like to thank Anna Moore of Routledge, who recognized the importance of this book for all who work and live with ASD children and teens.

Lawrence C. Rubin

About the Editors

Loretta Gallo-Lopez, MA, LMHC, RPT-S, RDT-BCT, is a play and drama therapist and a licensed mental health counselor in private practice in Tampa, Florida. Her practice is focused on providing creative and effective interventions for children, adolescents, and families with a wide range of issues, including trauma, loss, and transitions, as well as anxiety, mood, and behavior disorders. She specializes in working with children and adolescents with autism spectrum disorders, developmental disabilities, and other special needs. She is coeditor of the book *Play Therapy With Adolescents* (Jason Aronson, Inc., 2005), has authored numerous chapters related to her work, and has been an invited national conference presenter. In 2008 Gallo-Lopez established The ACT Project, a drama therapy and performance program for children and adolescents with autism spectrum disorders and other special needs.

Lawrence C. Rubin, PhD, LMHC, RPT-S, is a professor of counselor education at St. Thomas University in Miami, Florida, where he directs the mental health counseling program and is a psychologist, mental health counselor, and play therapist in private practice. Rubin is a former president of the Florida Association for Play Therapy and currently serves on the board of directors for the Association for Play Therapy. His research interests and publications lie at the intersection of psychology and popular culture. His other books are *Diagnosis and Treatment Planning Skills for Mental Health Professionals: A Popular Casebook Approach* (Sage, 2011); *Popular Culture in Counseling, Psychotherapy, and Play-Based Intervention* (Springer, 2008); *Using Superheroes in Counseling and Play Therapy* (Springer, 2007); *Psychotropic Drugs and Popular Culture: Medicine, Mental*

Health, and the Media (McFarland, 2006) (which won the 2006 Ray and Pat Browne award for best anthology); *Food for Thought: Essays on Eating and Culture* (McFarland, 2008); *Mental Illness and Popular Media: Essays on the Representation of Psychiatric Disorders* (McFarland, 2012); and *Messages: Self-Help Through Popular Culture* (Cambridge Scholars Press, 2009).

About the Contributors

Sarah Levin Allen, PhD, earned her clinical psychology doctorate from Drexel University with a concentration in pediatric neuropsychology. Her training has included neuropsychological and psychological testing as well as cognitive-behavioral therapy for children with neurological impairments, learning disabilities, and developmental delays. She specializes in generalizing neuropsychological, learning, and social recommendations to classroom settings.

Bonnie Badenoch, PhD, LMFT, is an in-the-trenches therapist, supervisor, teacher, and author who has spent the last 7 years integrating the discoveries of neuroscience into the art of therapy. In 2008 she cofounded the nonprofit agency Nurturing the Heart with the Brain in Mind in Portland, Oregon, and was formerly the founder and executive director of the Center for Hope and Healing in Irvine, California, for 17 years. Her work as a therapist has focused on helping trauma survivors and those with significant attachment wounds reshape their neural landscape to support a life of meaning and resilience. As a mentor and supervisor of marriage and family therapist interns for the past two decades, she supports their developing mental health side by side with helping them internalize the principles of interpersonal neurobiology as a guide to evidence-based practice. She is one of the founders of the Global Association for Interpersonal Neurobiology Studies (GAINS), a nonprofit organization dedicated to fostering application of the principles of interpersonal neurobiology (IPNB) to professional and personal life, and is editor-in-chief of its quarterly publication, *Connections & Reflections*. Badenoch currently teaches at Portland State University in the IPNB certificate program and speaks internationally about applying IPNB principles both personally and professionally. Her years of studying with Daniel J. Siegel and Allan Schore, coupled with her conviction that brain wisdom can transform human relationships, led to the publication of *Being a Brain-Wise Therapist: A Practical Guide to Interpersonal Neurobiology* (Norton IPNB Series, 2008) and *The Brain-Savvy Therapist's Workbook* (Norton, 2011). Therapists say that these books fill the gap between science and practice with clarity, compassion, and heart.

Nicole Bogdan, MA, LMFT, has 15 years of experience working with children who have developmental delays. Her early training started in Peabody College at Vanderbilt University where she worked with programs in the Nashville, Tennessee, metro area helping severely physically disabled children and children with developmental delays, including those on the autistic spectrum. Bodgan obtained further training working with children with developmental delays and autism in Southern California while obtaining a master's in clinical psychology from Pepperdine University. Her training and experience consisted of using relationally based interventions such as Greenspan's Developmental, Individual Difference, Relationship-Based (DIR®) model to work in the home, school, and social environment with children who have Asperger's and varying degrees of autism. Bogdan used this mode of treatment in play therapy sessions and facilitated play groups and became experienced with using facilitated communication (FC) with autistic children and adults who are nonverbal. She has had success at helping these individuals be able to express themselves after years of not being able to successfully communicate with others. In addition to her private practice in Irvine, California, she works for a nonprofit agency in Long Beach that is contracted with the U.S. Department of Mental Health to provide child development assessments and therapeutic services to at-risk children and their families.

Susan Bundy-Myrow, PhD, RPT-S, is a licensed psychologist in private practice, an autism consultant, and Certified Professor of Child Psychotherapists and Play Therapists (IBECPT-P). As an affiliate trainer of the Theraplay Institute, Bundy-Myrow has helped to bring Theraplay to professionals around the world and has developed a model for multiple family group Theraplay for children with autism. Together with David Myrow, she is a recipient of the 2011 Ann M. Jernberg Theraplay Award. As a clinical assistant professor at the State University of New York at Buffalo, Bundy-Myrow also teaches child and play therapy approaches to psychiatric residents.

Sarah E. Carlson, MA, LPC-Intern, is doctoral candidate in the counseling program at the University of North Texas specializing in play therapy and school counseling. Her clinical work focuses on the implementation of child-centered play therapy in schools with both children and teachers.

Cosmin Colţea, MA, has been training both dogs and their owners since 1991. He has bred and shown dogs in both conformation shows and in trials. In 2011, he received a master of arts in developmental psychology from Carleton University. His area of research, to be continued during his PhD, gravitates toward the relationships between families and their companion dogs. More specifically, Colţea is interested in the interactions between children with autism spectrum disorders (ASD) and their companion dogs, as well as the effects of companion dogs on parents of children with ASD. Currently, he combines his research and his experience in dog-training to develop programs designed to enhance the well-being of children with ASD and their families. In 2011, his dog communication program for children with ASD received an award for social innovation.

Janet A. Courtney, PhD, LCSW, RPT-S, is the director of Developmental Play & Attachment Therapies, a center in Palm Beach Gardens, Florida, established to promote more conscious and connected relationships among parents, caregivers, and children. Since 1998, Courtney has taught a variety of advanced practice courses as an adjunct professor at Barry University School of Social Work in Miami Shores, Florida. She has held the positions of president, vice president, and immediate past president with the Florida Association for Play Therapy (FAPT) from 1998 to 2008. She resides as the chair of the Viola Brody Committee through FAPT and is a member of the FAPT annual conference committee. She lectures nationally and internationally on the topic of developmental play therapy, art play therapy, family play therapy, eco-psychology, and Gestalt therapy. Courtney has acted as a consultant to several Florida-based children's agencies and supervises clinicians seeking Florida board licensure as well as those seeking certification as a registered play therapist with the Association for Play Therapy (APT).

Christina Devereaux, PhD, LCAT, LMHC, BC-DMT, NCC, is a board-certified dance/movement therapist. She received her doctorate in clinical psychology with a specialty in prenatal and perinatal psychology and currently serves as an assistant professor and director of clinical training in the dance/movement therapy (DMT) and counseling program at Antioch University New England and as an adjunct assistant professor at Pratt Institute in the Department of Creative Arts Therapy. In addition, she is supporting the development of Inspirees, a DMT-training program, in China as a senior trainer. Devereaux's research has focused on the early interactive experiences between mothers and their infant children who were later diagnosed with autism. She has extensive clinical experience with a variety of populations, including children with severe emotional disturbance and with pervasive developmental disorders, those with physical disabilities, victims of abuse and neglect, families in crisis, adults with mental illness and dual diagnosis, and supporting healthy attachment with mother–infant dyads. Devereaux currently serves as spokesperson for the American Dance Therapy Association (ADTA) and on the editorial board for the *American Journal of Dance Therapy*. She has presented nationally and internationally on topics such as the dance of attachment relationships, dance/movement therapy with autism, trauma and the body, and clinical writing. Further, she has published articles in the *American Journal of Dance Therapy* and the *Journal of Dance Education* and has been featured on the radio.

Cathy Goucher, MA, ATR-BC, LCPC, is a registered, board-certified art therapist and is a licensed clinical professional counselor in the state of Maryland. Goucher specializes in the treatment of adolescents and young adults with developmental disabilities and autism spectrum disorders (ASD). She is a graduate of the art therapy graduate degree program at George Washington University, one of the oldest art therapy programs in the country. She has over 14 years of clinical experience as an art therapist. Goucher currently works per diem at The Retreat at Sheppard Pratt, a premier self-funded psychiatric setting, and full-time as an art therapist at St. Elizabeth School in Baltimore, where she works with adolescents and young adults with multiple disabilities, including ASD. She also maintains a small private practice, providing in-home art therapy services to home-schooled ASD clients. Most recently, she has cofounded a nonprofit organization, Make Studio Art Program, Inc., the mission of which is to provide professional-grade work space, psychosocial supports, and sales opportunities for emerging adult artists with disabilities in Baltimore.

Eric J. Green, PhD, RPT-S, is an assistant professor of counseling and director of the counseling clinic at the University of North Texas at Dallas. He maintains a part-time private practice in child and family psychotherapy. Green is a member of the Jung Society of North Texas. He actively presents his research and clinical work on Jungian play therapy with children at peer-reviewed conferences and invited workshops across the United States.

Esther Hess, PhD, RPT-S, is a developmental psychologist who specializes in the assessment, diagnosis, and treatment of children with developmental delays, specifically autism, Asperger's disorder, and pervasive developmental disorder—not otherwise specified (PDD–NOS). Her expertise is in the use and application of a developmentally based psychotherapy—the Developmental, Individual Difference, Relationship-Based

(DIR®) model—devised by Stanley Greenspan. In addition to working with the impacted person, Hess interfaces with the entire family and coordinates the efforts of various members of team specialists who assist in boosting the impacted individual's developmental lag. She is certified in DIR/Floortime™ and has trained parents, interventionists, and clinicians throughout the United States in the developmental/relational method known as Floortime. Hess is the founder and executive director of Center for the Developing Mind, a multidisciplinary treatment facility for children, adolescents, and young adults impacted by developmental delays or regulatory disorders in West Los Angeles.

G. W. Krauss, PsyD, earned his doctorate in clinical psychology at Widener University with a specialization in neuropsychology. He previously studied community psychology at the University of Alaska. Krauss's internship years were spent working with children, adolescents, and young adults with Asperger's disorder and other social competence issues, including evaluations and individual and group therapy (Dr. Dan's LEGO therapy). He has previously worked with other clinical populations, including those with severe mental illness, forensic clients, and trauma/abuse issues.

Daniel B. LeGoff ("Dr. Dan"), PhD, is a child psychologist and developmental neuropsychologist who has been specializing in the assessment and treatment of neurodevelopmental conditions in infants, children, and adolescents for the past 24 years. His training and clinical experience have included specializations in neuropsychological assessments, functional behavioral assessments, school consultation, cognitive–behavioral and behavioral therapies, play therapy, and family therapy. LeGoff is perhaps best known for his work with LEGOs as a therapy medium for improving social development. He has collaborated on research for this therapy method with Simon Baron-Cohen and the Autism Research Centre at Cambridge University and Gina Gomez of the National Autism Service in the United Kingdom. More recently, LeGoff has also been collaborating with the Innovations and Education Divisions of LEGO Corp. in Denmark and England.

Dee C. Ray, PhD, LPC-S, NCC, RPT-S, is an associate professor in the counseling program and director of the Child and Family Resource Clinic at the University of North Texas. Ray has published over 40 articles, chapters, and books in the field of play therapy and over 15 research publications specifically examining the effects of child-centered play therapy. She is author of *Advanced Play Therapy: Essential Conditions, Knowledge, and Skills for Child Practice* (Routledge, 2011) and *Child-Centered Play Therapy Treatment Manual* (Self Esteem Shop, 2009), coeditor of *Child-Centered*

Play Therapy Research (Wiley, 2010), and former editor of the *International Journal of Play Therapy.*

Jane Ferris Richardson, LMHC, EdD, ATR-BC, is a registered play therapist and supervisor, a board-certified art therapist, and an art therapy educator at Lesley University, where she is a core faculty member. She holds an EdD from Boston University, where she was the managing editor of the *Journal of Education.* Her current research is focused on the use of expressive and play-based approaches to therapy for children with autism. This work has been inspired by the educational practices of Reggio Emilia and the idea of "100 Languages" for communication and understanding. She has a private practice working with children and families. Richardson has presented her work nationally and internationally. Most recently she shared Sandtray Worldplay with preschool educators in Khyalitsha Township in Cape Town, South Africa. She has also worked with creative arts therapists in Beijing, China, where she collaborated with creative arts therapists practicing there. Richardson is interested in international approaches to play and art therapy.

Richard Solomon, MD, is a medical director at the Ann Arbor Center for Developmental and Behavioral Pediatrics and an adjunct clinical associate professor at the University of Michigan. He is board-certified in pediatrics and developmental and behavioral pediatrics with special interests in the prevention of child abuse and community violence, pediatric pain management, and early intervention for children with autism. In 2000, while at the University of Michigan, he developed a community-based statewide training and early intervention project for young children with autism called The PLAY Project. The PLAY Project's train-the-trainer model coaches parents to provide intensive developmental intervention for their young children with autism. In the last 5 years, since leaving the university, the PLAY Project has expanded to become a national model. In 2007, an article that evaluated the PLAY Project was accepted for publication in the peer-reviewed journal *Autism*. In 2009 Solomon received a National Institute of Mental Health (NIMH) grant—a randomized, controlled trial—in collaboration with Easter Seals National and Michigan State University to study the project's effectiveness.

Jeffrey M. Sullivan, MS, NCC, LPC, is a doctoral candidate at the University of North Texas. His current focus lies in researching and providing child-centered play therapy for children on the autistic spectrum. His research addresses the extent to which teaching parents of children with high-functioning autism, Asperger's disorder, and pervasive developmental disorder—not otherwise specified (PDD–NOS) the skills of child-centered play therapy addresses and improves the child–parent relationship.

Lisa Powers Tricomi, MA, RDT-BCT, LCAT, is a practicing theater artist, drama therapist, and educator. While teaching theater performance as a visiting associate professor in the University of South Florida's College of the Arts, Tricomi has had the opportunity to introduce drama therapy to theater students through the ACT Project while working with children and adolescents diagnosed with autism spectrum disorders (ASD). Along with Gallo-Lopez, Tricomi presented the ACT Project at the NADT Conference and the Expressive Therapies Summit in 2010.

Risë VanFleet, PhD, is president of the Family Enhancement & Play Therapy Center in Boiling Springs, Pennsylvania, through which she trains and supervises clinicians in play therapy, filial therapy, and animal-assisted play therapy. She is a licensed psychologist, registered play therapist and supervisor, and certified dog behavior consultant with over 35 years of experience. VanFleet is the author of dozens of books, manuals, chapters, and articles on play therapy, filial therapy, and canine-related topics, and is featured on several DVDs. She has received several national awards—three recognizing her training programs and five for her professional writing. She has trained thousands of professionals internationally. VanFleet is the founder of the International Collaborative on Play Therapy and is past board chair of the Association for Play Therapy.

Darcy Walworth, PhD, MT-BC, directs the music therapy program at the University of Louisville and previously taught at Florida State University. She actively researches the effects of music therapy in medical and early childhood settings with emphases in medical procedural support, autism treatment, and developmental outcomes of premature infants. She has coauthored and contributed chapters to multiple books addressing varying client populations. Walworth has presented papers at regional, national, and international conferences and currently serves on the board of directors of the Certification Board for Music Therapists and the editorial board for the *Journal of Music Therapy*.

PART I

Foundations

Safety and Connection
The Neurobiology of Play

BONNIE BADENOCH AND NICOLE BOGDAN

Picturing the Brain With Bonnie Badenoch

The teacher leads the boy to the mat. He takes off his shoes. Then he takes off his socks. He begins walking a circle around the outer edge of the mat. I watch him closely and quietly. He lifts his elbows, pressing his thumbs rhythmically into his ears. He utters a stream of vowels and light consonants. I listen, feel the resonance of his sound in my body, and join him exploring the same sounds with my own throat and breathing. Then I lie down in the center of the mat on my back, the boy walking around me, occasionally peering down at me from the corner of his eye. I don't know why I lay down this way. I question it for a moment, but somehow it feels right. As the boy circles me, slowly his orbit comes closer. I gently extend my hand and follow his curving path. The next time around he lightly encircles my fingers with his and continues circling, but a little slower now. Then he comes right in and stands on my chest, holding both of my hands and looking down at me. I breathe. He rises and falls. I begin making sound with my breath. *Ha*s and *ho*s and *oo*s. Suddenly laughter bursts from me. His feet and knees soften, his toes grip my chest. He begins to bounce on my breath and my laugh. He watches me closer. Then he returns to his circling walk, still lightly holding my hand. Then right back on my chest, making his own sounds while bouncing gently. The two of us exchanging sound through his feet. A moment later he curls down into my lap. I sit up and wrap around him closely. He pushes his head into the crook of my elbow. I mirror the intensity of his curling and pushing with the pressure and firmness of my touch. After several cycles of nuzzling, curling in, and pushing, he relaxes, looks me clearly in the face, and we begin a round of squirming, close in, gentle play, scooching around the mat, swirling close around, over and under each other. Then he settles down against my body, gently touching my arm, my face, the back of my head. Then, clear as a bell, we're done playing. He gets up, puts his socks and shoes on, and returns to class with his teacher. Usually, this boy does not want to leave the play mat and will collapse in a slithering pile, but today he goes easily, calmly. Later, the teacher tells me that this boy had been having a tough morning. He was agitated and was being aggressive with his body and his touch. Walking to the play session, the boy repeatedly reached over to the teacher, pinching and scratching him. After the play session, the teacher reported that they walked quietly back to class, the boy reaching over to gently touch the teacher's arm and hold his hand. (M. Otto, personal communication, February 19, 2011)

It seems fitting to begin our exploration with the *experience* of pure play, even though these activities differ from what we usually think of as play therapy. Marc Otto and his wife, Melanya Helene, play with the children of Portland, Oregon*—including those on the autistic spectrum, like this young man. What do we see here? A child who enters the play space in a state of disconnection, lingering in his private world of agitation and discomfort, gradually coming forward into the invitation that Marc offers, one that is full of safety, interpersonal warmth, and resonance with this young boy's state every step of the way. In these few moments of play, this youngster moves from being dominated by his nervous system and emotional circuitry being in severe dysregulation to clear signs that both the social and regulatory systems in his brain are online and in the lead. As a result, he is able to flow back into his school day in a warm and connected way.

What do we know about the neurobiology of play that will help us understand this transformative shift? We can begin with the work of Jaak Panksepp (1998, 2008), a neuroscientist devoted to the study of the brain's

---

* Their nonprofit organization, The Center for the Art and Science of Attunement (formerly Play After Play), presents child-centered theater events followed by free play with parents and children. They are also invited into schools to work with classes and individual students who are having difficulties with emotional regulation, regardless of the cause.

motivational circuitry. Spending time with animals first and then children, he discovered seven flows of energy and information that are part of our genetic inheritance, all of them lying deep within the limbic region of the brain. Social creatures that we and our mammal compatriots are, the functions of these circuits all have to do with maintaining or regaining connection with one another. In childhood, six of the seven are present from the beginning of life. Three are available when we feel safe, comfortable, and connected—the seeking system (curiosity and exploration), the care and bonding system (attachment and empathy), and the play system (the free-flowing, full-bodied, uninhibited expression of joy). While one or another of these systems may be in the lead, they often blend in the richness of the space between two people. The other three flows of motivation manifest when we fall out of connection—fear, separation panic, and rage. They seem to be intended to signal so much distress that someone will read the need in our face, voice, and body and will feel moved to come to our aid through reconnecting with us. The joyous news about this is that we don't need to teach children to play but instead need to remove the obstacles so that the natural capacity can emerge.

In the actions of the previously described young boy, we can see some fear and rage in his exchange with his teacher on the way to the play mat, signs of him experiencing disconnection. As he comes into the room, Marc prepares a safe place for him—quiet, resonant with his state, moving in tandem with his need of the moment. This youngster is then able to gradually flow into sufficient connection to engage with Marc and then with his teacher. We intuitively sense that there is a link between safety and the capacity to move smoothly into sustained relationship. The neurobiology bears this out in a very clear way.

How do we know we are safe, and how does this increase our ability to connect? Stephen Porges's (2004, 2009b, 2011) work on the three branches of the autonomic nervous system (ANS) gives us clarity about the differences for our embodied and relational brain between the experience of a state of danger and a state of safety. We are using the term *embodied and relational brain* to keep our awareness on how the brain is not isolated in the head but instead is distributed throughout our bodies—in the muscles, gut, heart, nervous system, and skull brain and how the neural firing patterns in our brains are continually influenced by and influencing of the firing patterns in others' brains (Iacoboni, 2009). If my gut is in a knot, my skull brain senses threat. If I am in the presence of someone who is anxious, my nervous system will resonate to a greater or lesser degree with his or her anxiety. Keeping these close connections in mind can help us sense how we can enter this embodied and relational system at many levels to help stabilize another person's embodied experience as well as their interpersonal connectedness.

How do we know whether we are safe or in danger? Porges uses the word *neuroception* to mark the distinction between our conscious perception of danger or safety and our sense, often below the level of conscious awareness, of these states. We may find ourselves wanting to leave or actually leaving a room for no reason we can easily articulate, in response to a neuroception of threat, for example, or we may settle easily into our chair with a warm smile as we neuroceive safety. Each person's threshold for danger is different and also varies from day to day or moment to moment, depending on circumstances and which circuits in his or her brain are being activated. An example may clarify how these variations occur. In the presence of someone who reminds me of my delightful old grandmother, the memory circuits of being with her will be activated, leading to a low threshold for danger in this moment. However, when someone who reminds me of my critical father enters the room, those memory circuits will activate, putting me in touch with a pervasive sense of danger that radiates through this current situation. So safety and degrees of danger are always moving targets responding to both the interpersonal situation and the neural activations in our brains.

What is happening neurobiologically as we neuroceive the presence or absence of safety? The ANS has three branches that operate hierarchically, meaning that when we can no longer sustain one, the next one comes online: These are the ventral vagal parasympathetic (safety), the sympathetic (danger), and the dorsal vagal parasympathetic (life threat). The ANS does not operate alone but works together with circuits that recognize faces, assess intention, rapidly assess threat, and carry emotionally relevant information from the body to the limbic region (Adolphs, 2002; Critchley, 2005; Morris, Ohman, & Dolan, 1999; Winston, Strange, O'Doherty, & Dolan, 2002). Together, these are the very circuits that allow us to sense safety or danger in our world. As attachment-seeking human beings, our nervous system's preferred way of finding and maintaining safety is through connection with others. As a result, the first system in the hierarchy is the ventral vagal parasympathetic, a circuit that allows us to be still and stay engaged at the same time, a central requirement for sustained interpersonal connection—what Stephen Porges (1998) calls "love without fear" (p. 849). This circuit slows the heart (the vagal brake), decreases our fight–flight response, and reduces the stress hormone cortisol (Porges, 2009b). In short, it prevents the sympathetic branch from taking over.

Two people in this state can coregulate one another, even in stressful situations, largely because in the course of mammalian evolution the ventral vagus became integrated with the circuits that control the muscles of the face and head. These neural pathways govern eye gaze, prosody of the voice, ability to listen, and facial expression—in short, many of the nonverbal ways we invite connection with one another (Porges, 2009a). A calmly beating heart and relaxed yet animated face signals our readiness to engage. This calm, safe state rests at the foundation of all interpersonal connectedness, as we saw with the young boy at the beginning of this chapter.

Many children on the autistic spectrum find themselves without regular access to their ventral vagal circuitry for reasons we will explore below. Instead, they may be burdened with nervous systems that regularly respond to experiences we might perceive as neutral with a neuroception of danger or death threat, resulting in a move into one of the other two branches of the ANS. When our connection with others is insufficient to maintain a neuroception of safety, the sympathetic nervous system (SNS) takes over, telling us to fight or flee. In a state of safety, we can experience fluctuating levels of sympathetic arousal that support an active pursuit of attachment, curiosity, play, and other joyful quests. However, as our neuroception shifts from an assessment of safety to danger, the ventral vagal brake on the heart is removed, and the SNS is free to activate more fully to prepare us to defend ourselves (Porges, 2007). Our heart rate increases, the chemicals we need for action are released, and other metabolic shifts that prepare us for fight or flight unfold in our embodied brain. Most crucially, in the interests of survival, the circuits that connect us with others go offline so that we can focus on the threat, and, as a result, our capacity to take in new information is dramatically reduced. This means that others will not be able to regulate us until our neuroception of safety begins to be restored. This particular aspect of ANS functioning is vital information for therapists.

The third branch of the ANS, the dorsal vagal parasympathetic, comes online when we neuroceive even more dire circumstances—helplessness, which our embodied brains interpret as life threat. This shift reduces our heart rate, stops digestion, and shuts down other metabolic systems to move into death-feigning behavior—a freeze state that may be marked by dissociation or a collapse into stillness (Porges, 2007). Our bodies release endorphins to ensure a less painful death, as our entire organism prepares to die. Under extreme traumatic conditions, the SNS may not turn off completely as the dorsal vagal comes online, creating a state of extreme physiological stress akin to the strain on a car that results from revving the gas and slamming on the brakes at the same time. These two opposing processes produce an embodied state that is difficult to capture in words but might be partially described as a state of unmoving, wordless terror, or dissociated agitation. Perhaps some pictures of children on the autistic spectrum come to mind as we see them shift through their experience of all three branches of the ANS.

We can perhaps begin to sense that play and interpersonal connection work as a synergistic system so that play becomes more available when we feel connected and safe, with our ANS in that ventral vagal state, and once playing we are more able to sustain the interpersonal relationship. The potential for building the brain circuitry of bodily and emotional regulation, attuned communication, empathy, and fear reduction resides in these resonant states of connection (Schore, 2009; Siegel & Hartzell, 2003). The relational circuitry and the neural connections that provide for regulation both lie in the right hemisphere. They join the limbic region that monitors our internal and external environment for safety with the circuits in the prefrontal cortex that calm the limbic region and integrate information to slow our responses. As these circuits become woven together, we can more easily know our own inner state and sense the inner state of others, but only when we are having a neuroception of safety. The question for some children on the autistic spectrum is not whether they are able to use a safe space to bring their ANS into ventral vagal activity and their regulatory circuits online (we have seen that in the example of Marc's time with his young playmate), but whether these experiences are able to help the neural circuitry become woven together for long-term gains.

How can the new discoveries about the neurobiology of autism help us illuminate this question? While there are many avenues being explored to help us understand the brains of children on the autistic spectrum, we are going to focus on one strand that highlights difficulties in neural integration, since the degree to which our wiring functions in a connected, coherent way has everything to do with the quality of our lives in terms of relational goodness, mental coherence, and well-being (Siegel, 1999, 2006). We can think in terms of vertical integration that connects the regulatory circuits in the right hemisphere that we talked about before and bilateral integration that connects right and left hemispheres, allowing us to be aware of and tell the story of our internal world. As we will see, separation of these circuits contributes powerfully to the difficulties experienced by children on the autistic spectrum.

For children who are on the continuum of developmental differences that includes both autism and Asperger's syndrome, one substantial puzzle is the variability of symptoms, and particularly the difference in severity of symptoms within a given person. What might account for this? Michael Merzenich, a neuroscientist and leading student of neuroplasticity (the brain's capacity to change its wiring), has drawn together several pieces of the puzzle. He began to look for clues in the brain's remarkable plasticity right after birth to see what factors account for the opening and closing of critical periods of learning. Of the nerve growth factors, brain-derived neurotrophic factor (BDNF) seemed a likely candidate for difficulties because it reinforces new synaptic connections made during the critical period (Doidge, 2007). When we have an experience, neurons fire together and wire together, creating neural nets that hold memory and learning, emotional and relational, as well as cognitive. During the critical period, BDNF is released to consolidate the new synaptic connections so they will reliably fire together in the future. BDNF also promotes the growth of myelin, the white sheath that surrounds the axon, further stabilizing the new synaptic connections. During the critical period in infancy, BDNF also turns on the nucleus basalis, a part of the brain that automatically focuses attention, and "keeps it on throughout the entire critical period" (Doidge, p. 80). During this period, we learn effortlessly, with a flow of neural changes that are then stabilized by BDNF. Then, as the key pathways are completed, there is a need for decreased plasticity and increased stability, so a stronger release of BDNF shuts down the critical period. After that, the nucleus basalis only turns on "when something important, surprising, or novel occurs, or if we make the effort to pay close attention" (Doidge, p. 80).

With that basic process in mind, we now come to the part of the story that can help us see what happens differently in the brains of children who develop autism. One of the most important aspects of critical period plasticity is brain map differentiation. At birth, our brains are somewhat crude instruments, with large parts of the relevant section of the brain firing in response to a given experience. However, with repeated experience, the cortex becomes refined in its responses, using fewer and fewer neurons to respond to any familiar event. If we take the example of the auditory cortex, at the beginning of the critical period, large parts of the cortex fire in response to a single note, but with many experiences that note activates only a few neurons, producing a much more manageable degree of neural firing—and less brain noise.

Based on these understandings and reinforced by experiments with mice, Merzenich developed a theory suggesting that the widespread but unevenly distributed differences in children on the autistic spectrum may result, in part, from a genetic vulnerability that makes some but not other groups of neurons become overexcited when they are exposed to all the new experiences of infancy. In response to this neural activity, there is an excessive release of BDNF that first reinforces all connections rather than just the important ones and then prematurely ends the critical period before cortical brain maps have become adequately defined (Zhang, Bao, & Merzenich, 2002). This lack of differentiation would likely make the brain overfire in the presence of many kinds of incoming information, leading to possible patches of sensitivity to touch, sound, and sight as well as difficulty in modulating the intensity of relationships and organizing language learning. We might imagine that this is a frightening experience that would keep children in a state of sympathetic activation much of the time. For individual children, there may be more or less differentiation in various brain regions, leading to the variability in the degree of struggle in different aspects of development and different levels of fear when engaging in that activity.

While this is just one strand in Merzenich's research relating to the origins of autism, it correlates well with other discoveries about the brain. As we said already, the key to a well-functioning brain that supports a coherent mind and empathic relationships is the degree of neural integration (Siegel, 1999). However, before circuits can link, there must be adequate differentiation in the various regions of the brain. According to Merzenich's line of thought, this is precisely the step that gets short-circuited by the early foreclosure of the critical period. The circuits never differentiate sufficiently to allow for overall integration between brain regions. Instead, the individual circuits continue to overfire, stressing the system into a neuroception of danger, which then makes it harder to connect with others for regulation. For many children, even the core social circuits have not differentiated well, so the flood of relational information neurotypical children synthesize and process in microseconds, because of the overall integration of their circuitry, has to be gathered piece by piece and assembled by hand—the difference between computer calculations and doing math on an abacus. Instead of flows across the brain, these children have isolated silos that they struggle to connect.

This lack of differentiation has led Merzenich to wonder about the possibility of reopening the critical period, allowing children to revisit the era of effortless neuroplastic change so that brain maps can be adequately differentiated in preparation for integration. We know that brains are complex systems that are constantly seeking as much movement toward coherence and connection as possible, so simply starting this integrative process might lead to ongoing change in other brain circuits. There is one tantalizing bit of anecdotal information about this. Using a program with children with autism that was originally designed for young people with lesser learning challenges, Merzenich and his colleagues have seen instances where improvements in language (the targeted aspect of learning) were also accompanied by unexpected increases in social engagement for these youngsters (Doidge, 2007).

Porges's (2007) work with the ANS has also led him to think about how to help children with autism move from sympathetic to ventral vagal activation because, once there, the other brain circuits of social engagement naturally emerge. The Listening Project (Porges, 2008), based on Porges's work, employs five 45-minute listening sessions while children are engaged in free play in a setting designed to amplify the possibility of their neuroception of safety. They wear headphones, listening to various kinds of acoustic stimulation that is filtered to have a frequency similar to the human voice (a range that their undifferentiated auditory cortex may have difficulty picking out from the noisy world around them). If we can hear the modulated voices of those around us, our entire nervous system seeks to orient toward that safety. Listening in this range stimulates the ventral vagus nerve directly, and social engagement emerges as a matter of course. We humans are designed to flow into connection with one another, and our brains are always seeking greater integration. These are powerful allies in our work to help the brains of children on the autistic spectrum find connections between these crucial brain regions. In films of the Listening Project process, we see children move from frozen-faced inattention to joyous, smiling engagement with others in the midst of play. Additional study is ongoing to see how these gains can increasingly be amplified and sustained over longer periods of time. The best news is that this intervention shows that these circuits can be activated, so the relational difficulty is most likely not a function of missing or impaired circuitry but one of connectivity between the parts. Again, this is crucial information for therapists because our calm, attuned presence is the most powerful agent of neural integration.

Because of the close neurobiological connection among the circuitry of safety, play, and interpersonal connection, children on the autistic spectrum may find much benefit in conditions that bring these three together. For the remainder of our chapter, we will be spending time in the playroom to experience these principles in practice.

In the Playroom With Nicole Bogdan

The close connection among safety, play, and enriching interpersonal connection suggests that creating the safest possible environment from the first play session is always a primary concern. The more we can hold these particular children in our minds with clarity and warmth, the more we provide the underpinnings for the resonant experience that invites them into that ventral vagal space. The initial assessment period can help us gain a sense of the children before they arrive. Through the family interview, we can begin to determine the degree and quality of delay and functioning. The play techniques and style of interaction we therapists promote will be influenced by the level of overall functioning of the children and, in particular, by their speaking capacity. Children on the autistic spectrum range from being highly verbal and expressive to having very limited verbal skills, so they must rely on alternative means of communication such as computers or other facilitated communication devices. Using these devices during a play therapy session allows them to communicate their needs and wants during the play so they can be joined, acknowledged, and encouraged.

This initial assessment can also allow us to gain a sense of these children's sensory integration capacity. In what areas are they showing sensitivity—sound, light, textures, touch? What are these sensitivities like? I have found that many children have highly sensitized auditory channels, so they hear sounds from a distance and have a hard time filtering the noises, sounds, and vibrations in their immediate and extended environment, as Merzenich's and Porges's research would suggest. Others may have difficulty with fluorescent light, finding the brightness highly dysregulating. Textures and certain intensities of touch can exceed children's window of tolerance for sensory stimulation, leading to physical and emotional agitation, whereas others calm to the deep pressure of a toy or sand on their bodies. It is important to find out about certain tics or body and vocal movements they use for self-stimulation when they are experiencing sensory dysregulation so that we can accommodate these as part of the child's well-developed repertoire for self-regulation. As we are able to meet each child in the world he or she inhabits, we have a much better chance of creating the safe environment that facilitates interpersonally rich play.

Some of these young ones also have toys that they favor, fixating on them as a means of regulating themselves, particularly in an unfamiliar environment. By using this single focus as a way to limit the amount of new information they are taking in, it is likely that their brains are somewhat "less noisy" and frightening for them. This rigidity is both a sign of fear and a means of trying to ameliorate that fear. While ultimately we want to woo them away from this single focus, initially it can also provide a place of joining in what is a safer space for them.

Since the core deficits of these children are their inability or difficulty in engaging with others, showing appropriate affect, expressing thoughts and feelings, and understanding and applying the typical "rules of play," establishing the initial connection is the essential element of play therapy. Initially, this can be difficult; however, having internalized as much about these children as possible, we have a better chance of creating an environment in which they will experience safety and resonance from the beginning. Using exaggerated affect can help these children begin to see how emotion is expressed on the face, in the voice, and in the body, as long as the intensity stays within their safe range. Such a rich, affective drama may captivate these children and increase interest in the play.

When children direct the play for the most part, there is less chance of sympathetic activation than if the adult takes over, so this is an important component of maintaining the safety required for the limbic play circuitry and social circuits to come online. In addition to feeling trusted and respected, the children have the sense of being able to flow with their free play movements without interruption. In this way, they guide the therapist to a topic or play idea of interest, and then the therapist can follow.

In the big picture, the goal is to provide an environment that fosters the child and therapist remaining in engagement for the longest time possible. Our calmness with the flow of connection–disconnection–reconnection, rather than becoming anxious or overworking to bring the children back quickly, maintains the atmosphere of quiet acceptance and certainty that they are doing what they need to do in the moment. This creates a wide ventral vagal space within us that is a constant invitation for the children to come home to safety and to play.

Let me share two stories about interactions that unfolded according to these principles of safety, play, and connection. The first talks about our play over time, and the second describes a single session in the midst of the therapy. I spent about 2 years working with a 6-year-old boy who was considered to be high functioning on the autistic spectrum. His primary struggle was with integration of the regulatory circuits in his right hemisphere, manifesting as strongly heightened anxiety and rigid routines. When we started, he sought his "safe toys" and security object in every play session. Although he was highly verbal, expressive, and functioning at grade level academically, he struggled to expand his play ideas to include varied expressions of emotion, changes of scenario, and shared control of the storyline with anyone else. After seeing how easily he became severely dysregulated at the slightest change or frustration, I became aware of the importance of these controls for him at this stage of his neural development.

From then on, we used his safe mode of play to expand his expression of emotional wants and needs rather than trying to shift the way he was playing. Through use of his favored dolls, he was eventually able to conceptualize emotions and the idea that these dolls could have varied emotional expressions based on their interactions with each other and their environment. It seemed as though we were refining his social circuitry in a way that he might be able to include others in his emotional awareness, too. After a year of play sessions, he had created his own word code for certain feelings. For example, he called his happy feeling *dolly-lamas,* and he would use this reference when he was at play with same-aged peers in a school or social setting. Even though his peers did not always understand the meaning of the reference, he was blossoming in his connection to others because he had been able to identify emotions in himself. Soon it became a fun game with his peers as they became fascinated with manipulating vocabulary to create language for feelings. All of this was quite an achievement for a child who at the outset was unable to leave his play area with his lined-up toys and his rigid routine of solitary play with them.

I want to invite you into part of a session with Jamie from about 9 months into our therapy. Prior to this session, I had heard from her father that she was experiencing some rage at home and sometimes directing it toward her younger brother. As I went into the waiting room, I saw Jamie pacing anxiously with her fists full of her favorite plastic figurines. These toys were actually characters from her favorite TV show. Her eyes were on the floor, avoiding contact as I approached. Without any context or formal greeting, she immediately plunged into telling me a story about her figurines that was a continuation of a story she had started the week before. I calmly watched her, my eyes available for direct contact when she was ready, quietly narrating and validating the tale she was telling me. After 5 or 6 minutes of this, her eyes gradually glanced up and then locked with mine. A smile-like change shaped her face as she stopped her story and blurted out a remark about the bright pattern on my shirt. With this redirected focus, we were engaged, connecting over something that had to do with us, and this allowed me to bring her into my office.

Once she entered the play space, she immediately ran toward her favored beanbag chair. Her fists were still full of her precious figurines, which she could not release even though they seemed awkward in her hands. Jamie rolled her body around in this beanbag and said assertively that she wanted *squishes*. I knew this meant she was craving some sensory input, so I came over to manipulate the beanbag until she was surrounded by it like she was the center of a burrito. As she settled into this sensory regulation, our play opened out into a new game of "Burrito Girl." After I initiated this playful, spontaneous game, she followed with a smile and a giggle and asked for more. We went back and forth 9 or 10 times, responding to variations on the Burrito Girl theme. I asked her what kind of burrito she would like to be, and she responded with "A messy burrito!" "An ice cream burrito!" "A mommy burrito!' "A bike burrito!"

All of this was accompanied by strong connection and laughter for quite awhile, but eventually her interest decreased. Wanting to see if we could maintain our connection without Jamie returning her focus to the toys that were so often her regulators and were still in her hands, I introduced a variation on the play theme. Remembering that her father had mentioned Jamie's rage, I said, "Miss Burrito Girl seems to be mad today. I wonder what could make this Burrito Girl mad." I often chose feeling words that were interesting, strong, and that provoked curiosity such as *mad* and *sad*. Variations on anger words seem to resonate with these children because it is a common emotion they experience but do not get to address appropriately. This reference to Burrito Girl being angry really struck a chord with Jamie as she immediately said, "Yes! Burrito Girl is angry!" From there, I responded with continued animation, heightened affect in my character voice, "What could Burrito Girl possibly be angry at?" Jamie started laughing and rolling around more aggressively, roaring and kicking her legs in the air, as she struggled to connect with the personal relevance of this anger. We seemed to have exceeded her capacity to integrate the various circuits that hold her nervous system, the feeling, and the meaning of the feeling to her.

Before losing her in this play idea, I reflected about her roaring and asked if she was roaring like another animal. She seemed to connect to that idea, identifying as another character as she said, "Yes! I am not a Burrito Girl, but a lion!" She then put her fist full of figurines aside for the first time, got up from the beanbag, and crawled around like a lion. I tried to reintroduce the emotional piece by asking her what this lion could be mad about. Jamie said that the lion was mad about having to go to school. She then assigned me to be the character of the girl who did not want to go to school and herself as the "Mean, Lion Teacher with moldy green eyes." During the play, Jamie revealed her anger, showing it in her roar and aggression, but still not connecting to the affective circuits as she laughed while describing the teacher hitting all the students. Stuck in this idea, she continued to anxiously laugh while referring to "give time-outs and hit all the bad kids." Unable to exit this pattern, she began flapping her hands while running and jumping in an attempt to regulate the too-strong experience. I followed her, resonating with her rising tension, but holding both of us calmly in my own ventral vagal space.

She suddenly realized that her dolls were not in her immediate view and leapt to the conclusion that they were lost or stolen. Her anxiety peaked as she ran around, becoming tearful that they were gone. In an effort to keep Jamie engaged and bring her back to our play so she could reengage with her emotions, I modified my character to "Nice, Curious Cub," changing my body posture and tone of voice to reopen the safe interpersonal space for her. I told her that Nice, Curious Cub wanted to help her feel better and find her toys. Knowing where her dolls were and sensing that she needed some additional sensory regulation, I began to engage her in some back-and-forth communication as she slowly returned to connection, although her body and voice told me she was still anxious. She accepted my new role, we found her figurines, and I suggested that perhaps they could use a sand bath. She brought them to the sand tray for a dip, submerging her hands in the soothing sand, and this brought her back to a calm-alert state quite quickly as she made eye contact and shared a smile. We continued talking about how the figurines were now safe in the sand and soon Jamie played the role of the "protector" and "life saver."

What I feel as I write about this time with Jamie is our mutual efforts to find resonance with one another. As best I could, I read Jamie's sensorimotor, emotional, and physical cues and then joined with her in what play idea or activity she was craving, expanding it from there so she remained engaged and could elaborate her play to get to a place where she was expressing personalized emotion. Fueled by the safety and the ventral vagal space I sought to maintain, it was a constant dance of engagement, joining, playing, increasing expressed emotion, stepping a little bit beyond tolerance into dysregulation, finding one another again, and getting back to a calm-alert state. Over the course of this session and the entire therapy, the dysregulation was less both in duration and intensity. This day, Jamie ended our time by not associating with any of our characters or her precious figurines but by reconnecting with the pattern on my shirt and then offering a smile and a wave good-bye.

Seeing the gradually accumulating changes in these children's capacity for engagement and regulation makes this work rewarding. In my mind, I can envision how the social circuitry in the right hemisphere is gradually being woven into patterns that will make for a more connected and satisfying life to whatever extent they can. I find that as I am able to open a ventral vagal space and maintain it even when dysregulation floods the room, we do find our way back to a healing space and make small steps forward with each moment of connection.

In Conclusion

Neurobiology reassures us that we are first and foremost social creatures, seeking warm attachment from birth until our last breath. Using the science and joyous experience of safety, play, and interpersonally rich connection to foster new pathways of neural integration seems like an excellent process for drawing together the circuitry that brains struggling with autism are forced to keep separate. As regulation increases and calm becomes a more familiar state, behavior and learning will also improve.

Understanding these principles can help us see clearly what is happening with these youngsters and that can, in turn, grant us greater calm and stability in the midst of dysregulation. Our own capacity for holding these intense states becomes the primary tool in the playroom as we maintain the safety of the emotional environment, opening the door to play and to deeper and more sustained connection.

Dipping our toes again in the beautiful movement from disconnection and agitation to the flowing warmth of relational goodness, let's conclude with the delicious taste of play running through our bodies.

> He was a runner and easily spooked, so I found myself having to chase and grab at times, things I would never choose to do. Then I had a breakthrough with him. I brought him into the gym to play on the mats. He immediately avoided them and headed for the doors. Fortunately, some people walked in at that point and he felt he could not go that way. So, I could keep my distance—give him space and not have to stop him from going out of the building. He sat down on a bench. I sat down the next bench over—maybe 10 feet away. He

stood up and sat down in agitation, and I simply sat and attended to him. He started running his hands over a grate on the wall behind the bench he was on. I gently shifted closer so I sat on the same bench as him, watching closely for any signal that this disturbed him. He noted my movement but continued to run his hands over the grate. It made an interesting sound. I began to run my hands over the grate also. I felt the sensation of it and explored the sound of it in my own way. I wasn't just copying him; I was joining in an exploration of touch and sound. We did this for a while, and then he lay down on the bench with his feet toward me. He started pushing his feet against me. As he pushed me, I let myself slide away from him. And as he let up, I moved back to my original position. This started slowly and became a rhythmic game. But in the push, I began to feel he might fall off the bench. I very slowly and gently began to move off the bench onto the floor. He kept his feet on me the whole time. I placed myself on my hands and knees just below where he lay on the bench so if he fell my body would be there to catch him. He lay there with his feet on me and looked down at me. He seemed intrigued by this configuration with my entire body lower than his. He started to scooch over onto my body very slowly and gradually. I followed his movements—supporting him, attuning with him, not really knowing where we were going. I couldn't tell you how we got there, but we ended up lying on the floor together—me on my back and he lying close, curled into my side—his head resting on my arm and shoulder. We lay that way for a long time, maybe 15 minutes. He had no agitation; his body was soft and relaxed. And I took the opportunity to relax as well. It reminded me of when my children were babies: the contented glow of lying with them resting on my body, of just being together. That is the feeling I found with him that day. (M. Helene, personal communication, February 19, 2011).

References

Adolphs, R. (2002). Trust in the brain. *Nature Neuroscience, 5,* 192–193.

Critchley, H. D. (2005). Neural mechanisms of autonomic, affective, and cognitive integration. *Comparative Neurology, 493,* 154–166.

Doidge, N. (2007). *The brain that changes itself: Stories of personal triumph from the frontiers of brain science.* New York: Viking.

Iacoboni, M. (2009). Imitation, empathy, and mirror neurons. *Annual Review of Psychology, 60,* 653–670.

Morris, J. S., Ohman, A., & Dolan, R. J. (1999). A subcortical pathway to the right amygdala mediating "unseen" fear. *Proceedings of the National Academy of Science, USA, 96,* 1680–1685.

Panksepp, J. (1998). *Affective neuroscience: The foundations of human and animal emotions*. New York: Oxford University Press.

Panksepp, J. (2008). PLAY, ADHD and the construction of the social brain: Should the first class each day be recess? *American Journal of Play, 1*, 55–79.

Porges, S. W. (1998). Love: An emergent property of the mammalian autonomic nervous system. *Psychoneuroendocrinology, 23*(8), 837–861. doi:10.1016/50306-4530(98)00057-2

Porges, S. W. (2004). Neuroception: A subconscious system for detecting threat and safety. *Zero to Three: Bulletin of the National Center for Clinical Infant Programs, 24*(5), 19–24.

Porges, S. W. (2007). The polyvagal perspective. *Biological Psychology, 74*, 116–143.

Porges, S. W. (2008). The Listening Project. Retrieved from http://www.education.umd.edu/EDHD/faculty2/Porges/tlp/tlp.html

Porges, S. W. (2009a). Reciprocal influences between body and brain in the perception and expression of affect: A polyvagal perspective. In D. Fosha, D. J. Siegel, & M. F. Solomon (Eds.), *The healing power of emotion: Affective neuroscience, development, clinical practice* (pp. 27–54). New York: Norton.

Porges, S. W. (2009b). The polyvagal theory: New insights into adaptive reactions of the autonomic nervous system. *Cleveland Clinic Journal of Medicine, 76*(2), S86–90. doi:10.3949/ccjm.67.s2.17

Porges, S. W. (2011). *The polyvagal theory: Neurophysiological foundations of emotions, attachment, communication, and self-regulation*. W. W. Norton.

Schore, A. N. (2009). Right brain affect regulation: An essential mechanism of development, trauma, dissociation, and psychotherapy. In D. Fosha, D. J. Siegel, & M. Solomon (Eds.), *The healing power of emotion: Affective neuroscience, development, and clinical practice* (pp. 112–144). New York: Norton.

Siegel, D. J. (1999). *The developing mind: How relationship and the brain interact to shape who we are*. New York: Guilford.

Siegel, D. J. (2006). An interpersonal neurobiology approach to psychotherapy: Awareness, mirror neurons, and neural plasticity in the development of well-being. *Psychiatric Annals, 36*(4), 247–258.

Siegel, D. J., & Hartzell, M. (2003). *Parenting from the inside out: How a deeper self-understanding can help you raise children who thrive*. New York: Tarcher/Putnam.

Winston, J. S., Strange, B. A., O'Doherty, J., & Dolan, R. J. (2002). Automatic and intentional brain responses during evaluation of trustworthiness of faces. *Nature Neuroscience, 5*, 277–283.

Zhang, L. I., Bao, S., & Merzenich, M. M. (2002). *Disruption of primary auditory cortex by synchronous auditory inputs during a critical period*. Proceedings of National Academy of Sciences, USA, 99(4), 2309–2314.

CHAPTER 2

Playing on the Autism Spectrum

LAWRENCE C. RUBIN

Play is of serious importance.... It follows that the abnormalities of play in Autism are not just inconsequential epiphenomena. Rather, abnormal play in Autism has significant consequences for development (Boucher & Wolfberg, 2003, p. 341).

Introduction

As is the act itself, play is a rich and versatile construct. It can refer to the solitary behavior of a child and, as such, can provide a window into her fleeting interests as well as her compelling passions. As a shared activity, play can provide insight into the rules of social engagement as well as the common interests of a group of children. From a developmental life span perspective, play is a lens through which the different facets of growth and change—cognitive, moral, social, creative, and spiritual—can be observed and evaluated. On an even larger scale, play is an anthropological marker, a means of understanding the rules, roles, and beliefs of an entire people at either a point in time or across time.

The versatility and utility of play as both construct and developmental activity has been highlighted through the debate over whether the play activity of children with autism spectrum disorders (ASD) represents a difference to be appreciated or a deficiency to be remediated (Soldz, 1988). If the former, then children or adolescents so diagnosed become larger than their diagnosis, and their play becomes a window into their interests, challenges, and means of interacting with the world around them. If, on the other hand, the play of children with ASD is seen as deficient, then they grow smaller as our clinical gaze becomes tightly fixed on their play-based deficiency. *Playism*, which can be defined as the belief that abstract or symbolic play is the ideal form, takes hold, and we, the parents, teachers, and clinicians, focus solely on their play deficiency in the same way that their play often becomes rigidly fixed on a single object or activity.

The purpose of this chapter is to provide insight into both sides of this debate—first by discussing the broad spectrum of play and then by fine-tuning the lens so that we may better understand the varied experiences of play in children along the autism spectrum. This discussion begins with a description of two very different brothers at play, followed by a theoretical overview of play and then by a description of the play of children on the autism spectrum. The chapter ends with a focus on therapeutic efforts to enhance play with these children and offers suggestions for clinical practice.

The Many Facets of Play

Brothers at Play

Tyler and Austen are fraternal twins. Although only minutes apart in age and conspicuous in their physical similarities, they differ in profound ways, one of the most significant of which is the manner in which they play. Tyler, the *neuro-typical* one, loves superheroes, a passion that he shares with his uncle, a fan of superhero comics and movies and with whom he has long conversations about Superman and Spider Man's origins, powers, vulnerabilities, and missions. Tyler loves superhero television shows, comic books, and movies, reads everything he can about caped crusaders, and immerses himself in grand imaginary adventures, during which he dons cape and mask and travels through time and space to confront and ultimately defeat the forces of evil. Austen, the *neuro-atypical* one, has been diagnosed with autism and also loves superheroes; however, he expresses his passion quite differently from his brother. While the boys sit together watching superhero cartoons and movies, Tyler asks abstract questions about heroism and cowardice that pass right by his brother—who is wondering aloud what life would be like if he had super powers and whether he would use his powers for good and evil. He engages his superhero action figures in play that not only parallels what he is viewing in the moment but also takes off on a variety of tangents. He brings his characters alive with conversation.

Austen, who has a formidable collection of superhero T-shirts that he wears until threadbare and a vast array of action figures and comic books that sit neatly in piles organized by color, seems equally mesmerized by the rapidly changing images on the screen. He delights in the sound effects, which he has a knack for imitating. While Tyler adds his own narrative soundtrack to the unfolding stories, Austen sits on the floor playing intently and intensely with his superhero action figures, silently and mechanically crashing them together. As he does so, he effortlessly and rhythmically rattles off an impressive list of details about each of the superheroes; organizes and reorganizes them first by color, next by superpower, and finally by nemeses; and responds only perfunctorily, if at all, to his brothers queries about which superhero story is his favorite. While he occasionally glances in his brother's direction, Austen rarely makes sustained eye contact. Later in the day, when a few of Tyler's friends join them, Austen, without prompting, wanders off to a corner of the room and deepens his immersion into his action figure "play."

The "Meaning" of Play

Which boy, Austen or Tyler, is "truly" playing? Which boy plays "better" or at a "higher" level? Which of the two is genuinely enjoying himself, and perhaps using his engagement with superheroes to scale new cognitive, social, emotional, or even moral heights? To answer these questions and to ultimately understand what play means to each of these boys, we must first consider exactly what play is.

The range of voices that have spoken out in efforts to define play spans many disciplines—both theoretical and applied, including psychology, counseling, sociology, and anthropology. For some, play is a construct to be studied and for others an activity to be facilitated. Some study play from a philogenetic perspective—as it relates to the development and evolution of the species. Among these is play theorist and cultural anthropologist Brian Sutton-Smith (2008), who suggests that play, whether it be physical or mental, is an "existential [and] separately motivated reality" (p. 98), through which children transcend the bounds of their immediate world with all of its "stuffy and bossy" (p. 94) constraints. In so doing, each child is an evolutionary messenger of sorts, carrying forward the important knowledge and experiences of all children. For Sutton-Smith, play is elemental to social and evolutionary survival, in that it allows children to practice and master roles and challenges they will someday confront. Similarly, Henricks (2008) notes that play offers the "freedom of human beings to express themselves openly and to render creatively the conditions of their life" (p. 159). By acting in an unencumbered and creative way, playful activity exercises the unique elements of the human condition: free will. Social historian Mihaly Csikszentmihalyi (1976) evokes the notion of *flow* to describe the intrinsically motivating nature of creative and playful activities. Through the freeing-up-to be-in-the-moment process that is the basis of play, he argues that "human survival might depend on whether we learn to work synergistic forms of enjoyment into the structure of human motivation, while preserving their playful quality" (p. 9).

Others, typically clinicians and developmentally oriented psychologists (and psychiatrists), have focused on the ontogenetic nature of play as it relates to the growth and development of the individual. Among these, and most famous for his psychoanalytic interpretation of fairy tales, psychoanalyst Bruno Bettelheim (1987) fashioned play as a time machine of sorts, through which the player "was anchored in the present but also took up and tried to solve problems of the past [while being] offered future direction as well" (p. 40). For Bettelheim, play provided freedom from all but personally imposed rules and, in spite of providing an opportunity to engage in the most primitive forms of activity, also moved the child along a socializing trajectory. Along similar lines, Erik Erikson (1963) believed that "child's play is the infantile form of the human ability to deal with experience by creating model situations and to master reality by experimenting and planning" (p. 222). Erikson believed that play allows children to "step out" of everyday constraints such as time, gravity, social reality, and even fate so that they can "synchronize the bodily and social processes of the self" (p. 211). In this way, play acts as a stage on which life is rehearsed. Jean Piaget (1962) believed that play and playful activity, predicated on spontaneity and pleasure, subserved the mental processes of assimilation and accommodation. Whether playing sensorimotorically or symbolically, children playfully engaged are exercising their capacity for problem solving. Vygotsky (1978) also viewed play, particularly symbolic or representational play, as a vehicle both for the development of abstract thought and social connectedness. He believed that play "contains all developmental tendencies in a condensed form and is itself a major source of development" (p. 102), one crucial aspect of which is the capacity to encode social behavior through practice.

Each of these ontogenetic play theorists, if you will, offered a developmental foundation for clinicians who applied these principles in the playroom, such as Virginia Axline (1947), Clark Moustakas (1953), Haim Ginott (1961), and most recently Garry Landreth (2002). It was Landreth, speaking from a rich tradition, who said that "play is the singular central activity of childhood, occurring at all times and in all places...[and is] spontaneous, enjoyable, voluntary and non-goal-directed" (p. 10). He, like the others, believed and still does that play is not a privilege but a fundamental right, an active engagement with the world, both external and internal that forms the foundation of the self.

Tyler and Austen in Retrospect

Before moving on to the next section that explores the play world of children with ASD, it is important to consider how the previously described (small sampling of) play-related notions help us to better understand Tyler and Austen. Clearly, both boys enjoy their superheroes, engage playfully and spontaneously with them (whether through action figures or action adventures), and are in one way or another exercising motor and cognitive skills. While Tyler's play is also clearly social in nature, Austen's play lacks social responsivity and connection. Each is exercising his evolutionary prerogative to create order, structure, and meaning while "having fun," and both are experimenting with tangible reality as well as intangible possibilities. Each, according to the previous discussion, is exercising both philogenetic and ontogenetic muscles, so to speak, and is in every sense of the word... playing. While sociologists, anthropologists, and historians may look similarly upon them, teachers, clinicians, and parents clearly understand that Tyler and Austen play quite differently, and by clinical standards one is correct, or healthy or appropriate, and the other is not.

A Different Type of Play

To fully appreciate the play of children on the autism spectrum, it is important to consider the various developmental functions that play subserves. From a cognitive perspective, the manipulation, organization, and later use of objects to represent people, place, and things in the real and imaginary worlds helps children develop a working model for understanding and problem solving. From a social perspective, playing with objects and ideas, first alone and then with others, helps children to connect. As a vehicle for emotional development, play allows children to explore and express feelings, both positive and painful. In the context of language and literacy, play provides opportunities to develop narrative and storytelling skills, which contribute to autobiographical awareness (Habermas & Bluck, 2000) and which, in turn, contribute to social connection.

Across these developmental domains, play is, or at least has traditionally been, conceptualized in neuro-typical children as being a pleasurable, voluntary, flexible, and changing as well as an increasingly symbolic activity. It also progresses from simple to complex, routinized to flexible, literal to abstract, and external to internal (Wolfberg, 1999). In the case of Tyler and Austen, our superhero fans, Tyler has a far broader repertoire of activities from which to choose while playing with his action figures. Certainly, he enjoys collecting and categorizing them, clapping them together, and making noises as they fly and battle, and he is drawn to their brilliant primary colors. However, unlike Austen, whose action-figure play never quite moves beyond this literal and sensorimotor level of engagement, Tyler "makes" his action figures come alive by assigning human qualities to them, creating rich and elaborate narratives about their families, lives, and adventures, and even attributing false properties (Wolfberg) to them, (i.e., those that are neither evident or even possible). This latter skill is considered the hallmark of neuro-typical play and is thought to be absent in autistic play. When friends come over, it is Tyler who is quick to rush into joint action and symbolic play, offering up complex rules of engagement and orchestrating elaborate interpersonal adventures between the action figures, whereas Austen seems quite content to remain in his room, organizing his superheroes by power and reciting their adventures verbatim from comic books and Internet sites he regularly visits. Unlike his brother's spontaneous, enjoyable, flexible, complex, and interactive use of the action figures as a starting point for creative expression and engagement, Austen's play is private, ritualized, stereotypical, and concrete—the hallmarks of *autistic* play (Jordan, 2010; Stanley & Konstantareas, 2007).

A Closer Look at Cognitive and Social Development

Reflecting on Tyler and Austen, the earlier raised question of difference versus deficiency must now be reconsidered. Is Tyler truly playing while Austen is merely playing at? Is Tyler's play cognitively, linguistically, and socially ideal for a child his age and thus "healthy," whereas Austen's play suggests developmental delay? Is Tyler moving forward while Austen is, at best, standing still?

This simplistic dichotomization of the boys' play is misleading and predicated upon some rather common, yet not necessarily valid, presumptions about the play of children on the autism spectrum. Among these are the misconceptions that children with autism do not play in any real sense, are not capable of pretending (which would otherwise suggest symbolic capacity), and neither engage in social play nor "enjoy" playing in any observable way (Boucher & Wolfberg, 2003).

These misconceptions derive from decades of research into the nature of autistic play and the often complex and conflicting array of theories that have been advanced to explain it. They loosely divide into two camps: the social and cognitive. In the forefront of the cognitive domain is the notion of theory of mind (ToM) and its role in the development of mature, symbolic, and interactive play. Simply stated, ToM is a developmental capacity or ability to appreciate that others have unique thoughts and feelings and act in accordance with them (Wellman, Cross, & Watson, 2001). Children who have developed a theory of mind understand that other children may see the world differently from them and that their behavior may be motivated by thoughts and feelings very different from their own. Children who have not developed this capacity assume that everyone else thinks and feels as they do. They may not even be aware of their own sense of self and internal states. To do so, these children must be able to *decouple* (Leslie, 1987) or step back and reflect on the differences between themselves and the "other." These children must be able to appreciate that a whole is sometimes greater than the sum of its parts—sometimes referred to as central coherence—and that a toy can be used to stand for something other than itself or incorporated into a broader play activity. This latter ability allows children to move beyond functional play (i.e., the use of toys and objects based on their appearance or immediate sensory gratification) to symbolic engagement with that same toy (i.e., using it in a way that is creative and not bound by the immediate characteristics and qualities of that object; Baron-Cohen, 1987; Rutherford, Young, Hepburn, & Rogers, 2007). These children are able to engage in "as-if" play by understanding that context is multidimensional.

Children without, or who have a rudimentary, theory of mind may be able to fly a caped superhero action figure around a room but will not be able to engage that same toy in imaginary adventures or do so with other children. Baron-Cohen (1987) referred to this distinction as the difference between functional and symbolic pretend play. Pretend play, as opposed to functional play, requires that these children "set aside familiar schemas that are evoked by external objects...and instead to guide their actions by internal plan" (Jarrold, 2003; Jarrold, Boucher, & Smith, 1994, p. 1474). Children with autism's play are therefore limited by and to the most immediate and salient aspects of the object they are playing with. Lacking in the executive ability (Rutherford & Rogers, 2003) to plan ahead, to decenter (or decouple) from either the object of their play or its context, or to attribute false or imagined qualities to that object, children with autism are bound, rather than free, in their play. To the observer, this play indeed appears stereotypical, rigid, and uninventive.

In the context of the previous discussion, Tyler understands that his superhero action figures are a subset of a larger universe of toys and that they "stand for" fictional characters—the creation of comic book writers and movie makers. He understands that each of these characters has qualities and characteristics that are themselves creations, some his and others not, and that their stories can be modified. He positions himself as the conductor of a symphony of endless variation. He is unfettered. Austen, on the other hand, is but a member of that symphony, guided by notes on a page, incapable, or perhaps unwilling, to consider that those notes and the pages themselves can be altered.

The aforementioned possibility that Austen may be "unwilling" as opposed to unable is an interesting one, because it suggests that there may be an element of volition guiding Austen's struggle with symbolic play. Indeed some researchers have provided evidence that children on the autism spectrum can understand and even explain pretend play in others (Jarrold, 2003) as well as engage in symbolic play with prompting and shaping (Beyer & Gammeltoft, 2000; Charman & Baron-Cohen, 1997)

The differences between Tyler and Austen's superhero action figure play, and with it the differences between neuro-typical and atypical play, can also be understood from the perspective of social development. In the first scenario in which we met the boys, friends had just come to visit. Tyler was eager to greet them to share his newest acquisitions and to invite them to create new adventures. He has a theory about why super villains do such terrible things and why, in many ways, superheroes and their arch nemeses were alike in so many ways. Austen seemed overwhelmed by the flood of words and activities of the rambunctious group, and although he tried to show the boys his newest action figures, he had difficulty keeping up with the rapidly changing conversation and couldn't understand what they meant when they said that "superheroes like Superman and Spiderman are really jealous of Lex Luthor and Kingpin." While adept at functional activities with the action figures (Williams, Reddy, & Costall, 2001) like flying and smashing, he has great difficulty decoupling from his play to join in the play of the other boys. Once again, he retreats to his corner of the room and surrounds himself with familiar toys, talking to himself about the powers and abilities of super villains.

Capable of "seeing the larger picture" or context, of decoupling qualities such as heroism and villainy, and of possessing a theory of mind, Tyler easily brings his characters to life and, even more importantly, understands that his friends have their own theories about superheroes, which makes the shared play all the more interesting. Tyler possesses the capacity to engage in *joint attention*, which is defined as the "psychological coordination of self and other (here/there, whole/part) which is the basis for a more generalized capacity to adopt multiple orientations to an object or situation" (Charman, 1997, p. 9). Tyler recognizes that he is part of a group and as such plays a role in that group. He pays attention to his friends' facial expressions and body language, follows the rapidly shifting conversations, and understands the metaphors and symbolism in the play. He appreciates that the mutually shared activity is an as-if scenario and can easily move in and out of various roles. Capable of *affective sharing* (Kasari, Sigman, Mundy, & Yirmiya, 1990), Tyler adjusts his emotions to those of members of the group and is capable of shifting his attention from his own interests to those of others and back again (Gulsrud, Jahromi, & Kasari, 2010). Unlike his isolated brother, Tyler *plays with* rather than *playing at*. Austen, on the other hand, remains stuck in the moment.

It is very likely that this difference in the capacity for joint attention has always distinguished the boys from each other and dates to infancy. It was then, and during the period of early intense bonding, that Tyler was comfortable with face-to-face contact, enjoying extended shared gazing and social games such as peekaboo games. It was during these intimate interpersonal encounters that Tyler learned the subtle rules of social interaction and that play activities could be both self- and other-directed (Williams, 2010). People, for Tyler, were as enjoyable if not more so than toys. In contrast, Austen was far more comfortable, for reasons not yet understood, with objects and pieces rather than people and complex wholes.

Interestingly, both Tyler and Austen have excellent vocabularies, particularly when it comes to superheroes. Each can rattle off the names, powers, origin stories, nemeses, and vulnerabilities of scores of caped heroes. However, when it comes to applying their verbal skills to social situations such as the gathering of friends noted already, the differences in the boys' play becomes pronounced. As has been suggested (Honey, Leekam, Turner & McConachie, 2007; Lewis, 2003), language and play develop alongside each other, and nowhere in the course of development is this more obvious than in the relationship between symbolic play and symbolic language, both of which emerge around the same time in neuro-typical children. Both play and thought for these children become increasingly complex, abstract, and flexible, while the play and thought of the neuro-atypical child remains concrete, rigid, and object bound. Tyler creates rich stories that transcend time and place, whereas Austen's narration is intractably anchored to the action figures before him. He is not interested, or perhaps even aware, that the other boys in the room have lost interest in his repetitive and unchanging narration.

As Tyler and Austen's parents watch on, they ask each other what can be done to help their atypical son become a more "playful" player, one who can share his passion rather than wrap it around him like a protective cloak, one who can transcend the gravitational pull of objects to join in with others around him, one who can create and share stories rather than mechanically recite them.

Teaching the Child With ASD to Play

From a developmental perspective, play evolves throughout childhood— beginning in sensorimotor engagement with the physical world and culminating in the capacity to symbolically and internally represent the world, as a client might do in the sand tray, dollhouse, or through creative storytelling. Neuro-typical play, or what we call *normal* or *mature*, frees children from physical, temporal, and spatial constraints, providing them with limitless as-if possibilities. Coupled with the capacity to take another's perspective and to project human attributes onto inanimate objects, these children can engage reciprocally and creatively with other children.

Children with ASD have difficulties in all of these domains (Hess, 2006), resulting as we have seen in repetitive, stereotypical, unimaginative, and isolated play. The critical question is, "Can these children be taught to play?" Interestingly, a growing body of empirical research has suggested that under certain conditions—more specifically, prompting, shaping, and modeling—children with autism spectrum disorders can and do spontaneously engage in symbolic, pretend, and joint-imaginative play (Hobson, Lee, & Hobson, 2009; Libby, Powell, Messer, & Jordan, 1998). This research leads us back to the *deficiency-difference* question raised earlier and to wonder whether the play deficits in these children represent actual skill deficiency or lack of interest dictated by the possibility that the sensorimotor appeal of toys and activities may simply outstrip their symbolic and functional interest. A closer look at some of this research may help to better address this question.

Behavioral interventions centered on Lovaas's (1977) applied behavior analysis (ABA) have been successfully applied in teaching children with autism spectrum disorders to play symbolically and interactively. Noting the deficiency in joint attention that is central to autism, Jones and Carr (2004) discussed the importance of ABA in building eye contact as a basis for a series of interactive skills including pointing, requesting, responding, and commenting on their partner's play. Each of these fundamental joint attention skills was considered crucial by these authors to the development of shared play.

More specific forms of ABA that have been used to teach play to children with autism spectrum disorders include discrete trial training (Stahmer, Ingersoll, & Carter, 2003), a method of teaching and then reinforcing the elements of a symbolic play behavior, and then chaining them together to form sequences of play. Pivotal response training (PRT) (Stahmer, 1995) is the extension of discrete trial training to naturalistic settings in which a trainer combines incidental learning with direct reinforcement to shape interactive play behavior. Reciprocal imitation training (Stahmer et al., 2003) combines PRT with contingent imitation of spontaneous play by the facilitator followed by prompting and reinforcement of children's attempts to imitate the play action. Ingersoll has noted that young children can learn pretend play in this manner and that it generalizes across settings, materials, and children (Ingersoll, 2003). Importantly, and in contrast with the previous positive findings, it has been argued that behavioral interventions targeting play with children on the autism spectrum are most effective when they build on children's existing repertoire of play behaviors rather than when relying solely on external reward (Luckett, Bundy, & Roberts, 2007). Specific examples of this would include modeling and reinforcing initiating behavior using social stories, comic strip conversations, role playing, and cooperative games; using inclusive strategies such as circle of friends and peer mentors; and teaching perspective taking—all in the context of a safe and accepting classroom or play space (Mastrangelo, 2009).

In contrast to the highly individualized behavioral approaches noted already, efforts have been directed at using more holistic interventions to teach play in children's naturalistic environment. Foremost among these is the Developmental, Individual Difference, Relationship-Based (DIR) Floortime Model (Wieder & Greenspan, 2001) in which "adults follow the child's lead utilizing affectively toned interactions through gestures and words to move the child up the symbolic ladder by first establishing a foundation of shared attention, engagement, simple and complex gestures, and problem solving to usher the child into the world of ideas and abstract thinking" (Wieder & Greenspan, 2003, p. 425). More will be said about this popular mode of intervention later on in this volume in Chapter 12.

Within the school environment, the Integrated Play Group (IPG) Model has been successfully implemented. Based on Vygotsky's notion of scaffolding, or the use of others to encourage, guide, and teach, this model relies on structured and facilitated play sessions (Hess, 2006; Kok, Kong, & Bernard-Opitz, 2002) with both expert and novice players working together to coexperience and colearn symbolic and interactive play (Lantz, Nelson, & Loftin, 2004; Wolfberg & Schuler, 1993; Yang, Wolfberg, Wu, & Hwu, 2003). The use of more experienced or expert *peer players* is less threatening to socially isolated children and can be the focus around which the adult builds playful social interaction (Mastrangelo, 2009). A related intervention that can be used in the school setting is called *toy play* (Van Berckelaer-Onnes, 2003), in which the facilitator demonstrates various ways of playing with toys, building to a more symbolic level of engagement with them. This type of intervention is based on the observation that children with autism spectrum disorders lack a sense of *central coherence* that must be supplied through demonstration and supportive interaction. Along similar lines, a recently developed intervention made use of virtual reality activities to develop symbolic play in two boys, ages 8 and 15, with autism spectrum disorders (Herrera, Alcantud, Jordan, Blanquer, Labajo, & De Pablo, 2008).

Play Therapy

The affirmative response to the question of whether children with autism spectrum disorders can be taught to play is encouraging for parents, teachers, and clinicians. The next logical question would be, "Can play therapy be effectively used with these clients?" Such is the premise of this book, which suggests that although neuro-typical clients are capable and competent players who can use the varying materials of the playroom and the therapeutic relationship in increasingly flexible, abstract, and metaphoric ways, ASD clients are rigid, stereotypical, and sensorimotoric in their engagement with toys, games, play-based activities, and the play therapist.

As we have seen in this section, numerous empirically based and qualitative therapeutic research efforts have been successfully used to teach

ASD clients to play; however, little of this research has focused specifically on the use of play therapy with this population. There is a difference between using a play-based therapeutic approach during which play skills are taught, modeled, and reinforced and systematically implementing techniques of established play therapy treatment modalities such as cognitive-behavioral play therapy (Knell, 1993), client-centered play therapy (Landreth, 2002), developmental play therapy (Brody, 1993), Gestalt play therapy (Oaklander, 1988), and psychoanalytic play therapy (Bromfield, 1989).

A growing body of play therapy-based research has indeed been evolving over the last several years, as will be seen in the chapters to come. As examples, Kinney and Winnick (2000) effectively used an *integrative approach* to help an 11-year-old ASD girl improve her social and affective functioning in school and at home. Their approach incorporated elements of nondirective (i.e., client-centered) work. Relatedly, Solomon, Ono, Timmer, and Goodlin-Jones (2008) incorporated elements of client-centered play therapy into a manualized intervention called *parent–child interaction therapy* with 19 male clients ages 5–12 and found evidence of improved adaptability as well as parents' perceptions of decreased behavioral problems.

Using the creative metaphor of the *homonculus*, or little people inside the head, Greig and MacKay (2005) effectively applied the principles and techniques of cognitive behavior (play) therapy with a middle-school–age ASD child and observed measureable improvements in the areas of anxiety, depression, anger, and stress level. Similarly creative was the work of Legoff and Sherman (2006), who incorporated LEGO toys into the play therapeutic work with 60 ASD children over a 3-year period and found that in comparison with controls these subjects improved in social functioning. We shall revisit Legoff's work later on in this book. In yet another study using a play-based approach to counseling, Cashin (2008) drew upon the methods of narrative therapy to assist a 13-year-old boy diagnosed with ASD to externalize the "big bang" (his tempestuous feelings) to improve his social functioning and overall behavior. And finally, Herrera et al. (2008) incorporated virtual reality games into the play therapy of two ASD boys ages 8 and 15, who at the end of treatment showed improved symbolic play capacity and a generalization of this behavior into their daily lives.

Regardless of the many types of interventions designed to teach ASD children and teenagers to play as well as benefit from play therapy, the question remains as to whether newly acquired play skills or coping skills are practiced spontaneously or generalize across situations. One of the most encouraging studies to date was a meta-analysis conducted by Barton and Wolery (2008) of interventions that purported to teach symbolic play.

Their results indicated that "overall, the reports suggest that an increase in pretense behaviors are related to adult modeling or prompting in classrooms with materials found in early childhood classrooms" (p. 120). This study was particularly useful because it developed a "pretend play taxonomy" to better articulate the nature of the play behaviors being assessed. This taxonomy included categories such as functional play with pretense, object/absent-other substitution, sequencing, and verbalizations and, in so doing, provided empirical evidence for the remediability of play behaviors. To date, there is not yet a parallel analysis of play therapy interventions with ASD clients. It is our hope that the contributions to this book will form the foundation of such analysis and validation.

Closing Remarks—Playing It Forward

Returning for the final time to the question of whether the play of children on the autism spectrum (i.e., autistic play) is deficient or different, perhaps it makes the most sense to conclude that it is both. To the parents who worry that their child will be consigned to social isolation and constrained by objects, acts, and activities that offer little to no promise of cognitive or creative growth and versatility, autistic play is deficient. Similarly, to the teacher who struggles to integrate these children into the social milieu through joint attention and shared activities, their literal, functional, repetitive, and rigid play behavior represent an obstacle to overcome. To (play) therapists who perceive their role as change agents and their therapeutic engagement with children on the autism spectrum as repair work, conceptualizing autistic play solely as deficiency may deprive them of the opportunity to understand the interests, perceptions, and personality of these children. To children who play in an autistic way, there are no distinctions between deficiency and difference—there is only the moment.

And what of our superheroically inclined brothers Austen and Tyler? If we are to consider "helping" Austen to "play," his natural interest in superheroes and the previous research suggest enlisting Tyler, at least initially, as a peer-expert player who under the guidance of parents, teachers, and the clinician could model varying levels of symbolic play. Such play might begin with engaging two superhero action figures in conversation about their respective attributes already known to Austen such as costume, abilities, and enemies. Modeling these conversations could be a starting point for building inner conversation and could lead to higher levels of abstraction and symbolic interactions. Austen's teacher could capitalize on this foundation by enlisting more advanced peer players in school to continue modeling and reinforcing different levels of play both in the classroom and on the playground. Both in the classroom and at home, Austen and his play facilitator could engage in a variety of superhero activities including reading comics and watching television and movie depictions of super-heroes, all the while having conversations at increasingly higher levels of abstraction. These might center on the superhero origin stories, their inner conflicts, and the struggles they have leading two lives. Such guided conversations might help Austen to strengthen his theory of mind capability. These efforts may indeed have effect and may even generalize to other play situations, providing Austen with new skills for self-understanding, expression, and meaningful social connection.

References

Axline, V. (1947). *Play therapy*. Cambridge, MA: Houghton-Mifflin.
Baron-Cohen, S. (1987). Autism and symbolic play. *British Journal of Developmental Psychology, 5,* 139–148.
Barton, E. E., & Wolery, M. (2008). Teaching pretend play to children with disabilities: A review of the literature. *Topics in Early Childhood Special Education, 28*(2), 109–125.
Bettelheim, B. (1987). The importance of play. *Atlantic Monthly, 259,* 35–46.
Beyer, J., & Gammeltoft, L. (2000). *Autism and play*. Philadelphia, PA: Jessica Kingsley Publishers.
Boucher, J., & Wolfberg, P. (2003). Editorial. *Autism, 7*(4), 339–346.
Brody, V. (1993). The *dialog of touch: Developmental play therapy*. Northvale, NJ: Jason Aronson, Inc.
Bromfield, R. (1989). Psychodynamic play therapy with a high functioning autistic child. *Psychoanalytic Psychology, 6*(4), 439–453.
Cashin, A. (2008). Narrative therapy: A psychotherapeutic approach in the treatment of adolescents with Asperger's disorder. *Journal of Child and Adolescent Psychiatric Nursing, 2191,* 48–56.
Charman, T. (1997). The relationship between joint attention and pretend play in autism. *Development and Psychopathology, 9,* 1–16.
Charman, T., & Baron-Cohen, S. (1997). Brief report: Prompted pretend play in autism. *Journal of Autism and Developmental Disorders, 27*(3), 325–332.
Csikszentmihalyi, M. (1976). What play says about behaviour. *Ontario Psychologist, 8*(2), 5–11.
Erikson, E. (1963). *Childhood and society*. New York: W. W. Norton & Company.
Ginott, H. (1961). *Group psychotherapy with children*. New York: McGraw-Hill.
Greig, A., & MacKay, T. (2005). Asperger's syndrome and cognitive behavior therapy: New applications for educational psychologists. *Educational and Child Psychology, 22*(4), 1–13.
Gulsrud, A., Jahromi, L., & Kasari, C. (2010). The co-regulation of emotions between mothers and their children with autism. *Journal of Autism and Developmental Disabilities, 40*(2), 227–237.
Habermas, T., & Bluck, S. (2000). Getting a life: The emergence of the life story in adolescence. *Psychological Bulletin, 126,* 748–769.
Henricks, T. (2008). The nature of play. *American Journal of Play, 1*(2), 157–180.

Herrera, G., Alcantud, F., Jordan, R., Blanquer, A., Labajo, G., & De Pablo, C. (2008). Development of symbolic play through the use of virtual reality tools in children with autism spectrum disorders. *Autism, 12*(2), 143–157.

Hess, L. (2006). I would like to play but I don't know how: A case study of pretend play in autism. *Child Language Teaching and Therapy, 22*(1), 97–116.

Hobson, P., Lee, A., & Hobson, J. (2009). Qualities of symbolic play among children with autism: A social-developmental perspective. *Journal of Autism Development Disorders, 39*, 12–22.

Honey, E., Leekam, S., Turner, M., & McConachie, H. (2007). Repetitive behavior and play in typically developing children and children with autism spectrum disorder. *Journal of Autism and Developmental Disorders, 37*, 1107–1115.

Ingersoll, B. R. (2003). Teaching children with autism to imitate using a naturalistic treatment approach: Effects on imitation, language, play and social behaviors. *Dissertation Abstracts International: Section B: The Sciences and Engineering, 63*, 6120.

Jarrold, C. (2003). A review of research into pretend play in autism. *Autism, 7*(4), 379–390.

Jarrold, C., Boucher, J., & Smith, P. (1994). Executive function deficits and the pretend play of children with autism: A research note. *Journal of Child Psychology and Psychiatry, 35*(8), 1473–1482.

Jones, E. A., & Carr, E. G. (2004). Joint attention in children with autism: Theory and intervention. *Focus on Autism and Other Developmental Disabilities, 19*(1), 13–26.

Jordan, R. (2010). Social play and autistic spectrum disorders. *Autism, 7*(4), 347–360.

Kasari, C., Sigman, M., Mundy, P., & Yirmiya, N. (1990). Affective sharing in the context of joint attention interactions of normal, autistic and mentally retarded children. *Journal of Autism and Developmental Disorders, 20*, 87–100.

Kinney, M., & Winnick, C. (2000). An integrative approach to play therapy with an autistic girl. *International Journal of Play Therapy, 9*(1), 11–33.

Knell, S. (1993). *Cognitive-behavioral play therapy.* Northvale, NJ: Jason Aronson.

Kok, A., Kong, T. Y., & Bernard-Opitz, V. (2002). A comparison of the effects of structured play and facilitated play approaches on preschoolers with autism. *Autism, 6*(2), 181–196.

Landreth, G. (2002). *Play therapy: The art of the relationship.* New York: Brunner-Routledge.

Lantz, J., Nelson, J., & Loftin, R. (2004). Guiding children with autism in play: Applying the integrated play group model in school settings. *Teaching Exceptional Children, 37*(2), 8–14.

Legoff, D., & Sherman, M. (2006). Long-term outcome of social skills intervention based on interactive LEGO play. *Autism, 10*(4), 1–31.

Leslie, A. (1987). Pretense and representation: The origin of "Theory of Mind." *Psychological Review, 94*(4), 412–426.

Lewis, V. (2003). Play and language in children with autism. *Autism, 7*(4), 391–399.

Libby, S., Powell, S., Messer, D., & Jordan, R. (1998). Spontaneous play in children with autism: A reappraisal. *Journal of Autism and Developmental Disorders, 28*(6), 487–497.

Lovaas, O. I. (1977). *The Autistic child: language development through behavior modification.* New York: Irvington Publishers.

Luckett, T., Bundy, A., & Roberts, J. (2007). Do behavioural approaches teach children with autism to play or are they pretending. *Autism, 11*(4), 365–388.

Mastrangelo, S. (2009). Play and the child with autism spectrum disorder: From possibilities to practice. *International Journal of Play Therapy, 18*(1), 13–30.

Moustakas, C. (1953). *Children in play therapy.* New York: McGraw-Hill.

Oaklander, V. (1988). Windows to our children. Highland, NY: Real People Press.

Piaget, J. (1962). *Play, dreams and imitation in childhood.* New York: W.W. Norton.

Rutherford, M.D., & Rogers, S. (2003). Cognitive underpinnings of pretend play in autism. *Journal of Autism and Developmental Disorders, 33*(3), 289–302.

Rutherford, M. D., Young, G., Hepburn, S., & Rogers, S. (2007). A longitudinal study of pretend play in autism. *Journal of Autism and Developmental Disorders, 37,* 1024–1039.

Soldz, S. (1988). The deficiencies of deficiency theories: A critique of ideology in contemporary psychology. *Practice, 6,* 50–64.

Solomon, M., Ono, M., Timmer, S., & Goodlin-Jones, B. (2008). The effectiveness of parent–child interaction therapy for families of children on the autism spectrum. *Journal of Autism and Developmental Disorders, 38,* 1767–1776.

Stahmer, A. C. (1995). Teaching symbolic play skills to children with autism using pivotal response training. *Journal of Autism and Developmental Disorders, 25,* 123–141.

Stahmer, A. C., Ingersoll, B., & Carter, C. (2003). Behavioral approaches to promoting play. *Autism: The International Journal of Research and Practice, 7,* 401–413.

Stanley, G., & Konstantareas, M. M. (2007). Symbolic play in children with autism spectrum disorder. *Journal of Autism and Developmental Disorders, 37,* 1215–1223

Sutton-Smith, B. (2008). A personal journey and new thoughts. *American Journal of Play 1*(1), 80–103.

Van Berckelaer-Onnes, I. A. (2003). Promoting early play. *Autism, 7*(4), 415–423.

Vygotsky, L. (1978). *Mind in society: The development of higher psychological processes.* Cambridge, MA: Harvard University Press.

Wellman, H., Cross, D., & Watson, J. (2001). Meta-analysis of theory of mind development: The truth about false belief. *Child Development, 72*(3), 655–684.

Wieder, S., & Greenspan, S. I. (2003). Climbing the symbolic ladder in the DIR model through floor time/interactive play. *Autism, 7*(4), 425–435.

Wieder, S., & Greenspan, S. I. (2001). The DIR (developmental, individual-difference, relationship-based) approach to assessment and intervention planning. *Zero to Three, 21,* 11–19.

Williams, E. (2010). A comparative review of early forms of object-directed play and parent–infant play in typical infants and young children with autism. *Autism, 7*(4), 361–377.

Williams, E., Reddy, V., & Costall, A. (2001). Taking a closer look at functional play in children with autism. *Journal of Autism and Developmental Disorders, 31*(1), 67–77.

Wolfberg, P. (1999). *Play and imagination in children with autism.* New York: Teachers College Press.

Wolfberg, P., & Schuler, A. L. (1993). Integrated play groups: A model for promoting The social and cognitive dimensions of play in children with autism. *Journal of Autism and Developmental Disabilities, 23,* 467–489.

Yang, T-R., Wolfberg, P., Wu, S-C., & Hwu, P-Y. (2003). Supporting children on the autism spectrum in peer play at home and school. *Autism, 7*(4), 437–453.

PART II

Individualized Play-Based Interventions

CHAPTER **3**

Helping Children With ASD Through Canine-Assisted Play Therapy

RISË VANFLEET AND COSMIN COLŢEA

Introduction to Canine-Assisted Play Therapy

Animal-assisted play therapy (AAPT) represents an integration of play therapy and animal-assisted therapy (AAT). It systematically involves nonhuman animals in the play therapy process in a variety of ways. AAPT has been defined as "the involvement of animals in the context of play therapy, in which appropriately trained therapists and animals engage with children and families primarily through systematic play interventions, with the goal of improving the children's developmental and psychosocial health as well as the animal's well-being. Play and playfulness are essential ingredients of the interactions and the relationship" (VanFleet, 2008, p. 19). AAPT can be conducted with animals of several different species as cotherapists, but the field has been developed most completely with dogs and horses (VanFleet & Faa-Thompson, 2010). The current contribution focuses specifically on dogs, and the approach will heretofore be referred to as canine-assisted play therapy (CAPT). It should be noted that throughout this chapter the term *animals* will be used interchangeably with *nonhuman animals* for the sake of brevity.

CAPT differs from other forms of play therapy due to the presence and active involvement of a play therapy dog in the playroom. It differs from other forms of AAT in that it is conducted by or with a play therapist who uses play interventions as a means of communicating, understanding, relationship building, and helping children overcome social, emotional, and behavioral problems. The interactions have a decidedly active and playful flavor. The therapists and the dogs need specialized training beyond the typical play therapy and AAT training, respectively, which is described elsewhere (VanFleet, 2008).

The practice of CAPT has arisen from a variety of sources, as a number of play therapists independently began involving their dogs and other animals in play sessions. A total of 83 play therapists participated in a 2007 survey about the involvement of animals in their work, showing that therapists were uniformly enthusiastic about the impact on children of live animals participating in their sessions (VanFleet, 2007; see http:// play-therapy.com/playfulpooch/pets_study.html for full results). Several play therapists began developing a more systematic approach to AAPT, including Faa-Thompson in the United Kingdom (VanFleet & Faa-Thompson, 2010), Parish-Plass in Israel (2008), and Thompson (2009), Trotter and Chandler (Chandler, 2005; Trotter, Chandler, Goodwin-Bond, & Casey, 2008), and VanFleet (2004, 2008; VanFleet & Faa-Thompson, 2010) in the United States. The field continues to evolve.

Research in developmental psychology has clearly established the importance of animals in the lives and development of children across many cultures (Jalongo, 2004; Jalongo, Astorino, & Bomboy, 2004; McCardle, McCune, Griffin, Esposito, & Freund, 2011; Melson, 2001; Melson & Fine, 2006). Children are drawn to animals, think about them, enjoy stories about them, and dream about them. Anecdotal reports and a growing body of research have shown the benefits of family companion animals for children (Beck & Katcher, 1996; Chandler, 2005; Colţea 2011; Esteves & Stokes, 2008; Podberscek, Paul, & Serpell, 2000), including increased calmness and self-regulation, lowered blood pressure, improved empathy and caregiving behaviors, increased responsibility, development of prosocial behaviors, improved sense of security, and social lubricant effects in which shy children engage more readily with other people in the presence of a companion animal. Recent biological research has revealed that when humans touch or pet their family dogs, their oxytocin levels rise significantly, and so do the dogs' (Olmert, 2009). Oxytocin, known to mediate mother–infant attachment, is now believed to be the biological basis of the human–animal bond as well. Oxytocin, which operates as both a neurotransmitter and a hormone within the body, appears to be responsible for the ability of many animals to read emotions, relax in the presence of others, overcome fear, and seek contact with others, both physically and for companionship (Olmert, 2009). Interestingly, oxytocin production in both humans and canines is elevated when people pet their family dogs.

Play therapy has an established and growing empirical history (e.g., Bratton et al., 2005) that has shown it to be an effective approach in the treatment of children. Likewise, animal-assisted therapy has an emerging research basis (Nimer & Lundahl, 2007; Trotter et al., 2008). While the combination of these two fields has yet to be studied in a well-controlled fashion, initial research is promising (Thompson, 2009; VanFleet, 2008). One of the obstacles to the study of CAPT is the small, but quickly growing, number of practitioners who have been thoroughly trained in this modality. As more clinicians use CAPT in systematic ways, more research will become possible. Related to this, practice guidelines and a credentialing process that capture the unique qualities of CAPT are being developed (VanFleet, 2011).

Philosophy and Guiding Principles

Whenever nonhuman animals are asked to perform tasks under human direction, their welfare needs to be considered. Too many therapy animals are exposed to debilitating levels of emotional stress or exhaustion without any recognition by their owners, a state of affairs that disregards the dog's welfare and presents a very poor model of caring to children. Similarly, when therapists bring dogs into the playroom, they must think about additional factors that impact the child and the therapeutic process. To ensure the physical and emotional well-being of children and dogs as well as the therapy itself, the following principles have been developed (VanFleet & Faa-Thompson, 2010).

In short, to the fullest extent possible, CAPT ensures that canine needs are considered equally important to human needs and that therapists use education and limits to ensure safety of child and dog. Activities are selected that are pleasant and enjoyable for the dogs as well as the child. Therapists accept the children and the dogs for who they are and do not try to mold them into something different. Only positive training methods are employed, and the dogs are not overcontrolled. The dogs can be dogs as long as they behave politely and safely. While CAPT is used to achieve therapeutic goals, it is a process-oriented approach in which therapists facilitate interactions and metaphors in the moment, so they must have competence in play therapy as well as dog handling and communication.

Therapeutic Goals

Five major goal areas can be addressed by CAPT, and in many cases the same interventions can accomplish more than one objective (VanFleet, 2008; VanFleet & Faa-Thompson, 2010). Each broad goal area is now described briefly.

Self-Efficacy CAPT offers a unique way to develop children's capabilities, including their ability to protect themselves and participate in their own safety. Children first learn to stay safe with dogs and to avoid behaviors, such as hugging, that dogs typically do not like. Pelar (2007, 2009) clearly outlined safety features that can be incorporated easily into CAPT. Therapists help children develop competencies in animal welfare and handling and simple positive dog training methods, which in turn appear to build children's self-confidence.

Attachment/Relationship CAPT helps children learn how to develop healthy relationships with another living being. Children often comment how much the dogs "like" them. It is often easier for children to drop their defenses and create relationships with dogs than with humans (Gonski, 1985). Healthy human attachments and relationships bear many similarities to those between people and dogs (and other species) (Clothier, 2002). Because of this, CAPT can help children learn basic relationship skills in a fun way, such as taking turns and adjusting to meet the other's needs some of the time. Dogs also offer "social lubricant effects" whereby reticent children seem more willing to engage socially in the presence of a dog. For some children, an enjoyable relationship with the therapy dog is the first step toward the development of trusting and satisfying relationships with trustworthy humans.

Empathy CAPT offers a unique and effective way to help children develop empathy. In its simplest form, empathy involves looking at something from another's point of view. In CAPT, therapists can easily turn the child's attention to the dog: "How do you think Sparky is feeling right now?" Therapists can help children learn about animal emotions in this informal, facilitative manner, and they can also teach children to watch for and understand some basic canine communication signals. This includes learning to read the dog's entire body: ears, eyes, mouth, whiskers, stance, tail position, movement, and many other indicators of the dog's state of mind. When children develop their awareness of the play therapy dog's feelings, they can be encouraged to provide caregiving behaviors. For example, one young girl played ball with Kirrie, a CAPT dog, and asked the therapist, "Does Kirrie have a loose tooth? Her tooth felt loose to me!" The therapist responded, "You're worried about Kirrie's tooth. It's great that you are paying attention to how Kirrie feels. Let me check—I think her tooth is fine, but you did just the right thing; you paid close attention to her and then you told a grown-up about what Kirrie needed. That was wonderful, right Kirrie?" Other caregiving activities include feeding and watering the dog, gentle grooming, petting to help the dog relax, and simple massage. A 6-year-old boy poured water into a bowl for Kirrie after they engaged in some dog-training activities together. Kirrie lapped it all up. The boy's face broke into a wide smile as he commented, "How did she know to drink it all up? She was really thirsty!" He was thrilled to be able to perform this very simple act of caregiving for the dog. Evidence suggests that children who develop humane attitudes toward animals can transfer those empathic attitudes to humans (Ascione, 1992; Ascione & Weber, 1996).

Self-Regulation CAPT offers clinicians additional ways to help children develop better emotional and behavioral regulation. Therapeutic activities with the dog that require children to (1) remain calm (e.g., petting, simple grooming), (2) manage arousal levels in self and dog (e.g., tug or stop–go running games), (3) use patience (e.g., training the dog to perform a new trick), and (4) exercise tolerance (e.g., when the dog doesn't get it right or fails to do what the child asks) can help children apply improved self-regulation in the context of an enjoyable, noncritical situation.

Problem Resolution CAPT can be used to overcome a variety of specific problems that children experience. With the right training, dogs can learn a number of cues and behaviors that are useful in addressing different problems. Furthermore, an experienced play therapist can use the metaphors of play therapy and interactions with a dog to help children cope with their situations or difficulties. For example, children can teach a dog to make better eye contact while learning to do the same themselves. A dog taught to turn a light on and off with its paw can help a child overcome fear of the dark. Children with trauma histories can "give advice" to a dog who lived in a shelter and has some residual "problems." The possible ways to incorporate CAPT to address specific problem areas are nearly limitless, and many are detailed in VanFleet (2008) and VanFleet and Faa-Thompson (2010). CAPT is useful in addressing various emotional difficulties, social and communication problems, learning challenges, and animal abuse, to name a few.

Methods of CAPT

CAPT often is employed in conjunction with other mental health interventions, such as nondirective play therapy, directive and cognitive-behavioral play therapies, filial therapy, and other family play interventions and group therapy, and it can be applied in many different settings. The methods of CAPT are detailed elsewhere (VanFleet, 2008, 2009; VanFleet & Faa-Thompson, 2010), but the basic approaches for preparing and involving a dog in play therapy are outlined here.

Dog Training and Preparation   All dogs involved in CAPT must be well trained, although their personalities and abilities determine the form of play therapy for which they are best suited. Play therapy dogs must be trained using positive, relationship-oriented methods for basic obedience, safe play activities, and some tricks. For example, if therapists plan to use child–dog tug games with a long tug rope, the dog first must reliably drop the toy on cue. "Find it" games are useful for attachment and search-and-rescue play scenarios. Canine targeting, in which the dog learns to touch a part of its body (nose, paw) on objects, can be useful for many play activities with children. VanFleet (2011) outlined considerations in finding the right type of dog training. Furthermore, dogs need to be well socialized to people, children, movement, child and toy noises, and all items that are in the playroom.

Nondirective CAPT   The principles of nondirective, or child-centered, play therapy (VanFleet, 2006a; VanFleet, Sywulak, & Sniscak, 2010) are upheld during nondirective CAPT as much as possible. Children choose how to play and what to play with, and that may or may not include the dog. If children do not wish to involve the dog, the dog is permitted to rest in a special area within the playroom or in a separate room. If children want to include the dog, the therapist facilitates the process so that the dog behaves as they ask. If children ask the dog to do something that is not enjoyable or hurtful to the dog, the therapist sets a limit. Otherwise, the therapist includes the dog in some of the empathic reflections if children are playing by themselves: "Kirrie, Jake seems really angry at that bad guy. He's tying him up and putting him in jail so he can't hurt anyone anymore" or in the actual imaginary play if the child requests it: "Kirrie, Jake needs your help from the bad guys! He wants you to bark and scare them off. Kirrie, SPEAK to the bad guys! Speak!" (This assumes, of course, that Kirrie has learned to bark on the cue "Speak!"). Just as the therapist reflects children's play and feelings in nondirective play therapy and plays roles as asked, the therapist helps the canine cotherapist do the same. If a limit is needed, the therapist sets it in the usual way: "Jake, you want to ride Kirrie like a horse. One of the things you may not do is sit on Kirrie's back, but you can do almost anything else."

Directive CAPT   In directive forms of CAPT, the therapist makes more of the decisions about the activities or involvement of the dog. Directive CAPT might include training activities in which children learn some basic positive training methods and then teach the dog some new tricks, nurturance activities suggested by the therapist such as grooming and feeding, or playful interactions designed to address one or more of their specific goal areas.

For example, a therapist might suggest agility activities, either on an actual outdoor course where children learn to work in tandem with the dog, or *fake agility* in the playroom, in which they teach the dog to jump over chairs, crawl under an easel, or jump through a Hula-Hoop, all rewarded by the children with treats or play reinforcements for the dog. Therapists often permit children to interact with the dog on certain tasks, giving them a few moments to reflect on the metaphors or processes involved in their handling of the task, the dog's reactions, and their feelings about it all. Therapists might help children show the play therapy dog how to pick up the "bad guy" doll in its mouth and put him in "jail" (a bucket or box) or may ask them to give the dog some advice about a behavior they are both struggling with, such as stealing or angry outbursts or sharing.

Sometimes therapists might use both nondirective and directive CAPT, but the two forms are kept separate, either during different sessions or sequentially in which a nondirective segment is followed by a directive one. This is important because the basic assumptions, principles, activities, and level of therapist direction is so different between nondirective and directive approaches.

Family CAPT   Families can be incorporated into the CAPT process in several ways. After three or four individual sessions, children demonstrate the basic training, tricks, or games with the dog for their parents. Just recently, in her first CAPT session with Henry, a Labradoodle play therapy dog, 9-year-old Casey (with severe attention deficit disorder) taught him to spin in a circle by using a treat as both lure and reward. Henry learned quickly and soon was making a circle immediately upon given the hand cue. Casey then asked if she could demonstrate the Spin game for her parents, showing great pride in her accomplishment. Demonstrations often begin to shift parents' negative perceptions of their children.

Family CAPT involves the entire family in various directive interventions. For example, the therapist might task the entire family with helping the dog negotiate an obstacle course or with asking the dog to sit in his or her bed for 2 minutes without leaving. The therapist provides parameters to ensure the dog's safety and to add complexity to the task, such as no speaking aloud, no touching the dog, and permission to use treats or toys. Once the task is completed, the therapist discusses the process and dynamics with the family. These initiative games are similar to those sometimes used in group play therapy (Ashby, Kottman, & DeGraaf, 2008; VanFleet, 2006b), but with the canine cotherapist as an integral part.

Finally, when therapists acquire sufficient dog training and handling skills, they might involve the family's own pets in the process in the therapy setting or at home. The therapist facilitates the family's interactions with their companion dog to achieve therapeutic goals or to help them generalize prior therapeutic gains to daily life.

Problems and Populations Appropriate for CAPT

CAPT can be used for many of the same problems or types of children or families for which play therapy is typically employed. Because it can be incorporated into nondirective, directive, and family play therapy modalities, it has broad applicability. It has been used for children with anxiety, depression, attention or learning problems, sensory issues, communication challenges, oppositional behaviors and conduct disorders, social problems such as withdrawal or bullying, trauma reactions to disasters or abuse, attachment disruptions and problems, emotional regulation difficulties, and many more. Therapists report that using CAPT helps them engage children and adolescents more readily in the therapy process and reduces defensiveness. Creative involvement of properly trained dogs and therapist-handlers has tremendous potential as this emerging integration of play therapy and animal-assisted therapy continues to develop rapidly throughout the United States and abroad.

Risks, Benefits, and Outcomes

The risks of CAPT affect children, dogs, and therapists. For children, there are always risks of scratches, bites, or other injuries. These can be dramatically reduced by proper training and continual supervision. No matter how nice the dog or how nice the child, children and dogs should never be left alone together. Therapist supervision is critical, and therapists should be able to read the stress and communication signals of their dogs (Kalnajs, 2006; Pelar, 2009). Some people are allergic to dogs, and whereas some dog breeds are partially hypoallergenic this is an area that deserves serious consideration and management by therapists. Zoönoses, or diseases that are shared between dogs and people, are also a potential risk. Ill dogs should rest at home, and dogs should not be expected to work with ill children.

Dogs are also at risk. Children, deliberately or unintentionally, can step on, kick, push, pinch, hit, or otherwise hurt a dog. Toys used improperly can cause injury. Magic markers pose a temptation to creative children who think the dog might benefit from a change of color. Therapist supervision is just as critical for the dogs' welfare as for the children's.

Finally, although there is little physical risk for therapists, there is a risk of countertransference. Most therapists love their dogs, and when children attempt to do something harmful to the CAPT dog it is natural for therapists to feel protective. If left unchecked, such feelings can have an adverse impact on a child's therapy. Therapists must regularly consider the role that their feelings about their companion dogs might be playing in the therapeutic process.

The potential benefits of properly conducted CAPT far outweigh the risks. CAPT appears to break down resistance, engage children more fully, and offer social lubricant effects (i.e., help children with their social interactions in the therapy process and beyond). CAPT offers a wide range of methodologies—more tools—that can be applied to a wide range of problems. Children typically are very interested in dogs, so using them conveys a warm, friendly, and welcome environment for children. Children who have had negative experiences with dogs or who are afraid of them can be helped to overcome those fears through CAPT. CAPT seems to reduce stress levels for children during the therapy process and facilitates the accomplishment of therapeutic objectives. The five goal areas described earlier have evolved from the work of approximately 100 play therapists in North America and the United Kingdom who have been trained in CAPT and who have made clinical reports of such benefits. The award-winning book *Play Therapy With Kids & Canines* (VanFleet, 2008) details clinical and preliminary research evidence of the value of CAPT.

The fields of play therapy and animal-assisted therapy have growing bodies of empirical support (Bratton et al., 2005; Nimer & Lundahl, 2007). To date, however, there is little research conducted specifically on CAPT or its broader counterpart, animal-assisted play therapy, although some preliminary studies and reports have demonstrated its promise (Parish-Plass, 2008; Thompson, 2009; Weiss, 2009). As more people are trained in the responsible and systematic use of CAPT, more research will become possible. Some information about the most relevant and best-controlled studies follows.

Trotter et al. (2008) conducted a well-designed study comparing 12 weeks of equine-assisted counseling (EAC) with the empirically supported, award-winning Kid's Connection classroom counseling intervention, using 164 at-risk children and adolescents. They used a pretest–posttest experimental-comparison group design. The EAC group demonstrated statistically significant increases in positive behaviors and decreases in negative behaviors on well-established measures. The EAC group made statistically significant improvements in 17 behavioral areas, whereas the comparison group showed statistically significant improvements in five areas.

Thompson (2009) used a repeated-measures (ABAB) design with subjects serving as their own controls to explore the value of a therapy dog in nondirective play therapy with anxious children. The presence of the therapy dog yielded improved mood, facilitated rapport between therapist and child, increased the occurrence of thematic play, and reduced aggressive and disruptive behaviors during play therapy. VanFleet (2008) used posttherapy sand tray creations to demonstrate that nearly all children involved in CAPT placed a dog figurine in their final sand tray depicting the "important parts of therapy," whereas children without the CAPT experience did so significantly less often.

Further and better controlled research is needed to determine the extent to which these promising results will be maintained.

Theoretical and Empirical Rationale for Use With Children and Teens on the Autism Spectrum

Two main characteristics of autism spectrum disorders (ASD) are impairments in social interactions and communication as well as impairments in language development (APA, 2000). These impairments, associated with the fleeting eye contact also characteristic of children with ASD, negatively affect children's ability to function in social settings. Several studies, however, have suggested that children with ASD are receptive to companion animals, although it is unknown yet why. A possible explanation for this preference could be that, when interacting with animals, children are not forced into a conversation. Children's interactions with animals, in contrast to interactions with people, are not guided by time constraints nor by subtle facial expressions but rather by obvious body movements and by sensory experiences (e.g., touching the body of an animal).

Although the influences of animals on children with ASD are yet to be understood, it is known that typically developing children experience an array of benefits (e.g., Walsh, 2009). If children with ASD are as responsive to animals as typically developing children are, it would be fair to expect that they could enjoy some of the same benefits. New and colleagues (2009) concluded that, in their sample, children and young adults with ASD equaled the performances of typically developing children and adults in recognizing changes in images depicting people and animals. Similarly, Celani (2002) investigated the reactions of 36 children to images of objects, people, and animals. The children were divided into three groups: (1) neuro-typical; (2) with Down syndrome; and (c) with ASD. The participants were presented with several combinations of pictures. Similar to the typically developing children, the children with ASD displayed a preference for pictures of animals. They also displayed disinterest in pictures of people, hinting to the potential disinterest of children with ASD in people.

In conclusion, some children with ASD manifest interest in animals, which implies that presence of therapy animals could be beneficial to them. The following section reviews the current literature on the interactions between children with ASD and animals.

Children With ASD: Preference for Dogs

Martin and Farnum (2002) presented 10 children with ASD with (1) a live dog, (2) a plush dog, or (3) a ball for a period of 15 weeks in a within-participants repeated-measure design. After the initial assessment of children's developmental age using the Psychoeducational Profile–Revised (PEP-R; Schopler, Reicher, & Renner, 1990), Martin and Farnum evaluated children's behavior and verbal occurrences during the interventions. Based on analysis of videotapes recorded during the interventions, the authors concluded that in the live dog condition the children with ASD cooperated more with the person conducting the experiment and talked more about the dog. In addition, the results suggested that in the live dog condition the children talked more about topics related to the session rather than preferred subjects (which is usually more common for children with ASD). The developmental age of the children did not moderate the outcome. The outcomes of this study imply that presence of dogs during a therapy session could influence children's attention and that interventions using therapy dogs might benefit children with ASD of various ages.

Similarly to Martin and Farnum (2002), Prothmann, Ettrich, and Prothmann (2009) presented a sample of children with ASD with three concomitant stimuli: a live dog, a person, and an inanimate object. By simultaneously presenting these stimuli, the authors could measure children's preference among these stimuli as determined by the time spent with each stimulus. Prothmann and colleagues concluded that the children preferred to interact with the live dog twice as much than they did with the person, suggesting a type of communication between the children and the dog. While the results cannot be generalized easily to other children with ASD due to the unique characteristics of this disorder, they suggest that this population could be attentive and responsive to animals.

Welsh (2009), however, concluded that the joint attention (JA) of children with ASD is not influenced by the presence of a team composed of a therapy dog and its handler. Joint attention is a critical precursor to communication, and it typically manifests through eye contact with another person, alternating gazes between an object of interest and another person, and pointing. Welsh investigated children's JA in a crossover repeated measures design, involving 15 children with ASD between 2 and 8 years of age. The children were presented with two conditions, a live dog or a plush toy condition. Welsh found no differences between the two conditions, implying that the presence of a dog does not influence JA in children with ASD. Several factors might have influenced these results, however. First, the dog was presented in a static manner, and the children were not accustomed to the dog prior to the first exposure. In addition, although the children were allowed to pet the dog, they were not allowed to play with the dog. Further, these results could provide a cautionary tale for the importance of considering the individual characteristics of the dogs and the children with ASD. It is very likely that dogs are not a universal cure (see Colțea 2011; Serpell, 2009).

Most of the research investigating the interactions and effects between children with ASD and companion animals has focused on dogs (e.g., Nimer & Lundahl, 2007). The present literature concerning the interactions of children with ASD with dogs can be divided in three sections: service dogs, companion dogs, and therapy dogs. For the purpose of this chapter, the term *autism service dogs* refers to purposefully trained dogs to serve persons with ASD, *companion dogs* refers to family pet dogs (i.e., dogs who are not trained for certain services), and *therapy dogs* encompass all assistance dogs (e.g., assisting professionals such as psychologists, play therapists, social workers) as well as dogs who provide support to certain individuals through their presence in schools, hospitals, and other environments. The next section briefly reviews the most relevant research.

Effects of Autism Service Dogs on Children With ASD

Few studies have examined the role of service dogs for children with ASD. Unlike other service dogs, the autism service dogs work in a triadic relationship—although the dogs usually are attached to the child via a tethering system, they receive instructions from parents. Burrows, Adams, and Spiers (2008) investigated the effects of service dogs on 10 families of children with ASD over a period of 12 months. The authors used a qualitative ethological approach to analyze the data (i.e., video observations and semistructured interviews with parents). The presence of autism service dogs in these families was associated with several benefits for the children, such as improvements in children's gross motor skills as well as a decrease in the frequency of behavioral tantrums and anxiety. In addition, the dogs enhanced children's safety by preventing them from running away, which is common in some children with ASD. One of the negatives associated with the service dogs in this study was that two of the dogs had to be returned due to family issues and misbehavior of the dogs. Overall, the negative effects of the service dogs on the families were outweighed by the positive influences on the children with ASD.

Viau, Arsenault-Lapierre, Fecteau, Champagne, Walker, and Lupien (2010) examined the role of service dogs on children with ASD over a shorter period of time. Viau and colleagues assessed changes in children's behavior as well as changes in their cortisol levels based on the Cortisol Awakening Response (CAR). According to Clow, Thorn, Evans, and Hucklebridge (2004), in typically developing adults there is a substantial increase in the amount of cortisol after awakening. In addition, the CAR differs from the diurnal cycle of the stress hormone, cortisol. Viau and colleagues presumed that the influence of autism service dogs on children with ASD would be reflected in the levels of the CAR. The measures were administered for 2 weeks prior to introducing the dogs, over a period of 1 month while the dogs were present in children's families, and for 2 weeks after the dogs were removed. The results suggested that the CAR spiked on average 58% from children's average cortisol secretion when the dogs were not present. Presence of service dogs was associated with a sharp decrease in the CAR, from 58 to 10%, suggesting that the dogs had a calming effect on the children. The CAR scores increased back to 48% from the average cortisol secretion once the dogs were removed. In addition, presence of service dogs was associated with a decrease in the frequency of unwanted behaviors, based on parental report. In summary, these results suggest that the service dogs enhanced the well-being of the children with ASD, even if they were present for a short time.

Two other studies investigating the influences of autism service dogs concluded that presence of dogs was associated with increased safety for children outdoors, increased social acknowledgement of the disorder by other people, companionship, enhanced communication with others, and expanded children's social activities (Smyth & Slevin, 2010; Waldie, 2005). Of note for all the studies concerning service dogs was that the benefits associated with presence of the service dog reflected on the family as a whole. Parents reported an increase in family outings, companionship, and benefits due to children's better behavior, especially in public environments. The previously reviewed studies shed light as to how children with ASD can benefit from the presence of purposefully trained service dogs.

Effects of Companion Dogs on Children With ASD

Another area that provides information relevant to CAPT is the interaction of children with ASD with their own companion dogs (Figure 3.1). In an unpublished study, Colțea (2008) investigated the role of companion dogs in 12 families of children with ASD, of whom 9 had companion dogs. Using parent report, the authors included questionnaires designed to measure symptom severity, language, and social skills for children (modified Yes/No Autism Behavior Checklist; Krug, Arick, & Almond, 1980) and children's bond with their dogs (Lexington Attachment to Pets Scale, or LAPS; Johnson, Garrity, & Stallons, 1992). Last, the Companion Dog Interactions Questionnaire (CDIQ) was created for this study to assess the reciprocity of interactions between children and their companion dogs (e.g., How often does the dog follow your child with its eyes? How often does your child touch the dog? How often does the child follow the dog through the house?).

Based on the CDIQ, Colțea (2008) concluded, for the first time, that some children with ASD interacted and were responsive to their companion dogs and that the responsiveness of the companion dogs was positively correlated with children's bond with the dog. Moreover, children's scores on both the LAPS and CDIQ suggested that some children had a strong bond to their dogs. The existence of a bond between children and their

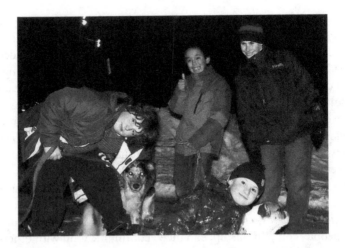

Figure 3.1 Group of children walking their companion dogs. (Courtesy of Cosmin Coltea, *My Companion Dog*, mycompaniondog.com.)

companion dogs implies the emotional availability of children with ASD. Age moderated children's bond to their dogs: Older children had a stronger bond with their dogs, interacted more with the dogs, and had better language skills, although their symptom severity was higher. The design of this study did not allow the authors to conclude whether presence of the dogs influenced children's language skills. While the findings of this study are limited by the small number of participants, it confirmed that children with ASD are responsive to their companion dogs and suggested that their bond with their companion dogs could influence their language.

In an ongoing follow-up study, Colţea (2011) has been investigating the interactions between children with and without ASD and their companion dogs. In-depth interviews were conducted with 14 families of children with ASD and 6 families with typically developing children. Of note was that the children with ASD varied in their attitudes toward their companion dogs, from indifferent to very interested in interacting with them. The *match* between certain characteristics of the children and of the companion dogs influenced the bond between children and dogs as well as the benefits based on presence of the dogs. This suggests that children's interactions with companion dogs are not universal and that factors such as child's personality and dog's personality should be considered for possible interventions. For example, some children did not develop a strong bond with a dog who is "always jumping, barking, trying to steal their food." Future research is needed to support or refute this theory, but this line of inquiry could provide useful information to clinicians considering the involvement of dogs to help children with ASD overcome some of their difficulties.

The author concluded that the companion dogs provided the children with ASD with direct social support (i.e., emotional support and companionship). For example, one participant mentioned that her daughter preferred the company of the dog to her family members:

> I think she likes to have him close against her, which is interesting because she won't touch anybody in the family. She's not demonstrative with people. If I sit next to her on the couch, no part of her body wants to touch my body. But she's very welcoming to say come sit on me Fido, put your head on me Fido, or crawls behind him.

In addition to providing direct social support, the companion dogs provided the children with indirect social support as well. For example, the dogs facilitated children's interactions with other people. One parent mentioned, "It [the dog] opened her up to have conversations with people when we're out for a walk. . . . She'll actually approach people and say, 'Can I pet your dog?' . . . She would never have approached people like that before— ever." While the design of the study does not permit conclusions about causality, it appeared that presence of dogs was conducive of language for the children with ASD. Another parent who participated in the study talked about the positive effect of the interactions between the companion dog and her 3-year-old daughter:

> Her language increased a lot, and most of her new language is around dogs. Like yesterday, she saw a picture of Fido, and my mother-in-law has two dogs, and she said the longest phrase she has ever said. She said, "It's a dog, it has ears, it's so cute, there's three of them."

In addition to these promising findings, parents of children with ASD reported that their children with ASD were able to understand certain social concepts easier if the concepts were related to the dogs. For example, explaining concepts about violence toward others was successful if explained in terms of violence toward the companion dog: "When I need to explain something to A., I use Fido as an example. If he does something to another human being he doesn't get it, but if I explain it in terms of Fido, he gets it. I'm like, 'Would you go and hit or kick Fido?'" In summary, for some children with ASD, presence of dogs was beneficial on multiple levels.

Effects of Therapy Dogs on Children With ASD

There are also studies that have attempted to look at the interactions and potential benefits of children with ASD and dogs in therapeutic settings. Levinson (1962) was one of the pioneers of animal therapy for children with ASD. During sessions involving his dog he made a series of observations related to the role of dogs for children. He suggested that dogs provided children with ASD with feelings of safety and with an affectionate presence and that they enhanced children's social interactions. Similar to the conclusions of Martin and Farnum (2002), Levinson concluded that presence of dogs in a therapy setting could anchor the children, therefore increasing their attention and focus. Further, Levinson (1965) suggested that dogs are beneficial in therapeutic settings because the children with ASD can communicate with them without language. While enhancing the language skills of children with ASD is in itself a goal of therapy, the non-verbal communication between child and dog could create a comfortable medium for the child, which in turn would contribute to development of language skills.

Although dogs have been included in therapy sessions with children with ASD since the 1960s, very little research has been conducted on this topic. Redefer and Goodman (1989) investigated the effects of a therapy dog on 12 children who exhibited autistic features. Children's ages ranged from 5 to 10 years, and although they did not receive a diagnosis they displayed autistic characteristics. Of note was that according to the authors the children were severely impaired. Measurements of children's behaviors were taken at the baseline (three 15-minute sessions), during the treatment phase (18 sessions of 20 minutes each), during the posttreatment phase (three 15-minute sessions), and a follow-up phase (three 15-minute sessions). The therapist was changed during the follow-up sessions, which tested for the generalization of the treatment. Of note was that unlike Welsh (2009), where the dog was kept stationary, Redefer and Goodman encouraged the children to interact with the dog. Importantly, children's introduction to the dog was gradual. The children started by talking about dogs and by petting them and gradually interacting more by feeding and playing with the dogs (e.g., ball throwing). The therapists also modeled these activities.

The therapists observed children's behavior in each phase and coded for *isolation*, described as activities directed at self, and *social interaction*, defined as either verbal or nonverbal interactions with the dog or the therapist (see Sullivan-Moricca, 1980/1981, for coding details). A sharp change was noted when the dog was introduced. When the dog was present, children's social interaction scores increased by 6.5 standard deviations, and their behavior isolation decreased by 5 standard deviations from the baseline. Further, children's autistic behaviors decreased as well.

During the follow-up a month later, the effects of the intervention diminished, but the effects were still present. Children's isolation scores were 2 standard deviations above the baseline, and their social interaction scores were 3 standard deviations above. These results suggested that although the effects tapered off in time the intervention with the dog clearly had a beneficial effect on children. Further, another important aspect of this study was that the therapist was actively involved by modeling and facilitating children's interactions with the dog. In addition, the gradual exposure to the dog might have strengthened children's trust in the dog and therapist, allowing the aforementioned effects to flourish.

Isaacs (1998) expanded on the previous study by using an ABAB design instead of the ABA design used by Redefer and Goodman (1989). Isaacs investigated the effect of dog therapy on five children with ASD, between 5 and 12 years old, using an observational coding procedure. The children's diagnoses varied from moderate to severe autism. Prior to conducting the interventions, extensive interviews with participants' parents were conducted to determine children's attention span and behavior in the presence of dogs. The observation protocol, based on the frequency of the targeted behaviors, was also based on the instrument designed by Sullivan-Moricca (1980/1981). The observed behaviors were "social verbal, social non-verbal, reciprocal interaction and social negative (which included isolative behaviors) (Isaacs, p. 60). The social verbal behavior consisted of words or sounds made by children in response to the therapist or in an effort to initiate interaction with the dog or therapist. The social nonverbal behavior included behaviors such as eye contact or imitations of gestures. The reciprocal interaction included, among other behaviors, any interactive play between the child and the therapist or dog. Last, the social negative behavior was any behavior that was inappropriate toward the therapist or the dog. Importantly, these behaviors were coded separately for the therapist and the dog.

Each child participated in nine sessions of 25 minutes each, over a period of 4 to 6 weeks. Although a protocol was used for each phase, slight deviations were necessary due to the individual characteristics of each child (e.g., if the child was nonresponsive). During the baseline phases, after the initial greeting period the child was engaged in turn-taking games such as walking around the room, ball rolling, blowing bubbles, and eating a piece of cookie. During the treatment phases the same activities were conducted, except that the dog was involved in each of them. Similar to Redefer and Goodman (1989), the children were gradually introduced to the dog by first encouraging identification of the dog's body parts, then talking about the dog, followed by modeling appropriate physical interactions with the dog. The child and the therapist took turns walking with the dog, identifying body parts on the dog, brushing the dog, and feeding the dog.

Isaacs (1989) concluded that several factors were important in the interventions. First, the activities were selected based on children's activity level. For example, more gross motor activities were conducted for hyperactive children, such as ball throwing. Second, some children preferred working on the floor whereas others preferred to stand. Third, the therapist's tone of voice was modulated in response to children's activity level (i.e., a soft voice was used with hyperactive children). Fourth, the individual characteristics of the children were also important (i.e., child's degree and nature of fear of the dog, if any, receptivity and tolerance to social intrusion by the dog and therapist, and ability to sustain focus during an activity) (p. 75).

The group-level results suggested that presence of the dog during the treatment phases resulted in less frequent social negative behaviors, increased social nonverbal and verbal behaviors, and increased frequency of reciprocal interactions. The author noted that the second phase of treatment resulted in higher scores, suggesting that increased interactions between children and dogs could result in higher benefits for the children. Because of the study design, which measured the behaviors separately for the therapist and for the dog, the author concluded that the children transferred their social interactions with the dog to the therapist.

At an individual level, the effects of dog therapy differed among the participant children (Isaacs, 1989). These results, similar to the recommendations of a few other researchers (e.g., Colţea, 2011; Serpell, 2009), highlight the importance of considering individual characteristics (i.e., personality, age, previous knowledge of dog behavior) in animal-assisted therapy.

Sams, Fortney, and Willenbring (2006) investigated the influence of animals on the language and social interaction skills of 22 children with ASD, between 7 and 13 years old. The children participated in two conditions: one involving only occupational therapy techniques and a second session where different animals (i.e., llamas, dogs, and rabbits) were present. The authors concluded that presence of animals resulted in better language and social interaction skills. The authors suggested that perhaps the nonjudgmental attitude of animals might encourage children's use of language and enhance their social interactions.

With regard to the social interaction of children with ASD, Solomon (2010) provided more evidence for the powerful role of therapy dogs. Solomon observed unscripted interactions among a 9-year-old child with ASD, her 4-year-old twin sisters, and a few therapy dogs and their handler. The observations concluded that presence of dogs helped the child with ASD engage in conversations with the handler and her two younger sisters. During the interactions with the dogs, the child with ASD learned several instructions, which she was later able to explain to her sisters. Further, she explained the "Speak" instruction to another child while in a park setting. The child with ASD had observed another child having difficulties getting her dog to respond to the instruction, after which the child with ASD spontaneously, without any prompting, offered information to the other child. The results of this case example suggest that, at least in this case, dogs do act as social facilitators and, more importantly, that children's skills in interacting with the dog can be transferred to social interactions with people.

In summary, several conclusions can be drawn from the previously reviewed studies. First, presence of companion animals seems to benefit children with ASD. Caution must be exercised, however, in making sweeping generalizations about these benefits, due to the spectrum effect of these disorders. Second, it is important to note that presence of dogs appears to generate most benefits, especially in social environments where presence of other animals is not readily available. Concerning this aspect, it is important for CAPT therapists to keep in mind that while interventions with therapy dogs are usually conducted indoors, the presence of a therapy dog in social settings could provide different benefits to children with ASD, such as acting as social facilitators and reducing anxiety levels in diverse environments. Last, the benefits appear to generalize from the interactions with animals to interactions with humans, suggesting that the nonverbal, furry, attention-catching presence of therapy dogs can play an important part in the social integration of children with ASD.

Specific Interventions Used With Children With ASD

Both authors of this chapter have involved dogs with children with ASD in somewhat different ways. VanFleet has helped develop the field of CAPT and, in so doing, has applied many of the specific interventions listed earlier and elsewhere (VanFleet, 2008) with children with ASD. These include (1) helping children learn to interact safely with play therapy dogs, (2) nondirective play therapy in which the therapist helps the dog play roles as designed by the children and reflects the child's feelings and intentions through the dog, and (3) a wide range of directive play therapy interventions such as training the dog, teaching the dog new tricks, playing ball or tug safely with the dog, agility work, and dramatic play involving child dress-up and special bandannas for the therapy dog as they enact social scenarios. There are vast possibilities in terms of specific methods that can be used to address areas of social and language functioning, and some of these are illustrated in the case examples that follow.

Coauthor Colţea has created a unique group program for children with ASD. The program is based on existing research on the value of companion dogs for typically developing children (e.g., Melson, 2003), his previous work and research with children with ASD (i.e., worked and volunteered with numerous children with ASD in situations that involved interactions with animals), and his experience as a dog trainer (professionally training other people to work with their dogs as well as training dogs directly since 1991).

The program is a recreational program, although it could easily be adapted by therapists with the proper skills for use in a play therapy setting as well. The program is a group class designed to enhance children's relationships with their companion dogs as well as children's interactions with peers during eight 1-hour weekly sessions. The requirements for participating in the program are that children have a diagnosis of ASD and have a companion dog (i.e., a family dog, not a specially trained service or therapy dog). The first time the program was offered, however, one of the children worked with one of author Colţea's dogs, due to the child's family not having a companion dog. This child's interactions with the dog were initially facilitated through subtle head signals from Colţea until the child had an opportunity to build a connection (Figure 3.2).

The first week of class is conducted without dogs present to allow for introductions and to learn about dog behavior based on pictures and on a live demonstration dog (one of the group leader's dogs). The group classes have been limited to three or four children to permit sufficient individual attention. Children who have participated to date have been 9 to 14 years old, and their symptoms were relatively mild (i.e., all children possessed some form of language) (Figure 3.3). Children's social skills were not observed without having at least one dog present.

The program has three core areas: (1) learning about dog behavior (i.e., dogs' communication style and their needs); (2) caretaking of the dogs (i.e., brushing and grooming, preparing their treats, and refilling the water bowl); (3) obedience and agility exercises, as well as diverse games (e.g., red light/green light, musical chairs, alternating the walking pace in different combinations—slow/normal/fast).

Children first participated in some obedience exercises, with emphasis placed on learning "Stop" (i.e., the child stops the dog in a standing

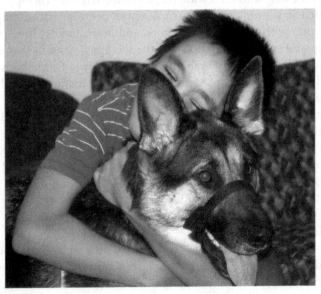

Figure 3.2 Emotional connection between a child and his companion dog. (Courtesy of Cosmin Coltea, *My Companion Dog*, mycompaniondog.com.)

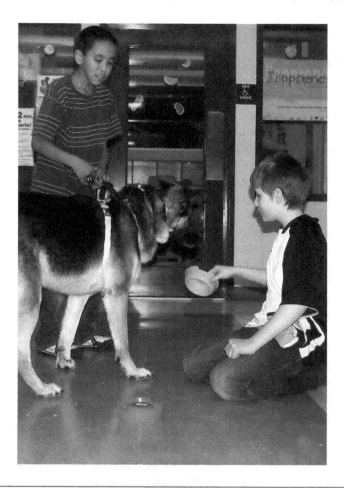

Figure 3.3 Companion dog facilitating child-to-child communication. (Courtesy of Cosmin Coltea, *My Companion Dog*, mycompaniondog.com.)

position by verbal instruction or by hand signal). This instruction was later integrated in the games. With regard to the games, the red light/green light consisted of having the children advance and stop with the dogs at their side. The children and the dogs moved both forward and backward to enhance children's gross motor skills (the goal was not to reach the person giving the instruction but rather to not get caught moving). For the musical chairs, the children walked around a circle of five or six chairs with the dogs at their side. The rules of the game stipulated that upon hearing an instruction from the group leader the children had to instruct the dog accordingly, and they themselves were to sit on the chairs. Similar to the previous game, no child was eliminated from the game; rather, the goal was on ensuring that the children were attentive to their dogs and that they were attentive to the instructions issued by the instructor. Depending on certain factors, such as dogs' training level and children's knowledge of dog behavior, the difficulty level of the games could be adjusted (e.g., the children have to advance in a line formation for the red light/green light game, which ensures that they are attentive to their peers).

In addition, the program targets certain areas of social functioning, such as turn taking, appropriate use of voices, problem solving, and organizational skills by involving the children in running the class. For example, in one group, the children decided the schedule for one of the classes—they had to discuss and agree on the exercises to be used. While this might not be possible with nonverbal children with ASD, in that instance it allowed the children to solve a difficult task, one that required independent thinking and social interaction.

So far, this program has been piloted successfully in advance of a research study slated to begin in fall 2011. The author's own observations and parental reports from the pilot programs have suggested that the group program offers some benefits for children. First, there was an improvement in children's awareness of the dog (e.g., discontinuing dragging the dog around while involved in discussions with other children). In addition, children's social interactions with each other became more fluent—although this could also be due to time spent together (i.e., the children talked more to each other, were learning about each other's interests, shared diverse personal stories). Second, there were improvements in children's eye contact with the group leader (author Colțea), probably because the children were encouraged to make eye contact with their dogs to ensure that their dogs were attentive to them. There were also improvements in children's posture, perhaps because they had to use different body positions when communicating with the dogs. Third, there were improvements in dogs' reactions to the children—they responded faster to instructions.

In addition to the authors' own observations, personal communication from parents confirmed the positive influence of this program on the children. One father mentioned that his son preferred this program in comparison with programs that did not have an animal component: "Out of all of them, yours was the one he loved the most. So much so that I believe he even sent an email to you. He referred to it as 'epic' and looked forward to each class."

Children's interactions with the dog during the program seemed to transfer to interactions at home. One parent reported, "My son has actually asked to take Fido out a few times this week and is doing well with talking to her. We are impressed so far with his increased understanding of what to do with her even though it sometimes takes a prompt or cue for him to step back and think about his attitude and how she is reacting." In another case, the parents, who acquired the dog for the child with ASD, had been somewhat disappointed that the dog had bonded better with them: "I think taking the course has helped with something we tried to foster—a little bit more of a bond with the dog where he takes the class, and my wife and I are completely gone, and it is just him and Fido doing this."

Case Examples

Three case studies are included here. The first represents an individual, in-home intervention by coauthor Colțea with the child's companion dog, and the second is an example from his group program for children with ASD. The third is a case example from coauthor VanFleet's play therapy practice involving a therapy dog. In all cases, identifying information has been changed to protect the privacy and identity of the children and families.

Jeremy

Jeremy was 9 years old when we started and had a diagnosis of autism. He was attending school with the help of an educational assistant. Although his language skills were good, his social skills (i.e., not looking and inter-acting with other people) and his rigidity in eating choices (i.e., certain fast-food products) were a cause of concern for his parents. Building rapport with Jeremy during the first session, I listened to Jeremy talk about his two companion dogs (two small cross-breeds, approximately 15 pounds each, and 6 and 8 years old). Although Jeremy interacted with the dogs inside his home (i.e., petting and playing with them), he did not inter-act with them outside, partly because his parents did not walk the dogs. Initially Jeremy and I played with the dogs inside the house and then in the backyard. Gradually, we took both dogs for walks in a nearby park and worked with them on a variety of obedience exercises. The exercises were meant to strengthen Jeremy's pronunciation and to enhance his self-confidence. In addition, the dogs seemed to welcome the exercises, given their exuberant attitudes.

After several sessions in which Jeremy became confident in walking with one dog after he clearly began enjoying running with his dogs in the park, the walks were scheduled during busy times in the park to meet other people. I modeled interactions with other people for several sessions (e.g., casually talking about dogs with other dog guardians in the vicin-ity) and continued introducing games designed to enhance Jeremy's inter-est in the dog (e.g., tobogganing with one of the dogs who enjoyed this activity). Gradually, Jeremy started to respond to people's questions about his dogs' names, and Jeremy furthered the conversations by mentioning his dogs' unusual activities (e.g., tobogganing). In the beginning, Jeremy's responses were "thrown," without looking or speaking in the direction of the other person. The "Watch Game" proved successful in having Jeremy make better eye contact with me and possibly others. The Watch Game required nonverbal communication only. I mentioned to Jeremy that it was important to get the dog's attention for any instructions and that eye contact told us that the dog was paying attention. Before practicing with the Watch Game with one of his dogs, Jeremy practiced making eye contact with me. After approximately 5 months of work on this with the dogs and me, Jeremy was consistently responding to questions from passersby about his dogs and looking in their direction while so doing.

With regard to Jeremy's eating habits, two methods were used to diversify his menu. First, I discussed with Jeremy about the varied menu of the dogs (as part of the program, parents were encouraged to feed their dogs a varied diet of dry food and vegetables). During these discussions, the variety of food was associated with dogs' speed and apparently inexhaustible energy, values that were desired by Jeremy. The second method involved walking with the dogs for longer periods of time and stopping strategically next to food establishments that were not initially favored by Jeremy. Gradually, by combining modeling of dog eating habits and proximity to certain establishments, Jeremy began to expand his restricted diet by including other foods. His parents reported, however, that while his meals were more varied during these sessions Jeremy maintained his strict diet with them.

Marcel

Marcel participated in one of the group classes. He was 10 years old, and his dog was 6 months old. During the first few classes, Marcel neglected the dog and focused on a Rubik's Cube puzzle, which his parents reported went everywhere with him. During these first classes Marcel participated in all activities, but his attention was still on the Rubik's Cube (i.e., at every opportunity he would play with it instead of focusing on the dog). In addition, his interactions with the dog were unfocused; he liked to run with the dog, but he did not know how to reward the dog or how to calm the dog if need be.

During the classes, one of the goals was to remove the Rubik's Cube and to increase Marcel's attention to his dog. One of the strategies I used to reduce the use of the Rubik's Cube was to ensure that Marcel, as well as the other children in the group, practiced heeling, which in turn requires rewarding the dog very often, by either petting or using treats. Rewarding the dog meant that both of Marcel's hands were occupied and that he was attentive to the dog. Further, the heeling exercises were conducted at different paces, from a very slow pace to a fast pace.

Another strategy was based on using games and activities that were engaging to deter Marcel from playing with the Rubik's Cube. Games such as maintaining a line formation while heeling ensured that Marcel's attention was focused on his peers and his dog rather than on the Rubik's Cube. In addition, running the agility course also made certain that Marcel did not have time to engage in playing with the puzzle. Another factor that contributed to Marcel eventually leaving his Rubik's Cube outside of class was an incident during which his dog grabbed one of the plastic pieces from the Cube after Marcel accidentally dropped it. After I discussed with the children the consequences of dogs swallowing foreign objects, Marcel began petting his dog.

During the following sessions, Marcel was more focused on his dog and no longer brought his Cube to class. Although it is unknown what caused him to stop bringing his favorite object to the class, I believe that it was due to Marcel's growing emotional attachment to his dog and his desire to protect his dog from being hurt. His parents noted that Marcel appeared to be more emotionally open about his dog, and he had shown them that he was able to care for another being.

Macy

Macy was a 9-year-old girl diagnosed with high-functioning autism, post-traumatic stress disorder, and attention-deficit/hyperactivity disorder. Due to her mother's drug addiction problems and her father's complete absence, Macy had been adopted at age 4 and raised by her aunt and uncle. She was seen in play therapy for her trauma and worsening behavior problems at home and school. She was unable to handle angry or fearful feelings and became destructive and extremely distraught when she experienced those emotions.

Macy had made progress through the use of play therapy and filial therapy in terms of her relationship with her adoptive parents. Disruptive behaviors had lessened, but Macy continued to struggle with her feelings and social relationships. She had no real friends, was unable to talk about her feelings, and had low frustration tolerance. She spoke rarely, made almost no eye contact, had very poor social skills, and had difficulty focusing on auditory information.

Macy readily admitted that she loved animals and much preferred their company to that of humans. She gravitated toward her primary therapist's office dog, Henry, a rescued Labradoodle, and enjoyed petting him and lying on the floor with him. Because Macy was seen at the practice affiliated with the first author (VanFleet), CAPT sessions were added to the services she was already receiving. Because Macy already had a relationship with Henry, I began CAPT with Henry, and the primary play therapist joined us for those sessions to ensure continuity. Later, I introduced Macy to two of my own play therapy dogs.

Henry was a good choice because he had some similar difficulties to Macy's. Although he was a very social dog, his attention drifted from one toy to another, and his focus on people was fleeting unless they were offering him food or rubbing his belly. He had a calm demeanor and relatively low energy while in the office, which made him seem safe and relaxed.

For Macy, the goals of CAPT were to increase her ability to focus, to help her learn more about recognizing and expressing feelings, to develop her self-confidence, and to improve her social and communication capabilities. She sometimes had been physically intrusive with Henry, resulting in his moving away from her or becoming too excited, so I hoped that CAPT would also show her how to create a relationship with him that was respectful of his space and body.

Macy: Early CAPT Sessions In her first three CAPT sessions with Henry, Macy said almost nothing. She had trouble following instructions and was distracted by the toys. During these early CAPT sessions, I chose simple dog-training activities that I thought would keep Macy's and Henry's attention while resulting in some success for both of them. They are briefly described herein.

First, I taught Macy about clicker training, during which she used a small device that made a click sound (conditioned reinforcer) just prior to her giving the dog a treat. The click communicates clearly to the dog that the current behavior is good. It also makes the interactions with the dog quite concrete and helps children focus more on the dog's behavior (they must watch for the right moments to click). Macy enjoyed this and mastered the clicker quickly. She chose not to talk and used the clicker to communicate with Henry. Next, in an eye contact game, Macy gave Henry treats whenever he made eye contact with her. Soon, Henry and Macy were making regular eye contact with each other. I offered encouragement and praise, with a few suggestions to help her succeed.

During the third session as Macy taught Henry a new trick, she accidentally tossed a toy so that it nearly hit me in the stomach. When I laughed, Macy began giggling. It was the first time I or her primary therapist had seen her smile. There was a brief moment of laughing together—a significant social connection—before our attentions turned back to the dog. The third session ended with a hide-and-seek game. Macy hid and Henry searched until he found her, rewarded by treats when he did. Each time I asked if she wanted to play this game again, she nodded and found a new place to hide.

When I suggested that Macy provide some verbal cues to Henry, she declined, and I accepted her decision. Pushing her would not yield the outcomes that we desired.

Macy: Middle CAPT Sessions Macy improved during the fourth and fifth CAPT sessions, entering the room with more confidence, taking the clicker and preparing the treats with new initiative. Macy taught Henry to turn in a circle, smiling frequently at Henry's attempts to learn this trick. She glanced and smiled slightly at me and at her primary therapist (still observing the sessions) several times. She offered several soft but audible comments to both therapists about Henry's behavior.

During the fifth CAPT session, Macy laughed openly several times. She obviously found Henry's antics funny, but of real significance was the frequency of her eye contact with me. Macy used hand gestures and whistles to prompt Henry to do one of his tricks, then looked at me and smiled, then returned her attention to Henry. Her acknowledgment of me seemed to convey her sense of joy in being able to play the games with Henry as well as a shared component; that is, she was sharing with me specifically her pleasure in the activity (a bit like two parents whose eyes meet and who smile when their child does something cute). This was a new behavior for Macy and seemed to be an indication of the social lubricant effects of the work with Henry. This socially engaging glance increased in frequency and duration with each session that followed.

At this time I introduced a canine puzzle game to Macy and Henry. Other than showing Macy how to work the game, I gave few instructions, allowing her to teach Henry as she wanted. Henry was particularly distractible during this session, so Macy first had to get his attention to show him that there were treats hidden in the puzzle. She tried several strategies to do this, and I was able to reinforce her persistence and problem-solving skills. When Henry walked away several times, I asked Macy how he might be feeling, and she was able to identify possible frustration and boredom. I reinforced her recognition of his feelings. Eventually, Macy helped Henry focus on the puzzle and gave him hints about how to solve it. Throughout this 20-minute sequence, Macy was fully engaged, showed complete focus on the task, and demonstrated more patience than would be expected of most people! She smiled when Henry succeeded and quietly waited when Henry seemed to forget what he was doing and became distracted. From a therapeutic perspective, Macy was showing significant progress and interest in what she was doing. She was pleased with Henry's (and her) eventual success and asked to demonstrate the puzzle game for her parents.

Macy: Later CAPT Sessions From this point forward, Macy made much progress. She increasingly was able to identify Henry's feelings when prompted, and she listened carefully to my instructions or prompts. She began using spoken language spontaneously and more frequently. Her focus was on the work she was doing with Henry, and it seemed to reduce her self-consciousness and discomfort when interacting with people.

During her eighth CAPT session, we made a DVD that demonstrated the things that she had taught Henry, and during a family session her primary therapist helped her decide to share it with some extended family members. They worked out the details so there was no pressure on Macy to talk about what she was doing—she simply could show the DVD, which I had edited to remove any sense of "therapy" from it.

During all of the CAPT sessions, I emphasized the metaphors as they arose: "It's hard to keep focused on things sometimes. Gee, Henry keeps trying and he can't figure it out. He's frustrated, but you're helping him take it a step at a time. Sometimes with tough problems, Henry has to keep trying different things, and he doesn't always get it the first time." I made little effort to "teach" these lessons to Macy, as that would have made the process much too cognitive. I knew she was absorbing much more through her own experiences with the dogs.

Macy also began to work with two of my own dogs during the later sessions, and she confidently was able to teach them some new tricks as well. This required her to have flexibility in teaching the dogs, as they did not react quite the same way that Henry did. Again, she was able to demonstrate focus, patience, and caring.

Some rather remarkable progress occurred during two sessions with Kirrie, my border collie/hound play therapy dog. Kirrie is very energetic and quick to learn, and she enjoys physical games. I brought in a 10-foot flexible fabric tunnel similar to those used in canine agility. Macy helped teach Kirrie to run through the tunnel, and Macy ran to the other end of the tunnel to meet Kirrie with a treat. Kirrie came to the end and stuck just her head out to get the treat from Macy. Macy began laughing at this, as did both of us therapists in the room. Soon thereafter, Macy began climbing through the tunnel herself, followed by Kirrie. Macy was trying to beat Kirrie to the end. Several times Kirrie came out of the tunnel and began licking Macy's face. Although she had some negative reactions to licking before this, Macy laughed even harder, clearly enjoying it. At the end of this session, I gave Macy a choice regarding which dog she would like to play with for the next session. She chose Kirrie.

When Macy came into the playroom for the next session, she was extremely talkative about school, a sports game she had played, and dogs. Neither her therapist nor I had seen her talk this much. There was much more tunnel play with Kirrie, including the "races," and Macy also found ways to "fool" Kirrie so she could get a head start in the tunnel. She laughed aloud during all of this play, highly engaged with the dog but also with us. Kirrie is also an expert hide-and-seek player, so I suggested this game, knowing that Macy had been interested in it before and because it fit well with some of her attachment needs. Macy hid in several locations and was always pleased when Kirrie almost immediately found her. After 40 minutes, I took Kirrie to my office and then met with Macy's aunt and uncle to review progress while Macy's primary therapist held a short play session with her.

Macy's uncle told me that in the waiting room just prior to this session with Kirrie Macy had initiated a conversation with him for the first time ever. He was very pleased. Macy's aunt and uncle also reported that her newfound confidence seemed to be spreading to the home and school settings, where there were fewer emotional or behavioral outbursts. Her verbal conversations were also on the rise.

As we talked, Macy and her therapist came from the playroom, and Macy asked me to come back to see "a surprise." This social initiation was also new for her, not seen before by her therapist, aunt, or uncle. She showed me a sand tray she had created, with people's houses neatly arranged around the edges and all the "courtyard" space in between filled with animal figures. There were also birds perched on the top of some of the houses. Macy proudly showed me her creation and commented about how it was such a fun place where animals could feel free and play! Macy seemed to be reaching out through the animals to some of the humans in her life.

After 12 CAPT sessions, I invited Macy to bring in her own family dog for us to work with part of the time. She was pleased to do this, and this part of the CAPT process is continuing. Her parents now join us for some sessions, as they are learning how to facilitate the canine interactions at home in ways consistent with the CAPT sessions.

In summary, CAPT helped open doors for Macy. She was able to develop her own skills and confidence. She began to communicate more appropriately with people while sharing social interactions involving the dogs. Her primary play therapist reported that she was able to relax more during play sessions and make greater progress than she had. Her parents reported that she seemed to demonstrate more interest in family life, especially when they included their dog in more activities (something I had worked with the entire family on).

Guidelines and Specific Levels of Client Functioning

The use of CAPT with children with ASD is a newly emerging practice. More research and clinical experience will help define its applications and limitations. Because the relative strengths and difficulties of children with ASD vary significantly across the spectrum and for each individual child, specific guidelines for the use of CAPT are not yet available. It does appear that CAPT is probably not appropriate for all children with ASD, and individual children may benefit from the involvement of specific dogs and types of interactions with them. A thorough knowledge of children with ASD and their needs is critical, and an accomplished and perceptive play therapist properly trained in the methods of CAPT can probably make some good decisions based on the guiding principles of child development, clinical child work, play therapy, and CAPT. It is hoped that future research and experience will begin to define the circumstances under which CAPT can facilitate therapeutic interventions and offer the most benefits.

It seems likely that forms of CAPT might be beneficial for children with ASD who are functioning at all levels. Dogs offer a tactile, living presence that does not require language or fine-tuned social skills. They provide a metaphor for attachment, communication, social skills, problem solving, and many other features of productive relationships. Interactions can be as simple as petting a willing dog and as complex as teaching the dog a new trick or game. When therapists facilitate interactions between children with ASD and dogs, they can capitalize on whatever interactions and metaphors along this continuum that best meet the needs of each individual child.

Given the special needs and symptoms of children with ASD, however, there are some special considerations to ensure that the use of CAPT is appropriate and helpful to all involved. First, it is absolutely essential that therapists have full training in play therapy and in CAPT. It is inappropriate to take one's own companion dog into a play session without preparing the dog and oneself fully for this eventuality. Supervision during initial use of CAPT is also very important to ensure professional skill development in the use of the method.

Second, therapists must develop competencies in positive dog training, handling, and relationship. Use of any force- or dominance-oriented equipment or methods is completely inappropriate, not only for its negative impact on the dog but also for the poor model it presents to children. Perhaps of greatest importance is to become fluent in canine communication and body language. Dogs communicate a great deal about their emotional states and their stress levels through their nonverbal signals, and therapists must be able to monitor the dog's reactions at all times before, during, and after therapy sessions to ensure that the dog is enjoying the interactions and to prevent negative outcomes for child or dog. Too often, in their enthusiasm to harness the potential benefits of canine involvement, therapists and researchers overlook the needs of the dog. This is counterproductive for the dog, the child, and the therapy process. Attentiveness to canine communications allows therapists to ensure the best possible experiences for all. Even if a child with ASD is enjoying an interaction with a dog, the therapist must be prepared to stop that interaction in the instant it turns negative for the dog. Therapists use their clinical skills to do this in a nondisruptive and therapeutic manner. In addition, fluency in canine communication allows therapists to foresee dogs' reactions and thus allows them to better guide the therapeutic process by knowing how the dogs will react to children's behaviors.

Third, children with ASD sometimes exhibit behaviors that can trigger dogs' instinctive reactions or that can startle or frighten dogs. These include children's sudden or erratic movements, laughing or talking very loudly, hitting or kicking when frustrated, talking in a pressured manner, squeezing or touching too hard, yelling, trying to keep things in a particular order, strong reactions to some sensory input, incoordination, intolerance of normal dog behaviors, and others. Any dog who works with children needs to be socialized for a wide range of unpredictable child behaviors, and this is especially true of dogs who work with children with ASD. Not all dogs have the right temperament for this type of work, and this fact needs to be taken seriously. For dogs who can tolerate varied and unexpected child movements and noises, the therapist still must be aware of canine reactions and know how to help adjust the child's behaviors or the activities to ensure calm, smooth interactions. Again, solid knowledge of dog behavioral communications is required to understand the dog's behavior as well as to reliably anticipate the dog's behavior when the children might exhibit certain threatening behaviors.

The use of CAPT has much potential to help children with ASD break through some of their difficulties and to facilitate their social development and communication abilities. The use of CAPT must be handled carefully and in conjunction with research and program evaluation so that the methods can be refined and expanded in the best interests of children with ASD, their families, and the dogs. The work involving autism service dogs, companion dogs in families of children with ASD, and CAPT can be complementary, and what is learned in one endeavor can benefit the others. This chapter represents an attempt to highlight key theory, research, and practice in the involvement of dogs in the lives of children with ASD, with the hope that more play therapists, child clinicians, and researchers will explore its considerable potential.

References

American Psychiatric Association. (APA). (2000). *Diagnostic and statistical manual of mental disorders* (4th ed., text rev.). Washington, DC: Author.

Ascione, F. R. (1992). Enhancing children's attitudes about the humane treatment of animals: Generalization to human-directed empathy. *Anthrozoös, 5*, 176–191.

Ascione, F. R., & Weber, C. V. (1996). Children's attitudes about the human treatment of animals and empathy: One year follow-up of a school-based intervention. *Anthrozoös, 9*, 188–195.

Ashby, J. S., Kottman, T., & DeGraaf, D. G. (2008). *Active interventions for kids and teens: Adding adventure and fun to counseling!* Alexandria, VA: American Counseling Association.

Beck, A. M., & Katcher, A. H. (1996). *Between pets and people: The importance of animal companionship* (rev. ed.). West Lafayette, IN: Purdue University Press.

Bratton, S. C., Ray, D., Rhine, T., & Jones, L. (2005). The efficacy of play therapy with children: A meta-analytic review of treatment outcomes. *Professional Psychology: Research and Practice, 36*(4), 376–390.

Burrows, K. E., Adams, C. L., & Spiers, J. (2008). Sentinels of safety: Service dogs ensure safety and enhance freedom and well-being for families with autistic children. *Qualitative Health Research, 18*, 1642–1649.

Celani, G. (2002). Human beings, animals and inanimate objects: What do people with autism like? *Autism, 6*(1), 93–102.

Chandler, C. K. (2005). *Animal assisted therapy in counseling.* New York: Routledge.

Clothier, S. (2002). *Bones would rain from the sky: Deepening our relationships with dogs.* New York: Grand Central Publishing.

Clow, A., Thorn, L., Evans, P., & Hucklebridge, F., (2004). The awakening cortisol response: Methodological issues and significance. *Stress, 7*(1), 29–37.

Colţea, C. G. (2008). *The effects of companion animals on families of children with autism spectrum disorders.* Unpublished honor's thesis, Carleton University, Canada.

Colţea, G. C. (2011). *Companion dogs could influence families with and without children with autism.* Unpublished master's thesis, Carleton University, Canada.

Esteves, S. W., & Stokes, T. (2008). Social effects of a dog's presence on children with disabilities. *Anthrozoös, 21*(1), 5–15.

Gonski, Y. A. (1985). The therapeutic utilization of canines in a child welfare setting. *Child and Adolescent Social Work Journal, 2*, 93–105.

Isaacs, J. M. (1998). *The effects of pet-facilitated therapy on the social and interactive behaviors of autistic children.* Unpublished master's thesis, California State University.

Jalongo, M. R. (Ed.). (2004). *The world's children and their companion animals: Developmental and educational significance of the child/pet bond.* Olney, MD: Association for Childhood Education International.

Jalongo, M. R., Astorino, T., & Bomboy, N. (2004). Canine visitors: The influence of therapy dogs on young children's learning and well-being in classrooms and hospitals. *Early Childhood Education Journal, 32*(1), 9–16.

Johnson, T. P., Garrity, T. F., & Stallons, L. (1992). Psychometric evaluation of the Lexington Attachment to Pets Scale (LAPS). *Anthrozoös, 5*, 160–175.

Kalnajs, S. (2006). *The language of dogs: Understanding canine body language and other communication signals* [DVD set]. Madison, WI: Blue Dog Training and Behavior.

Krug, D. A., Arick, J. R., & Almond, P. J. (1980). Behavior checklist for identifying severely handicapped individuals with high levels of autistic behavior. *Journal of Child Psychology and Psychiatry, 21*, 221–229.

Levinson, B. M. (1962). The dog as a "co-therapist." *Mental Hygiene, 46*, 59–65.

Levinson, B. M. (1965). Pet psychotherapy: Use of household pets in the treatment of behavior disorders in childhood. *Psychological Reports, 17*, 695–698.

Martin, F., & Farnum, J. (2002). Animal-assisted therapy for children with pervasive developmental disorders. *Western Journal of Nursing Research, 24*(6), 657–670.

McCardle, P., McCune, S., Griffin, J. A., Esposito, L., & Freund, L. S. (2011). *Animals in our lives: Human–animal interaction in family, community, & therapeutic settings.* Baltimore: Paul H. Brookes.

Melson, G. F. (2001). *Why the wild things are: Animals in the lives of children.* Cambridge, MA: Harvard University Press.

Melson, G. (2003). Child development and the human–companion animal bond. *American Behavioral Scientist, 47*(1), 31–39. doi: 10.1177/0002764203255210.

Melson, G. F., & Fine, A. H. (2006). Animals in the lives of children. In A. H. Fine (Ed.), *Animal-assisted therapy: Theoretical foundations and guidelines for practice* (2nd ed., pp. 207–226). San Diego: Academic Press.

New, J. J., Schultz, R. T., Wolf, J., Niehaus, J. L., Klin, A., German, T. G., et al. (2009). The scope of social attention deficits in autism: Prioritized orienting to people and animals in static natural scenes. *Neuropshychologia, 48,* 51–59.

Nimer, J., & Lundahl, B. (2007). Animal-assisted therapy: A meta-analysis. *Anthrozoös 20*(3), 225–238. doi:10.2752/089279307X224773.

Odendall, J. S. J. (2000). Animal-assisted therapy: Magic or medicine. *Journal of Psychosomatic Research, 49*(4), 275–280.

Olmert, M. D. (2009). *Made for each other: The biology of the human-animal bond.* Cambridge, MA: Da Capo Press.

Parish-Plass, N. (2008). Animal-assisted therapy with children suffering from insecure attachment due to abuse and neglect: A method to lower the risk of intergenerational transmission of abuse? *Clinical Child Psychology and Psychiatry, 13*(1), 7–30.

Pelar, C. (2007). *Living with kids and dogs... Without losing your mind.* Woodbridge, VA: C&R Publishing.

Pelar, C. (2009). *Kids and dogs: A professional's guide to helping families.* Woodbridge, VA: DreamDog Productions.

Pavlides, M. (2008). *Animal-assisted interventions for individuals with autism.* London: Jessica Kingsley Publishers.

Podberscek, A. L., Paul, E. S., & Serpell, J. (Eds.). (2000). *Companion animals and us: Exploring the relationships between people and pets.* Cambridge, England: Cambridge University Press.

Prothmann, A., Ettrich, C., & Prothmann, S. (2009). Preference for, and responsiveness to, people, dogs and objects in children with autism. *Anthrozoös, 22*(2), 161–171.

Redefer, L. A., & Goodman, J. F. (1989). Brief report: Pet-facilitated therapy with autistic children. *Journal of Autism & Developmental Disorders, 19*(3), 461–467.

Sams, M. J., Fortney, E. V., & Willenbring, S. (2006). Occupational therapy incorporating animals for children with Autism: A pilot investigation. *American Occupational Therapy Association, 60,* 268–274.

Schopler, E., Reicher, R. J., & Renner, B. R. (1990). *Individualized assessment and treatment for autistic and developmentally disabled children. Vol. 1: Psychoeducational Profile revised.* Austin, TX: Pro-ed.

Serpell, J. (2009). Having our dogs and eating them too: Why animals are a social issue. *Journal of Social Issues, 65*(3), 633–644.

Smyth, C., & Slevin, E. (2010). Experiences of family life with an autism assistance dog. *Learning Disability Practice, 13*(4), 12–18.

Solomon, O. (2010). What a dog can do: Children with autism and therapy dogs in social interaction. *Ethos, 38*(1), 143–166.

Sullivan-Moricca, K. (1980/1981). Autistic children: A theoretical and practical approach toward the psychological maturation of object relations (California School of Professional Psychology). *Dissertation Abstracts International, 41,* 1903B-3904B.

Thompson, M. J. (2009). Animal-assisted play therapy: Canines as co-therapists. In G. R. Walz, J. C. Bleuer, & R. K. Yep (Eds.), *Compelling counseling interventions: VISTAS 2009* (pp. 199–209). Alexandria, VA: American Counseling Association.

Trotter, K. S., Chandler, C. K., Goodwin-Bond, D., & Casey, J. (2008). A comparative study of the efficacy of group equine assisted counseling with at-risk children and adolescents. *Journal of Creativity in Mental Health, 3*(3), 254–284.

VanFleet, R. (2004). *Pets in play therapy: A training manual.* Boiling Springs, PA: Play Therapy Press.

VanFleet, R. (2006a). *Group play therapy techniques: Training manual.* Boiling Springs, PA: Play Therapy Press.

VanFleet, R. (2006b). *Child-centered play therapy* [DVD set]. Boiling Springs, PA: Play Therapy Press.

VanFleet, R. (2007). *Preliminary results from the ongoing pet play therapy study.* Boiling Springs, PA: Play Therapy Press. Full report available at http://playtherapy.com/playfulpooch/pets_study.html

VanFleet, R. (2008). *Play therapy with kids & canines: Benefits for children's developmental and psychosocial health.* Sarasota, FL: Professional Resource Press.

VanFleet, R. (2009). *Canine assisted play therapy: Theory, research, and practice training manual.* Boiling Springs, PA: Play Therapy Press.

VanFleet, R. (2011). *Practice guidelines and credentialing in animal assisted play therapy.* Unpublished document.

VanFleet, R., & Faa-Thompson, T. (2010). The case for using animal assisted play therapy. *British Journal of Play Therapy, 6,* 4–18.

VanFleet, R., Sywulak, A. E., & Sniscak, C. S. (2010). *Child-centered play therapy.* New York: Guilford.

Viau, R., Arsenault-Lapierre, G., Fecteau, S., Champagne, N., Walker, C-D., & Lupien, S. (2010). Effect of service dogs on salivary cortisol secretion in autistic children. *Psychoneuroendocrinology, 35*(8), 1187–1193.

Waldie, J. (2005). *The role of service dogs for two children with autism spectrum disorder.* Unpublished master's thesis, Lakehead University, Canada.

Walsh, F. (2009). Human–animal bonds I: The relational significance of companion animals. *Family Process, 48*(4), 462–480.

Weiss, D. (2009). Equine assisted therapy and Theraplay. In E. Munns (Ed.), *Applications of family and group Theraplay* (pp. 225–233). Lanham, MD: Jason Aronson.

Welsh, K. C. (2009). *The use of dogs to impact joint attention in children with autism spectrum disorders.* Unpublished dissertation, Walden University.

CHAPTER 4

Family Theraplay

Connecting With Children on the Autism Spectrum

SUSAN BUNDY-MYROW

A 5-year-old sits cross-legged atop two large pillows as he faces his smiling mom. Their hands are entwined, clasped together. A second adult sits close by with a supportive hand on the child's shoulder. As the mom signals, "Pokémon!" the child lunges forward, launching himself toward his "play-mate." Squeals of laughter erupt from the boy and feigned resistance from the mom, who says, "Push! More!" The adult guides her airborne child to her chest as she rolls backward. They each take a deep breath as their eyes meet. "Again!" announces the child. The second adult, the therapist, smiles at the parent and says, "You know just the way to make it fun for him!" This scene may not resemble the expected interactions of a child with autism. It happens in Theraplay® treatment, though, and parents are integral to this hands-on, attachment-based play therapy.

The synchrony and delight inherent in the secure attachment relationship of a mother and her baby is the cornerstone of Theraplay treatment. In the context of attuned, often joy-filled, sensorimotor-based play activities, the Theraplay therapist joins and leads children with autism spectrum disorder (ASD) to experiences that they can comprehend—experiences that promote the desire to relate. Theraplay builds the foundation to integrate awareness of self and others, communicative intent, regulation, and modulation. When children receive the right "dose" of multisensory "face time" to build basic connections, they want to respond—and do. The interpersonal dance of attuned play begins.

Theraplay includes parents each step of the way: assessment of parent–child play interactions, goal setting, treatment, and evaluation. Theraplay therapists have the unique opportunity to first establish direct, attuned play with the child and then share that therapeutic experience with parents as they increasingly assume a leadership role in the playroom. Parents first become therapeutic partners by viewing videos of Theraplay sessions with the therapist. Then they are included in role play, modeling in the playroom and direct coaching. Just as the therapist and parents "fill" the child's Theraplay prescription for specified doses of structure, engagement, nurture, and challenge (SENC) in the playroom, Theraplay can, further, inspire and guide healthy relationships at home. This chapter describes Family Theraplay and its application for children with ASD and illustrates the method via the treatment of a 5-year-old boy with autism. Modifications follow for children with higher-functioning ASD, such as Asperger's disorder, and those with cognitive delays as well.

Theraplay: Origin and Theory

Developed by Ann Jernberg in 1967, updated and expanded by Phyllis Booth (Booth & Jernberg, 2010; Jernberg, & Booth, 1999) and maintained by contributors at the Theraplay Institute (Chicago, IL), Theraplay is a trademarked method, with clinical certifications in Group Theraplay and Individual and Family Theraplay and practiced in more than 20 countries and instructed by national and international trainers. The interested reader is referred to the Theraplay website (http://www.theraplay.org) and the third edition of *Theraplay: Helping Parents and Children Build Better Relationships Through Attachment-Based Play* (Booth & Jernberg, 2010).

Theraplay is a developmentally based play therapy influenced by Jernberg's hands-on work with two colleagues. Psychiatrist Austin M. Des Lauriers emphasized the need to actively engage children, to make focused eye contact in their present-focused work together. From Viola Brody, Jernberg adopted the nurturing aspect of the therapist–child relationship with its characteristic touch, rocking, and singing. Brody continued to develop her own dyadic approach, known as developmental play. The observer of a session will note similar roots (Jernberg, 1979).

Booth (2003, p.4) defined the method: "Theraplay is a structured play therapy for children and their parents. Its goal is to enhance attachment, self-esteem, trust in others and joyful engagement. The method is fun, physical, personal and interactive and replicates the natural, healthy interaction between parents and young children." Children have been referred with overactive-aggressive behavior, withdrawn or depressed behavior, phobias, tantrums, and difficulty socializing. Children with learning and developmental disabilities may also exhibit various behavioral and interpersonal difficulties. Given that Theraplay is an attachment-based therapy, families with foster and adoptive children find it to be a logical and valuable choice for their needs. Theraplay also serves as a preventive program to strengthen parent–child relationships when faced with family or environmental stressors.

Myrow (2000) noted that Theraplay's focus on the *emotional* age of the child, coupled with an emphasis on physical closeness and warmth, expedites the building of a therapeutic alliance whether or not the attachment bond is the focus of treatment. Unlike traditional child-centered approaches, the Theraplay therapist is the primary playroom object and the method is tailored to give corrective experiences that organize the sensory system in an experiential-dependent way. Mäkela (2003) maintains that the result of Theraplay is change in the multiple systems of the child and parent's experience of self, other, and world.

Roots in Attachment Theory, Self Psychology, and Object Relations

1. Theraplay is based on the assumption that the self and personality develop out of early parent–child interactions that result in an inner representation of self that is either positive or negative. Consistent with Winnicott's (1987) concept of a *holding environment*, Theraplay is guided by the adult.

2. The kind of responsiveness from the parent is playful, empathic, and attuned for children to develop a strong sense of self, feelings of self-worth, as well as the capacity to understand and empathize with others. As discussed by Booth, not only is it the playful interactions between parent and child, but of primary importance also is the attunement (Stern), contingent response (Ainsworth), regulation of internal states (Schore), and reflexive function or mind reading (Fonagy) (Booth & Jernberg, 2010; Bundy-Myrow & Booth, 2009).

3. One's adult capacity for self-regulation depends on early experiences between mother and child regarding coregulation of affect (Booth & Jernberg, 2010; Bundy-Myrow & Booth, 2009). Their communication with each other is largely nonverbal; an interactive "dance" between their right brains, managing arousal and emotion (Schore, 1994; Siegel, 1999).

4. When care giving is attuned, children develop an "inner working model" (Bowlby, 1973, 1988) of themselves as lovable, valued by his primary attachment figure, who has provided a secure base from which to explore the world (Booth & Jernberg, 2010). Siegel and Hartzell (2003) suggest that positive *emotional* interactions may allow for neuronal growth in the hippocampus and synaptic development in the prefrontal and orbitofrontal cortex of the

right (emotional) hemisphere of the brain. For children who have missed the experiences of attuned care giving, the corrective nature of Theraplay provides with and for children an opportunity to access the relevant brain structures (Mäkela, 2003). This is accomplished via guided positive sensorimotor-based play, regulating optimal arousal and dyadic "now" moments for self-affirming stimulation.

Theraplay Research

Anecdotal case studies and qualitative research over a 50-year period have documented its use with diverse populations, from babies to senior citizens. Recent quantitative evidence of the effectiveness of Theraplay includes children presenting with attachment disorders, autism, speech and language disorders, and internalizing and externalizing behaviors such as social anxiety and aggression (Booth & Jernberg, 2010; Coleman, 2010; Wettig, Coleman, & Geider, 2011).

During Theraplay's early years of Head Start psychological services, outcome interviews of 23 teachers regarding the progress of 41 children found progress in social relationships with adults (87%), peers (73%), overall behavior (87%), and pretest–posttest predictions of success in kindergarten for the upcoming year (Myrow, 2000). Another means of documenting change in functioning as a result of early Theraplay treatment was the creation of two films, each with a 3-year follow-up and interview (Coleman, 2010).

Mäkela and Vierikko (2004) reported significant decreases in social problems and internalizing and externalizing behaviors in children who had experienced abuse, neglect, and loss. The study assessed Family Theraplay as the primary treatment for 20 children ages 4 to 13 and their community of foster parents in Finland.

The work of Siu (2007, 2009) addressed experimental design weaknesses of some previous studies in research where second- to fourth-grade boys and girls with elevated internalizing scores on the child behavior checklist (CBCL) participated in group Theraplay with their mothers (Coleman, 2010). The eight sessions of this Hong Kong project resulted in significant pre–post improvement for somatic symptoms, anxiety-depression, withdrawal, and self-esteem. Two additional experimental studies described by Coleman (2010) and conducted by Theraplay therapists in Korea further support the efficacy of Theraplay as a short-term group treatment to improve self-esteem and social relationships.

The most extensive experimental work to date is that conducted by Ulrike Franke and Herbert Wettig using Family Theraplay to treat dually diagnosed children with language disorder and shyness/social anxiety in Germany and Austria (Wettig et al., 2011). This well-controlled, two-part study first addressed 22 children ranging in age from 2 years 6 months, to 6 years 11 months at a single institution by one therapist. The second study investigated generalizability across nine sites ($N = 167$ children). Results indicated statistically significant improvements in assertiveness, self-confidence, and trust, improved expressive and receptive language skills, and maintenance of gains at a 2-year follow-up. The finding of similar results across nine sites suggests that Theraplay is replicable across settings and therapists, given consistent training. Following treatment, social behavior was within normal limits, typical of nonclinical peers. Receptive and expressive language skills improved as part of the Theraplay experience, which appeared developmentally sensitive for children as young as 2.5 years old. Theraplay required a relatively brief treatment phase of an average of 18 sessions.

Theraplay Dimensions

Structure, engagement, nurture, and challenge are necessary components in all healthy parent–child relationships and are consistent with the essential parenting tasks discussed by Sroufe, Egeland, Carlson, and Collins (2005). From this base, Jernberg, and later, Booth derived the Theraplay treatment "prescription" (Booth & Jernberg, 2010; Jernberg, 1979). When parents and children participate in Theraplay's structured interpersonal assessment, the Marschak Interaction Method (MIM), the therapist similarly considers the extent to which the parent *provides* and the child can *receive* structuring, engaging, nurturing, and challenging interactions. A description of the dimensions follows.

Structure   The essence of structure in the healthy parent–infant relationship is safety, organization, and regulation. The parent is trustworthy and predictable; activities have a beginning, middle, and end. Time is sequenced, planned, and finite. Songs and Rhymes have a rhythm. In treatment, the fact that the adult is in charge is reassuring, teaching the child to be in control of self, also assuring the child of order if the environment is unruly or chaotic. Structure, therefore, addresses inner and outer disorder. Rather than being about control, structure in Theraplay conveys a comforting assurance that a trustworthy adult can provide safety and predictability, especially for children who are overactive, undirected, or overstimulated or who anxiously try to control their world. Parents who can benefit from structure in their Family Theraplay work find it difficult to be regulated, follow through with directions, or to effectively lead their children (Booth & Jernberg, 2010).

Engagement   The essence of engagement in the parent–infant relationship is the synchronous emotional connection that happens when the parent entices the baby into joyful interaction. The parent is attuned to the intensity, type, and length of stimulation and maintains an optimal level of arousal. The result is that the baby is able to regulate and integrate physical and feeling states. In Theraplay treatment the therapist focuses on the child in an intensive and personal way using what the child says and does to maintain engagement. Empathic persistence draws the child into interaction and is helpful for children who are withdrawn, avoidant of contact, or too rigidly structured.

Nurture The essence of nurture in the parent–infant relationship is the responsive care that calms, soothes, and communicates a reassuring presence when needed. Rocking, feeding, cuddling, and holding make the world feel safe, warm, and secure. In treatment, nurture meets children's unfilled younger-child needs and helps them relax and "receive" care. Children who are overactive, aggressive, or pseudo-mature start to feel lovable and valued.

Challenge The essence of challenge in the parent–infant relationship is twofold. The parent helps the child take mild, developmentally appropriate risks, a kind of successful "stretching," whereby the child masters the "newness" and uncertainty of experiences. Second, parents support the child's independence and competence, communicating pleasure and support of the child's mastery. Similarly, in treatment, the therapist introduces mild, age-appropriate risks via two-person activities that support the child's sense of competence (Booth & Jernberg, 2010).

The Marschak Interaction Method

The MIM is a structured technique for observing and assessing the relationship between two people such as biological parent and child, foster or adoptive parent and child, or grandparent and child. It is the assessment tool unique to Theraplay that drives the treatment planning process. The adult is given a series of cards with instructions for tasks designed to elicit interactions in the four Theraplay dimensions. The MIM evaluates the parent's capacities to provide and the child's capacities to receive structure, engagement, nurture, and challenge. Additional MIM information is available in Booth and Jernberg, (2010, pp. 115–135).

The Family Theraplay Treatment Plan

A typical Family Theraplay protocol is presented as follows (Jernberg & Booth, 1999):

> Session 1: Initial interview with parents, gathering history, presenting problem, family dynamics to ultimately assess the parent–child relationship.

Session 2: One parent and child participate in the Marschak Interaction Method. The Theraplay therapist observes and makes a video recording of this interaction.

Session 3: MIM 2—In two-parent families the MIM is administered to the other parent.

Session 4: Feedback session with the parents in which the MIM observations are viewed and discussed, followed by a plan for treatment.

Session 5–8: Theraplay—parent and child apart. The therapist interacts with the child for a 30-minute session followed by consultation with the parents as they view the video of the session together. Alternatively, when two therapists are present, the "interpreting" therapist observes the session with the parents as it is occurring. In either format, the therapist and parents discuss the rationale for the SENC activities, link history and dynamics to present-day behavior, and discuss how parents can begin to apply these components to home.

Session 9–15 (or more when needed): Theraplay—parent and child together. Sessions continue as before, except that parents now join the child and therapist in the playroom for the last 15 minutes of the session. Parents receive guidance from the therapists, frequently in the form of coaching and role play. The final session ends with favorite activities and a good-bye party.

Session 16–19: Additional sessions or quarterly follow-up sessions occur with parents and child over the next year. Children with ASD often require more sessions.

Why Family Theraplay for Children With Autism?

The prevalence of autism in the United States, now at 1 in every 110 births (ASA, 2011), reflects the nature of the disorder as a spectrum, with mild, moderate, and severe cases. The core issues are neurologically based social communication deficits in the child's ability to engage and regulate (Tanguay, 1990). What differentiates Theraplay for children with ASD from other play therapy approaches is twofold: As the primary playroom object, the Theraplay therapist uses sensorimotor-based play to engage the child and counter autistic patterns. To empower parents as therapeutic partners, the Theraplay therapist demonstrates and guides parents to provide the unique relationship building blocks their child needs for development. In addition to the primary work of Family Theraplay, children with ASD can benefit from the shared sense of belonging with peers that Group Theraplay provides.

Primary Relationship Deficits and Theraplay Treatment Goals

Lindaman and Booth (2010) describe how basic neurological deficits associated with autism spectrum disorders result in difficulties in engagement and regulation:

1. Deficits related to sensory-affect-motor coordination make it difficult to establish regulation, rhythm, resonance, and synchrony with another. A Theraplay treatment goal is to link sensations, movement, and emotion to basic regulated patterns.
2. With mirror neuron deficits, the child is less able to imitate and anticipate others' actions. The goal is to read and respond to verbal and nonverbal cues contingently.
3. Difficulty communicating (e.g., emotional signaling, gestures, and language), engaging attention, and then shifting attention make it difficult to predictably identify feelings, thoughts, and wants. The goal is to express feelings and thoughts.
4. To varying degrees, processing deficits in motor planning, auditory, visual-spatial abilities, and sensory modulation may be present. The child may receive or process information differently and be hypo- or hyper-reactive to sensory input. Sensory differences may further complicate developmental experiences, making the child less able to feel comfortable, perceive the world as safe, achieve routines, and develop warm reciprocity with parents in typical activities such as holding or rocking (Bundy-Myrow, 2005). The goal in Theraplay is to establish physical engagement with optimal sensory arousal. In the context of the attachment relationship, the child can be helped to modulate responses to sensory stimuli and thereby increase attention and regulation (Kiermaier, 2010).
5. A deficit in core synchronization interferes with further development of connection, coregulation, and relatedness. Theory of mind, joint attention, higher-level abstract thinking, emotional reciprocity, and problem solving rely on the basic foundational skills to develop. In their review of executive functions (EFs) in preschoolers, Garon, Bryson, and Smith (2008) defined EFs as adaptive goal-directed behaviors (i.e., components of a central attention system strongly associated with the prefrontal cortex) that serve to override more automatic or established thoughts and responses. Particularly salient for children with ASD, EFs such as working memory, response inhibition, and shifting attention may be amenable to environmental remediation (Garon et al.). Theraplay may provide an important step in this regard via its

focus on establishing basic patterns of attention, regulation, and relating.

6. The child's difficulties make it challenging for the parent to attune to them and to coregulate interactions, which in turn may increase additional withdrawal of the child. The Theraplay goal is to guide parents to establish synchrony and mutually rewarding interactions.

Autism and Theraplay: Evidenced-Based Studies

Recent research has added experimental rigor to the case studies of children with ASD. Coleman (2010) described a recent experimental study of eight children with either pervasive developmental disorder (PDD) or mild autism. Texas Christian University conducted the intensive, daily, 2-week study with parents and their children. The behavioral measures to assess treatment effectiveness included the Gilliam Autism Rating Scale-2 (GARS-2; Gilliam, 2006), Parenting Stress Index (PSI; Abidin, 1995), the Sensory Profile (Dunn, 1999), and the MIM. This study included biological indicators of change; neurotransmitter assays were obtained from the children via urine samples. Specifically, epinephrine levels were assessed for both children and parents. The participants received daily Theraplay treatment conducted by certified Theraplay therapists over a 2-week period. Although results indicated no change on the standardized measures of autism, the PSI, or the Sensory Profile, significant improvements across MIM dimensions were found as well as normalization of epinephrine levels for both the children and parents. Changes in the children were consistent with stress reduction and included proximity seeking with the parent, gaze fixation, vocalization, and acceptance of parent support. Parents increased positive affect, eye contact, and ability to guide their children. The normalized epinephrine levels underscore the depth of relationship change experienced by both children and parents after their brief attachment-enhancing experiences, and further study was encouraged (Coleman, 2010).

The extensive, two-part, evidence-based Theraplay study by Wettig, Franke, and Fjordbak (2006) included a subset of children with autism. Treatment for the ASD group consisted of an average of 26 30-minute Family Theraplay sessions, somewhat greater than the mean of 20 sessions for children without neurologically based disorders. Results indicated that children originally identified with mild symptoms improved to levels similar to the interactive behavior of clinically nonsymptomatic controls. Those originally rated with moderate to severe symptoms improved at the end of therapy to mild or mild-moderate levels. The reduction of symptoms was clinically and statistically significant for children with ASD ($p < .0001$ to $p = .0009$). In the follow-up group, the treatment effect was maintained at 2 years. The authors noted that these studies meet stringent A-minus and B level codes of the American Psychiatric Association evidence-based therapies criteria (Wettig et al.).

Next is Theraplay for a young boy with autism and his parents. Identifying information has been changed to protect confidentiality.

Case Study: Jack   Five-year-old Jack was nothing like his older sister had been, reported Mrs. N. "I know boys are different, but he's like a loose cannon on deck!" Her wry smile veiled her distress: "We never know when he's going to fire. . . ." Frequent tantrums, pinching and hitting his sister, sleep dysregulation, and food selectivity were stressful enough. Given his preference for isolated play and strong resistance to preschool group activities, she worried in anticipation of a stormy kindergarten experience for Jack. As will be seen, the goals that were developed for Jack's Family Theraplay were to help him engage, regulate, and relate to others. For Mom and Dad to assist Jack in his current development, Family Theraplay was designed to help *them* to attune physically and affectively to him at his sensorimotor stage; to recognize and act upon his need to have both environmental stress reduced as well as to help him calm; and to help him focus and extend his positive interactions in Theraplay to his home.

Assessment

Assessment included family, developmental, and attachment history; educational and medical records review; school observation and consult with his teacher; and administration of the MIM with Jack and each parent followed by two parent feedback and planning sessions.

Birth and Developmental History   Mrs. N. reported having a normal pregnancy, labor, and delivery with Jack. As an infant he was very contented, smiled and liked to be held, but didn't sleep much. He was not as active and "verbally advanced" as his older sister Morgan, but Mom knew boys could develop speech later than girls. He became interested in cars and trucks: he liked the buttons and sound effects of toys and became content to be alone. Mom recalled that as a toddler Jack did not yet anticipate routines, wave bye-bye, show interest in other children from playgroup, or show Mommy and Daddy his toys. A speech evaluation showed that a slight delay was present but that Jack was progressing nicely with more words. Heartened by the fact that his "learning" seemed okay, Mr. and Mrs. N. chalked his oddities up to being strong-willed. As Jack neared age 4, his primary care physician referred him for a developmental evaluation. Results indicated "Asperger-like" tendencies and recommendation for a structured preschool.

At the intake session, Mrs. N. reported Jack's repetitiveness, expressive language delays, and narrow range of emotions. He didn't follow or imitate and would often push others away. For sleep he took clonidine 1 mg tablets; his mother said the medicine now enabled Jack and her to sleep until 5 a.m. Mrs. N. wanted assistance to help him calm and develop to his potential. Mr. N. repeated *his* family story of being a late talker who liked to play by himself. Now a successful engineer, he thought Jack might "grow out of it." He was concerned, however, about Jack's intermittent aggression to peers, disinterest in learning, and poor attention. Regarding home tantrum behavior, Dad would simply lift and carry Jack to a different location.

Both parents came from intact families of origin with no psychiatric histories. Mrs. N. described a very close relationship with her mother and two sisters. Her father had worked hard for the family and was often busy. Mr. N. described his mother as "a very good mother who covered all the bases" and his father as "smart and responsible." Mr. N.'s sister is married and lives 3 hours away, near his parents. They visit twice per year. Mrs. N. described Mr. N. as "a very good father who plays with the kids." Mr. N. described his wife as "a very good mother. The kids can get to her sometimes, though."

School and Peer Behavior   Jack had entered his 4-year-old preschool program midyear and was relatively strong academically. His teacher said his sense of humor emerged after about a month, and he often became very silly. She was puzzled by the fact, however, that it was difficult to find motivators that worked for any length of time. His solitary play focused on green cars—moving and gathering them. Jack also enjoyed pushing and pulling vacuums and sweeping the rug. Giving him this "heavy work" and large motor activities seemed to help when he needed a break. At times Jack's "silliness" became too disruptive, and a distant beanbag chair helped him calm. Staff learned, however, that he was finished with the beanbag when he would dash to touch and turn off the classroom lights! Teachers were beginning to teach him positive "Go" behaviors in which he worked for another car versus "Stop" behaviors, such as the classroom lights.

Marschak Interaction Method   MIMs were scheduled for Jack and each parent. General observations follow. It was often difficult to differentiate among what Jack was saying, what he understood to be happening, and his reaction to what was occurring because his facial expressions, movements, and gestures seldom matched his words. When frustrated or overwhelmed, Jack might laugh loudly or giggle uncontrollably. His difficulty "reading faces," tone of voice, and discerning body language prevented him from anticipating a fun activity or a serious concern. The words, "Jack, come here!" were either ignored or returned with a "Nooo!" despite the fact that the words pertained to something he enjoyed. However, if Mom or Dad persisted in attempting a task after Jack's initial, "No!" he would attempt it, as in trying on hats with dad. In general, Jack appeared motivated to end or avoid interactions. When something was familiar, however, he would interact longer and initiate more. Following are two specific MIM examples.

1. *Squeaky animals: Adult and child each take one squeaky animal. Make the two play together.* This is both an engagement and structure task. Mom pursued Jack verbally and consistently to engage him by attempting to both gain and *keep* his attention. Both were hard work. As Mom asked questions, Jack withdrew and attempted to leave the chair. He held the squeaky toy to his ear, squeaking it continuously. When Mom touched his arm and moved closer to him saying in her own squeaky voice, "Hi squeaky," he turned briefly toward her and smiled. She started to return her toy to the bag when, as an afterthought said, "Remember this little piggy?" The most intimate moment in the MIM between Jack and Mom occurred when she initiated the "This little piggy" game. With the expectation that Jack would finish the phrase, he smiled, made eye contact, and participated with her. Once the song ended, however, Jack was ready to end as well. Their brief but satisfying moment of interaction was a nourishing morsel for Mom.

2. *Adult leaves the room for 1 minute:* Mrs. N. clearly prepared Jack with eye contact, words, and touch. She kissed him on the cheek and told him he could play with the toys she had brought along. Both his toys and Mom were comforting as suggested by his eye contact and smile upon her return. On Dad's comparable separation task, he told Jack he'd be back and to "stay in your chair." Without the diversion of preferred activities, Jack clearly became anxious, called out to Dad while swinging his arms and legs, tossed the instruction cards off the table, and began to rub his shirt and to hum. He made eye contact when Dad returned, who inquired how the cards had "jumped" off the table. In this moment, Jack expressed his feeling, "All done!"

Treatment Goals and Methods

1. *Using Theraplay techniques, engage Jack in his world*—a sensorimotor world where actions are louder than words, where simple words support and clarify actions, where the actions are interper-

sonal, fun, and regulated for maximum registration and comprehension, where he can ask directly for more, where he can trust someone to extend a scaffold of support when he feels uncertain.

2. *Discover with Jack, how to calm him*—to use his visual strengths, strong memory, and humor to make interactions predictable with familiar beginnings, middles, and ends; help Jack calm his body, modulate his voice, guide him through transitions to familiar sequences, and help him "pack and transport" (Bundy-Myrow, 2005) the safe strategies to home.

3. *In the process of engaging and calming Jack*, he will be achieving the goals associated with the Theraplay dimensions (Booth & Jernberg, 2010):
   a. Accept and respond to his parents' attuned attempts to engage him.
   b. Accept his parents' limit setting, order, and direction (structure).
   c. Accept his parents' calming and comforting efforts (nurture).
   d. Participate in activities that support his developmental advancement (challenge).

4. *Support Mom's structuring activities with Jack*, guiding him to increase interactions and reciprocity. Help Mom set clear expectations and lead Jack, providing the consistent level of support he needs. Encourage Mom to develop ways to care for her own needs for emotional growth. As discussed by Lindaman and Booth (2010), the Theraplay therapist creates the following conditions with Jack and then guides Mom to take the lead to:
   a. Assist Jack to achieve an optimal level of arousal; neither under- or overstimulated.
   b. Lead Jack through simple, organized, and playful sequences.
   c. Increase Jack's ability to continue interactions for longer periods of time.
   d. Increase Jack's ability to transition between activities in a regulated way.

5. *Support father's efforts to be attuned to Jack's feeling states*—entice and lead Jack in achieving regulated, playful interactions (engagement). Assist Dad in determining Jack's behavioral signals indicating his need for regulation, calming, and comfort (nurture). Mr. N. wants Jack to be more grown up and enjoy his independence. Recognize when support is needed to encourage Jack's efforts to be successful at his developmental level (challenge). As discussed by Lindaman and Booth (2010), the Theraplay therapist creates the following conditions with Jack and then guides Dad to take the lead to:

    a. Focus intensely on Jack, noticing his special physical and interaction qualities.

    b. Acknowledge Jack's reactions, distress and pleasure, likes and dislikes.

    c. Determine what kind of touch is comfortable for Jack and soothe him when upset.

    d. Help Jack attend to Dad's face, expressions, and gestures.

    e. Imitate Jack to transform his behavior into communication.

    f. Involve Jack to develop turn taking, to anticipate other's actions, and to make predictions.

    g. Increase Jack's ability to continue interactions for longer periods of time by marking time with beginnings, middles, and endings.

    h. Encourage Jack's expression of nonverbal and verbal communication.

    i. Encourage Jack's ability to develop an assortment of play routines that *he* can initiate.

Treatment Description

Session 1 For the initial Theraplay session, Mom escorted Jack into the playroom with the therapist who said, "Mom, let's hold Jack's hands and run together so he can jump on top of those two pillows. Ready, set, go!" Jack liked the sensory input of the jumping and said, "Again?" The therapist noted, "You like jumping! Mom, we're going to do more jumping and other fun things. We'll get you when we're done!" Jack tolerated the separation well and helped to carry another big pillow to add to the stack. The therapist held his hand and ensured his eye contact and calm body before the structuring signal "Ready, set, go!" Once atop the three pillows, the therapist announced, "One more jump to me. Ready?" She then gave him a cuddle squeeze, like Mom had done last session, and guided his body to sit knee to knee facing each other. The Theraplay therapist engaged Jack in alternating quiet activities (checking for hurts or boo-boos and giving a "soft touch" with cotton ball around any hurts) with more active activities (e.g., "Row the boat"). The activities form a context within which to do the work of Theraplay. Jack was able to attend briefly with optimal arousal and began to follow the therapist's lead in simple play sequences. As the therapist focused intently and exclusively on Jack, she noticed his special attributes and showed these to him in a mirror (e.g., his blue crayon-colored eyes and the letter C-shaped dimple when he laughed). When Jack said, "No lotion!" the therapist acknowledged his discomfort: "You don't like the lotion today. Something about the lotion. Maybe the smell? Let's check." The therapist put a tiny amount on her finger so he could smell it and then surprisingly left a dab on her own nose when *she* smelled it. The therapist helped Jack to notice this funny moment, and he connected with his therapist in laughter.

Session 2, 3, and 4   When the therapist warmly greeted Mom and Jack in the waiting room, she said, "We're going to have fun today! This is our plan," and proceeded to write the numbers 1, 2, 3, 4 since Jack liked numbers: Number 1—Jack and Dr. S.; Number 2—Jack plays with cars and Dr. S. talks with Mommy; Number 3—Jack, Mommy, and Dr. S.; Number 4—Go home. The goals were to use Jack's visual strengths to increase comprehension and his ability to prolong interactions and to transition smoothly between activities. He joined the therapist and was able to follow this new sequence. Mrs. N. reported that aggression was decreasing over the past 2 weeks and some transitions at home were easier. The parents would track aggression at home and school.

Session 5: Parent Preparation With Mother   We discussed and role played Jack's reactions, including that he might pull away and protest with renewed "Nooos!" as he does at home. Mrs. N. practiced responding by soothing and was prepared to comfort him in her lap while demonstrating with the therapist to show Jack how the game would go. She would focus on leading in a reassuring, patient manner.

Sessions 6–8: Family Theraplay With Mother   Jack engaged in greeting and checkups with his therapist, and then Mrs. N. entered the session and assumed increasing responsibility to engage and lead Jack in his activities. She realized Jack seeks "a lot" of sensory input—loves to be picked up, swung, and squeezed. While he did not protest, it was difficult for Mom to lead him in a new, regulated way. The therapist modeled for Mom to "check to see if his body is calm and ready," and cued Jack with "Ready position!" In a stop/go game, he giggled as the soap bubbles rose in the cup when Mom blew air into a straw. The therapist guided him as a social translator to stop the bubbles from overflowing by yelling, "Stop!" Mom thoroughly enjoyed their shared attention to the bubbles, and at the end Jack spontaneously said, "Thank you!"

Notable in succeeding sessions was when Jack started to loudly perseverate about the toy cars. The therapist asked, "Jack, do you have a question?" He managed to say, "May I green car Jack?" He discovered he could make an impact on the adult in a new way and through turn taking could anticipate what would happen. Jack also asked Mom for a Theraplay game at home, the spinning airplane, then settled into bed to let her rub his back.

Session 9: Parent Preparation With Father   Both Mr. and Mrs. N. attended to be able to plan together. Mrs. N. had been surprised and pleased to note that by "hanging in" and trying to calm Jack he actually recovered *more* quickly and her relationship with him deepened. Mom and Dad had practiced a game called "Tunnels," where two adults suspend a sheet under which the child crawls. Jack wasn't sure about this new game at home— with Mom, Dad, and sister Morgan playing as well. He was both smiling and protesting simultaneously. Dad thought Jack was perhaps being stubborn. We discussed how his change could be overwhelming. Jack needed the grown-ups to "pack and port" the calming strategies of the playroom to home. The task was to continue to support him, not remove him, and be patiently persistent and reassuring in our expectation that this will be enjoyable, too.

Sessions 10–12: Family Theraplay With Father　For Dad to attune to Jack, the Theraplay therapist guided him to focus intently and exclusively on Jack, noticing first his physical attributes and how he looked when he interacted. As part of a checkup activity, the therapist had coached Dad to examine and measure how strong and big Jack's muscles were becoming. Mr. N. knew his son liked numbers, as did he, and enjoyed showing Jack the measuring tape. "Let's see what number your arms are," he said. Measuring Jack's biceps, Dad noted, "Your right arm is a little bigger—getting strong!" The therapist then helped the pair increase their shared positive affect by suggesting Jack's favorite push-push game, now using those strong muscles. Dad was coached to proactively ensure Jack's "ready position" by helping his arms and legs be just the right way for success.

Another kind of *noticing* that was important to their relationship was Jack's likes, dislikes, fears, and giggles. The therapist instructed Dad to observe Jack between sessions to determine whether Jack had any feelings other than contentment with his cars and stubbornness. The here-and-now experience with the therapist, however, was ultimately more useful for Dad to help identify and modulate Jack's excitement as well as his refusals. For example, Dad realized that Jack giggled so much he couldn't climb the tower of pillows until Dad hugged him, made sure his body was ready, and gave just enough help for Jack to be successful. Dad noticed in session that Jack could "stay longer" when he responded this different way. At one significant point when Jack started to disengage, Dad successfully kept his voice low and hands touching Jack, which helped the boy reconnect. Jack loved jumping to and hugging Dad. When Jack said, "Again jumping, Daddy?" Dad smiled and *met his eyes*, saying, "Let's get ready." At home Dad practiced helping Jack "get his body ready," meeting Jack's eyes and monitoring his own voice volume.

Sessions 13–14: Consult and Planning With Parents, Family Theraplay With Whole Family　With Dad's new skills in attuning to Jack's affect and Mom's new expectations that Jack can follow directions with support, they were excited to share their "mechanical gear" theory about Jack's resistance. He needed time to "switch gears," and the gears needed to be greased and "lined up" to shift smoothly. They understood their boy better, were enjoying their interactions with him, and felt hopeful about future transitions.

To mark the end of weekly sessions, there was a Theraplay family party. Jack got to pick his favorite activities and snacks, with Mom, Dad, and sister Morgan present. Jack helped Mom and Dad say "Ready, set, go," when it was Morgan's turn to go through the "tunnel sheet." He shared laughter with everyone when it was Daddy's turn to crawl under the sheet.

Monthly Sessions Over the Next 6 Months   Goals during this period addressed maintaining and supporting Jack's regulated states when changes occurred, such as Mom being away for a weekend and dealing with "resistance in the gears" such as transitions from "No!" to "Yes!" In Theraplay a green "Yes" square with attached pipe cleaners served as the portable gas station for Jack to follow Mom and Dad's game directions. *His* Theraplay fuel was cuddle squeezes and spin arounds. The "Yes" station became a "pack and port" tool to also help Jack at home.

Following formal Theraplay treatment, families with children with ASD know that they can check in with their therapist at any time. Theraplay reminds them how to reconnect joyfully, attune, and provide the structure and assurance often needed. Jack's parents have scheduled a follow-up MIM to see, on tape, evidence of the change they have experienced in their lives.

Guidelines for Family Theraplay Across the Spectrum

Because Theraplay is intensive, hands-on, and provides developmental and corrective parent–child experiences, specific training and supervisory experiences are required to prepare the practitioner to effectively and ethically address the needs of the child and family. To ensure consistency of training and proficiency of its practitioners, Theraplay is a registered service mark of The Theraplay® Institute (TTI). Introductory and intermediate coursework plus a supervision practicum lead to the credential of Certified Theraplay therapist. These practitioners may refer to their practice as Theraplay. There is also certification as Group Theraplay Specialist. The reader is referred to The Theraplay Institute in Chicago, Illinois (http://www.theraplay.org).

Determining When Family Theraplay Should Be Used

Family Theraplay may be modified, deferred, or combined with other treatments depending on the presenting concerns, strengths, and resources of the parents. Issues such as substance abuse, domestic violence, and parental mental illness may prevent the parent from ensuring the child's safety and consequently may require interagency service, parent therapy, support, and coordination prior to Theraplay. Enlisting the assistance and involvement of family members and others who can support the health-promoting work of Theraplay may also be possible.

Children who are dangerously acting out or actively psychotic may first require psychiatric consult and medication to experience sufficient safety and stability to benefit from Theraplay. In modified form, Theraplay is an important aspect of treatment for children with abuse, loss, and trauma histories. The Theraplay therapist recommends a course of treatment that meets the needs and capacities of both parent and child (Booth & Jernberg, 2010).

Theraplay Across the Spectrum

Unlike other disabilities with cognitive impairments, IQ and degree of relatedness will vary across people with ASD. The fact that Theraplay's treatment prescription is always individualized prepares the therapist for creative ways to connect with the child with ASD. Theraplay for school-age children with high versus low IQ and degree of autism symptoms follows.

High Cognitive Level and Mild Symptomatology   Higher IQ is often associated with relatively mild autism symptoms in children with ASD. In their work regarding uneven cognitive profiles of children in the autism spectrum, Black and his colleagues (Black, Wallace, Sokoloff, & Kenworthy, 2009) reported that although high-functioning children with fewer communication deficits often exhibit strong verbal abilities as measured by verbal IQ (VIQ), as the differences between verbal and nonverbal IQ increase notable *social* difficulties increase as well. A strong vocabulary, verbal usage, and fluency do not ensure social relevance, reciprocity, and the ability to process the multiple nonverbal cues associated with social competence. In addition to studying the social deficits associated with a diagnosis of autism, Klin, Saulnier, Sparrow, Cicchetti, Volkmar, and Lord (2007) also recommend focus on *adaptive social functioning* associated with specific cognitive abilities as these may have implications for treatment intervention and be associated with markers of functioning. Children with high-functioning ASD can benefit from both Family Theraplay and Group Theraplay. The following strategies are likely to be helpful:

1. Use the child's relative verbal strength and interests to engage interactively.
2. Provide clear, verbal, functional rules, in context, to clarify roles and expectations.

3. Rehearse steps of an activity, increase memory with key phrases; e.g., "Ready, set, go!" Check verbally for comprehension by saying, "OK, tell me the plan."

4. This child will more likely have intact basic interaction skills such as the ability to answer and ask questions, attend, wait, comment, and evaluate information. Particularly for older children, increase initiation and reciprocity by adding challenge to the Theraplay activities, such as, "Great! Let's see if you can do that on one foot!" "Now, you be the leader!" When one child saw that his therapist had the same koala bear as his "friend" at home, he identified the new one as "Fake bear junior!" and brought his own to add to the next session.

5. Empower the child to provide feedback, design social games, problem solve, vote, and provide opportunities to develop judgment in sessions.

6. Theraplay activities can address higher executive control functions specifically related to ASD social symptoms, such as semantic fluency and auditory divided attention (Kenworthy, Black, Harrison, della Rosa, & Wallace, 2009).

Executive Function and Theraplay Activities   Two activities designed to engage and provide practice in semantic fluency and auditory divided attention follow. Semantic fluency taps language organization by asking the child to orally name as many words as possible that belong to a certain category (e.g., foods or animals). Auditory divided attention requires a child to simultaneously divide attention and working memory between two stimuli (e.g., listening to music and waiting for the phone to ring). It may have implications for social reciprocity and general social interactions (Kenworthy et al., 2009).

Activity: Toll Booth: Family or Group Theraplay Activity to Increase Semantic Fluency

Materials

> Eight index cards with a consecutive number between 1 and 8 on each
> Eight paper plates each marked with a number from 1 to 8

Directions

Place eight numbered paper plates (i.e., the "stations") on the floor around the perimeter of a room. Person 1 is the toll collector who stands, arm extended, next to plate number 1. The toll collector holds the eight index cards in the other hand. He tells the traveler: "I'm thinking of a category (e.g., food items, Pokemon characters, weather-related items). Pick a card to see how many items you must tell me to move on." Person 1 picks a number and attempts to recite the number of items in the category. (If child cannot recall the exact number, he can ask a friend or family member for help. The helper joins the child at the station, and they together then advance forward from the new position). Children or family members take turns being the toll collector by moving to the spot of the next traveler. The therapist tracks the numbered spot of each player. The first member to reach plate number 8 reaches his destination and becomes the snack leader—offering a snack to the next person.

Variations to maintain attention of younger children include adding a bell or buzzer for the toll collector, who sounds the bell for every word spoken by the traveler. Simplify category items by providing a visual cue of the word for the traveler to say or point to relevant items in an array. Work in teams or decrease the number of items required.

Involve older children and young teens in establishing the categories and items for the set, such as video games, pop bands, or sports. Write on separate cards (in case the adults are unfamiliar). Consider working in dyads. Distribute snack for all when the entire group reaches station number 8. How quickly can the entire group reach their destination?

Activity: Awesome Name Ball: A Theraplay Activity to Increase Auditory Divided Attention

Materials

Ball
Chair for each person
List of positive adjectives for therapist to read

Directions

Family or group generates and records a list of positive words associated with each person, such as compliments. The Theraplay therapist selects a word from the list as the key word to "grab" during a concurrent game of name ball. Members toss a ball around the circle making eye contact and calling the member's name before throwing the ball. At the same time, the therapist slowly reads the list of words with the embedded key word. The member who recognizes and "grabs" the key word chooses the next key word for the following round. To vary this activity, members track the number of times a bell sounds during Name Ball until the therapist says, "Freeze!"

High Nonverbal Cognitive Level and Marked Symptomatology   Children with these characteristics often have severe language, social comprehension, and interaction deficits with relative strengths in nonverbal abilities. Family Theraplay and Group Theraplay can be provided:

1. Similar to the case of Jack, it is important to engage children in warm physical interactions via imitation and repetition of simple sequences. Assist children to regulate by tailoring the stimulation

to meet their emotional and physiological needs. Stay connected and patiently persist in being "present and felt."

2. Increase comprehension and clarify expectations by dividing the session into sections with obvious beginning, middle, and end rhythm and patterns. Avoid power struggles and questions to children; use fewer words and emphasize success by adjusting developmental expectations—where appropriate (Booth & Jernberg, 2010; Bundy-Myrow, 2005).

3. In Group Theraplay it is helpful to have a smaller number of children and more adults to engage and to provide physical guidance when needed and visual cues such as pictures, words, and objects. The therapist modifies the pace and duration of activities to meet limited attending skills and leads the children in both predictable and new fun ways to be together (Booth & Jernberg, 2010; Bundy-Myrow, 2000; Rubin & Tregay, 1989).

Low Cognitive Level and Autistic Symptomatology   Children with moderate cognitive impairment but mild symptoms of autism may more readily be able to calm and engage and to sustain attention and optimal level of arousal. More often, however, lower cognitive functioning is also associated with more moderate symptomatology. Emphasize simple skills and directions and increase structure and rehearsal to address receptive, expressive language delays and regulation issues.

Because children with ASD who are considered lower functioning often have strengths in visual, nonverbal learning, they can be surprising in their comprehension and enjoyment of Theraplay activities. A group of middle school students with moderate to severe academic delays were champs at an interactive game of cup stacking and removal. To stack the large plastic drinking cups, two peers had to cooperate in using a special device (four pipe cleaners twisted as spokes around a thick rubber band) to lift and move the cups without touching them with their hands. Max held the end of a green pipe cleaner in each hand. His partner, John, chose two red pipe cleaners for his hands. The boys sat knee to knee, and their therapist secured the pipe cleaners to a large rubber band by twisting the remaining ends to the rubber band. The boys could then work together to stretch and shrink the rubber band around the cups. Using the boys' visual strengths proved helpful to coordinate their motor skills. The therapist observed that to release the rubber band from the cup a *square* shape was formed as students pulled their pipe cleaners toward their respective bodies. In contrast, a *circle* was formed around the cup as it was carried to the stacked pile. The boys soon understood the coaching commands, "Circle!" and "Square!" As the team grasped and moved the cups, the peers counted them, seeing how many could be stacked. As a variation, the entire class tried to "beat their own record" as they became proficient.

Summary

Theraplay therapists have the unique opportunity to first establish direct, attuned play with the child and then share that therapeutic experience with parents as they, in turn, increasingly assume a leadership role in the playroom. Just as the therapist and parents "fill" the child's Theraplay prescription for specified doses of structure, engagement, nurture, and challenge in the playroom, Theraplay also inspires and guides healthy relationships at home. Theraplay can also be used in its group format as a stand-alone treatment or to help generalize gains from family work. This chapter described Family Theraplay and its evidence-based effectiveness and application for children with ASD and illustrated the method via the treatment of a 5-year-old boy with autism. Modifications followed for children with higher-functioning ASD, such as Asperger's disorder, and those with cognitive delays as well. Theraplay engages the power of the affective world of the child while prescriptively and systematically integrating it with the child's cognitive potential. Theraplay is rewarding to children with ASD and their families, but the *play therapist* may also find great satisfaction in exploring it for parents and their children with ASD.

References

Abidin, R. R. (1995). *Parenting Stress Index: Professional Manual* (3rd ed.). Odessa, FL: Psychological Assessment Resources.

Autism Society of America. (ASA). (n.d.). *About autism*. Retrieved February 28, 2011 from http://www.autism-society.org/about-autism/

Black, D. O., Wallace, G. L., Sokoloff, J. L., & Kenworthy, L. (2009). Brief report: IQ split predicts social symptoms and communication abilities in high-functioning children with Autism Spectrum Disorders. *Journal of Autism & Developmental Disorders, 39*(11), 1613–1619.

Booth, P. B. (2003). *The role of touch in Theraplay*. Paper presented at the First International Theraplay Conference, June 27, 2003, Chicago, IL.

Booth, P. B., & Jernberg, A. M. (2010). *Theraplay: Helping parents and children build better relationships through attachment-based play* (3rd ed.). San Francisco: Jossey-Bass.

Bowlby, J. (1973). *Attachment and loss. Vol. II: Separation, anxiety and anger.* London: Hogarth Press.

Bowlby, J. (1988). *A secure base: Parent–child healthy human development.* New York: Basic Books.

Bundy-Myrow, S. (2000). Group Theraplay for children with autism and pervasive developmental disorder. In E. Munns (Ed.), *Theraplay: Innovations in attachment—Enhancing play therapy* (pp. 301–320). Lanham, MD: Jason Aronson.

Bundy-Myrow, S. (2005). Theraplay for children with self-regulation problems. In C. Schaefer, J. McCormick, & A. Ohnogi (Eds.), *International handbook of play therapy: Advances in assessment, theory, research, and practice* (pp. 35–64). New York: Jason Aronson.

Bundy-Myrow, S., & Booth, P. B. (2009). Theraplay: Supporting attachment relationships. In K. J. O'Connor & L. D. Braverman (Eds.), *Play therapy theory and practice: Comparing theories and techniques.* (pp. 315–366). Hoboken, NJ: John Wiley & Sons.

Coleman, R. (2010). Research findings that support the effectiveness of Theraplay. In P.B. Booth & A.M. Jernberg, (Eds.), *Theraplay: helping parents and children build better relationships through attachment-based play* (3rd ed.). San Francisco: Jossey-Bass.

Dunn, W. (1999). *The sensory profile manual.* San Antonio, TX: The Psychological Corporation.

Garon, N., Bryson, S. E., & Smith, I. M. (2008). Executive function in preschoolers: A review using an integrative framework. *Psychological Bulletin, 134*(1), 3–60.

Gilliam, J. E. (2006). *Gilliam Autism Rating Scale* (2nd ed.). Austin, TX: Pro-Ed.

Jernberg, A. M. (1979). *Theraplay: A new treatment using structured play for problem children and their families.* San Francisco: Jossey-Bass.

Jernberg, A. M., & Booth, P. B. (1999). *Theraplay: Helping parents and children build better relationships through attachment-based play* (2nd ed.). San Francisco: Jossey-Bass.

Kenworthy, L., Black, D. O., Harrison, B., della Rosa, A. , & Wallace, G. L. (2009). Are executive control functions related to autism symptoms in high-functioning children? [Electronic version]. *Child Neuropsychology, 15,* 425–444.

Kiermaier, A. (2010). Theraplay for Children with regulation disorders. In P. B. Booth & A. M. Jernberg (Eds.), *Theraplay: Helping parents and children build better relationships through attachment-based play* (3rd ed.). San Francisco: Jossey-Bass.

Klin, A., Saulnier, C. A., Sparrow, S. S., Cicchetti, D. V., Volkmar, F. R., & Lord, C. (2007). Social and communication abilities and disabilities in higher functioning individuals with autism spectrum disorders: The Vineland and the ADOS. *Journal of Autism and Developmental Disorders, 37,* 748–759.

Lindaman, S., & Booth, P. B. (2010). Theraplay for children with autism spectrum disorders. In P. B. Booth & A. M. Jernberg (Eds.), *Theraplay: Helping parents and children build better relationships through attachment-based play* (3rd ed.). San Francisco: Jossey-Bass.

Mäkela, J. (2003). What makes Theraplay effective: Insights from developmental sciences. *The Theraplay Institute Newsletter,* Fall/Winter.

Mäkela, J., & Vierikko, I. (2004). *From heart to heart: Interactive therapy for children in care. Report on the Theraplay project in SOS Children's Village, Finland.* Retrieved February 28, 2011 from http://www.theraplay.org/18432.html

Myrow, D. L. (2000). Applications for the attachment-fostering aspects of Theraplay. In E. Munns (Ed.), *Theraplay: innovations in attachment-enhancing play therapy.* Lanham, MD: Jason Aronson.

Rubin, P. B., & Tregay, J. (1989). *Play with them—Theraplay groups in the classroom.* Springfield, IL: Charles C. Thomas.

Schore, A. N. (1994). *Affect regulation and the origin of the self: The neurobiology of emotional development.* Hillsdale, NJ: Erlbaum.

Siegel, D. J. (1999). *The developing mind.* New York: The Guilford Press.

Siegel, D. J., & Hartzell, M. (2003). *Parenting from the inside out.* New York: Jeremy P. Tarcher /Putnam.

Siu, A. (2007, July). *Theraplay for elementary school children with internalizing problems: The Hong Kong experience.* Poster presented at the International Theraplay Conference, Chicago, IL.

Siu, A. (2009). Theraplay in the Chinese world: An intervention program for Hong Kong children with internalizing problems. *International Journal of Play Therapy, 18*(1), 1–12.

Sroufe, L. A., Egeland, B., Carlson, E., & Collins, W. A. (2005). *The development of the person: The Minnesota study of risk and adaptation from birth to adulthood.* New York: The Guilford Press.

Tanguay, P. (1990). Infantile autism and social communication spectrum disorder. *Journal of the American Academy of Child and Adolescent Psychiatry, 29*, 854.

Wettig, H. H. G., Franke, U., & Fjordbak, B. S. (2006). Evaluating the effectiveness of Theraplay. In C. E. Schaefer & H. G. Kaduson (Eds.), *Contemporary play therapy: Theory, research, and practice* (pp. 103–135). New York: The Guilford Press.

Wettig, H. H. G., Coleman, A. R., & Geider, F. J. (2011). Evaluating the effectiveness of Theraplay in treating shy, socially withdrawn children. *International Journal of Play Therapy, 20*(1), 26–37.

Winnicott, D. W. (1987). *Babies and their mothers.* New York: Addison-Wesley.

CHAPTER 5

From Monologue to Dialogue

The Use of Play and Drama Therapy for
Children With Autism Spectrum Disorders

LORETTA GALLO-LOPEZ

...My life has been spent in a perpetual state of parallel play, alongside but distinctly apart from, the rest of humanity. Tim Page (2009, p. 3)

In his memoir *Parallel Play*, Tim Page (2009) chronicles his life growing up with undiagnosed Asperger's disorder and in so doing provides the reader with a rare glimpse into the social and overall life challenges of individuals with autism spectrum disorders (ASD). That Page chose the title *Parallel Play* to describe his experience is at once telling and poignant. The term parallel play so clearly describes what we often see when observing a child with autism spectrum disorder engaged in play—a child playing "alongside but distinctly apart" from others.

The word *autism* is derived from the Greek word *autos* meaning "self." This sense of children rarely relating beyond the self—disconnected from the world and the people around them—is arguably the most profound and significant description of autism. In searching for a way to reach and connect with these children, it is obvious that the most effective and purposeful approaches would (and should) somehow move them beyond the solitary and toward the shared experience. Toward this goal and in this context, drama and drama therapy are interactive in nature, providing an experience that has at its core interpersonal and social interplay. In theater, we use the term *monologue* when referring to an individual speaking alone. The term *dialogue*, on the other hand, refers to a conversation between two or more people, a discussion, an exchange of ideas—requiring relating, connecting, or joining with others. It is this lack of a capacity for dialogue, not just through language but through experience as well, that embodies the core deficit of children with autism spectrum disorders. And so it must be the mandate of those seeking to assist these children to transport them from an existence limited by monologue to a life as rich as possible with dialogue.

It is the intention of this chapter to present an approach to working with children with autism spectrum disorders that uses drama therapy to specifically address the core deficits and needs of this population. As an introduction, a brief look at autism will be offered, including a discussion of the increase in the numbers of individuals being diagnosed with ASD as well as the most common symptoms and behaviors that typically characterize this very diverse group of individuals. Drama therapy will then be defined, and an overview will be presented. The significance of dramatic play in child development and a rationale for the use of drama therapy with children diagnosed with ASD will be examined. A drama therapy treatment protocol based on the continuum of dramatic play skills will be explained. Finally, a case presentation will be offered to provide a clear example of the use and effectiveness of this protocol with children diagnosed with ASD.

Autism Spectrum Disorders

As recently as 30 years ago, autism was considered a rare condition diagnosed in only 4 of 10,000 children (Baron-Cohen, 2008). However, in 2006, the Centers for Disease Control and Prevention (CDC, 2009) reported that approximately 1 8-year-old child in every 110 was classified as having an autism spectrum disorder. The CDC report postulates that the marked increase over time may be due to several factors including a change in terminology. Prior to the 1980s, statistics were based on the single diagnosis of *autism*. The current statistics refer to three different diagnostic categories that comprise ASD: autistic disorder, Asperger's disorder, and pervasive developmental disorder—not otherwise specified (PDD-NOS).

There are several categories of characteristics that span the "spectrum." Those considered the essential triad are social difficulties, communication deficits, and a third category including narrow, sometimes unusual interests or fixations as well as repetitive behavior (Baron-Cohen, 2008). Another key deficit that many children on the autism spectrum share is that of theory of mind (ToM). ToM refers to "the ability to put oneself in someone else's shoes, to imagine their thoughts and feelings, so as to be able to make sense of and predict their behaviour" (Baron-Cohen, p. 57).

Baron-Cohen maintains that the ToM deficit may lead to anxiety and confusion in individuals with ASD due to the fact that they are unable to predict, understand, or interpret the behavior of others. Individuals with ASD often have difficulty understanding what behaviors or actions on their part, or that of others, may hurt someone else as well as difficulty directly experiencing or understanding empathy or interpreting facial or bodily expressions. These skills are prerequisites to successfully engaging in social interaction and initiating and maintaining social relationships.

A second deficit area that many children with ASD share is that of *joint attention* skills. This refers to the ability to follow another person's gaze, to show interest in what another person is interested in, or to share a play experience. Many young children with ASD exhibit significant deficits in this skill area (Kasari, Freeman, & Paparella, 2006). Kasari et al. report study results that indicate the importance of teaching joint attention and symbolic play skills to children with ASD. They also postulate that under the right circumstances children with autism can learn these skills. Even more significantly, they note that these skills can be generalized from the treatment milieu to the home or school environment. They go on to urge that to affect changes in children with ASD both joint attention and symbolic play skills should be a significant focus of any intervention.

Most non-ASD, or *neuro-typical*, 2- to 3-year-old children are capable of pretend play. They demonstrate at least a basic understanding of the idea that both they and the person they are playing with are pretending. Pretend play involves at least to some extent the use of symbolic play—the representational use of objects. In symbolic play we accept that one object represents another as a box becomes a jail—or that inanimate objects such as dolls and toys can engage in human activities, can express language, and can feel emotion (Kasari et al., 2006; Lewis, 2003). Because many young children with ASD do not have an inherent understanding of symbolic play, they would benefit from interventions that provide pretend play experiences and practice.

The importance of pretend play experiences for children cannot be overstated, as it is through such play that children learn what is culturally and socially significant. Pretend play affords children the opportunity to explore and experiment with activities that prepare them for life. The fact that children with ASD often miss out on these experiences is highly relevant when examining the deficits in social competency that so many individuals with ASD share. With the increasing numbers of children being diagnosed with autism spectrum disorders, it is even more imperative that we identify effective and purposeful interventions. Most typical interventions are adult led and directed, such as those that rely on principals of applied behavioral analysis (Stahmer, Ingersoll, & Carter, 2003) or the use of social stories (Gray, 1994). Such approaches have been shown to be effective in extinguishing certain problem behaviors and in learning skills such as activities of daily living (Attwood, 2007; Baron-Cohen, 2008).

Play, however, because of its spontaneous and inherent nature, may not be truly teachable through techniques such as social stories and imitative play. It would seem that the most effective means of enhancing play skills in children with ASD would be an approach that is primarily informed by the social significance of play and the implications of play deficits on a child's ability to engage in social interaction and to form relationships. Such an approach would recognize the developmental nature of play and the progressive nature of the acquisition of play skills and offer a comprehensive conceptual framework incorporating focus on each of the areas of the play continuum.

Drama therapy is one such approach that encompasses both the developmental and social aspects of play, enables a more internalized participation in actual play, and relies on intrinsic as opposed to external motivation and reinforcement. An overview of drama therapy is provided next, along with support for the use of drama therapy with children with ASD. The framework for a drama therapy approach that supports the social nature of play within a developmental context is then presented.

Drama Therapy

According to the National Association for Drama Therapy, drama therapy involves the intentional use of drama and theater techniques by professionals trained in the field of drama therapy to bring about healing, growth, and therapeutic change. Drama therapy is practiced in a wide variety of settings including inpatient and outpatient mental health facilities, prisons, schools, and private practices and with a broad range of client populations including children, teens, adults, and the elderly. Drama therapy is used in individual, group, and family therapy. Drama therapists employ an expansive array of techniques and interventions including role play, improvisation, enactment, storytelling, puppet, and mask work (http://www.nadt.org). Drama therapy is based at its most organic core on the prehistoric human need and instinct for connection and for engaging in rituals and storytelling to explain and explore our world and celebrate our history (Courtney, 1974).

In drama therapy, the child is the creator, the actor, the director—while the therapist may at once take on the role of actor, observer, and audience. Although the child is typically the director of the drama, at times the therapist/actor may attempt a divergent path to support the child's move along the developmental play continuum. As a play partner, drama therapists offer total acceptance of the child relying not only on their clinical competence but also on the skills of a creative and spontaneous player

(Cattanach, 1994). Whenever the therapist is actor—taking on a role in play as assigned by the child—it is important that the therapist clearly distinguish between playing and not playing, between being in and out of role, so as not to confuse the child. The boundaries between self and role, between me and not me, should always remain clear. The therapist can accomplish this by speaking about the character in third person or asking specific questions about how a particular character should be played. As therapists enlist the child in explaining what their character should say or do, they help the child to determine when they are in and out of role. For example, in a drama where the therapist is assigned the role of an alien who has just landed on Earth, the therapist might ask the child to demonstrate how the alien character moves and speaks and what he might say when confronting the earthlings for the first time.

Drama therapy supports the use of symbolism and projection in play "as the child endows the object with properties of himself and represents his view of reality through his projective play" (Landy, 1986, p. 12). Similarly, Jennings (1993, 1995) affirms the relevance of dramatic imagination in child development, asserting that it is through dramatic imagination that we gain understanding of why we behave as we do. She argues that "the creative imagination is the most important attribute that we can foster in children" (1993, p. 20).

Drama Therapy and Autism Spectrum Disorders

Drama therapy is for the most part a child-led and child-inspired intervention, making it well suited to therapy with children with ASD. Such an approach is supported by Rogers and Vismara (2008), who cite a 2001 National Research Council (NRC) report on interventions for young children with autism that identifies as best practice those "approaches that begin with child choice and use intrinsic reinforcers, foster child motivation and generalization" (pp. 32–33). Another element of drama therapy that supports its use with individuals with ASD is that it is an interactive process that fosters interpersonal interaction and growth (Irwin, 2005; Sandberg, 1981). Interactive and shared play experiences provide opportunities for the development of cognitive, social, and communication skills in ways that solitary play experiences cannot (Chasen, 2011; Lewis, 2003). Wolfberg (2009) asserts that "peer play is an especially important social and cultural context within which children acquire various skills equated with social competence" (p. 34).

When considering most neuro-typical children, independent and peer play is widely acknowledged as their primary means of communicating about, experimenting with, exploring, and understanding their world (Cattanach, 1994). This is often not the case, however, for children with ASD, whose play typically is less exploratory and more rigid and repetitive.

Schuler and Wolfberg (2000) coined the term *echoplaylia* to compare the often literal and highly repetitive quality of the play of children with autism to the mimicking and imitative speech that defines echolalia. They maintain that the play of children with ASD is often limited to repetitive manipulation of objects or play materials, engagement in complex and intricate routines or rituals, and obsessive focus on specific topics or ideas. Without direction and guidance, children with ASD may not participate in pretend play, may not use toys and play materials in imaginary, functional, or symbolic ways, and will rarely engage in role play or enactment in a flexible or spontaneous manner. Likewise, without adult intervention children with ASD do not typically or spontaneously engage in free play with peers or siblings, instead choosing to play in a solitary or parallel fashion (Wolfberg, 2009).

Shared pretend play is a primary vehicle for the social development of children. The social world and social behavior inspire and inform collaborative play. Through shared pretend play, children's social communication skills are strengthened, and the participants engage in an exchange of ideas that leads to a deepening of understanding of the social world, social behavior and relationships (Attwood, 2007; Chasen, 2011).

Along related developmental lines, Irwin (2005) describes the significance of role play in the evolution of empathy skills. She notes, "When one plays a role, for example, one is asked to think, talk, and be like someone else. In this way, one can develop an appreciation, perhaps even empathy, for another's point of view" (p. 21). Greenspan and Wieder (2006) strongly advocate the use of drama to communicate affect in play. Through drama, children can begin to experience the expressive and receptive communication of a broad range of emotions and begin to truly understand their significance. As we take on a role, we are experiencing the "me and not me"—the similarities and differences between self and others, the joining that brings about connection. Sandberg (1981) maintains that "the ability to see things from another's point of view is central to our understanding of the self and others" (p. 39). Role taking and role playing, understanding the role as separate from the self, not only allows the development of empathy and perspective but also supports a clear sense of self-identity. Cattanach (1994) emphasizes the connection between role play and the development of perspective-taking abilities, a key element necessary for deepening skills related to ToM. She maintains that "to re-experience the world from the others point of view is the very meat of role taking" (p. 24). The development of plot and adapting the space to establish the "where" in an improvisation enhances the use of imagination and guides the sense of the "as if," the use of symbolism and projection that is central to drama.

For children with ASD, drama therapy provides a purposeful intervention that affords a unique opportunity to address many of the significant areas of need via a single medium. Meaningful communication, shared experience, social connection, and social understanding are each developed and enhanced through joyful, child-initiated dramatic play.

Toys and Materials for Facilitating Dramatic Play

Over the years, I have successfully engaged children in dramatic play without props or costumes and in spaces that were hardly conducive to imaginary and spontaneous play. Such an approach may be adequate for more typically functioning children whose play skills develop in a more natural fashion. When fashioning a drama therapy experience for children with autism spectrum disorders, however, it is helpful to provide materials that enhance the play experience and help to move children along the dramatic play continuum. Toys and materials should be purposeful and deliberately chosen to support the identified goals. Typical play therapy toys such as dollhouses, people, and animal figures, baby dolls and accessories, vehicles, and a sand tray are all basic necessities. These materials support the development of symbolic and projective play skills. Materials and an environment that promotes sociodramatic play are equally important elements and include hats, capes, masks, and fabric for creating costumes and defining space—all of which support the development of imaginative play and improvisation. Telephones for communicating, a cash register and pretend food items, household items such as brooms and dust pans, and props such as keys, doctor kits, and flashlights are helpful tools when engaging in play related to typical daily activities. Materials such as wands, swords, shields, crowns, and animal ears enrich and inspire fantasy play. A full-length mirror and large dry erase board are helpful additions. A final key ingredient is a space that provides both the level of safety and freedom necessary to facilitate the drama effectively.

The Dramatic Play Continuum

Jordan (2003) emphasizes the concept that as children move through and develop skills related to the various developmental stages of play they acquire a repertoire of play skills that they will continue to use throughout their lives. The dramatic play continuum is based on a similar concept—the idea that children must experience and master play skills in a developmentally significant manner, moving from one level to the next as mastery is achieved. For neuro-typical children, this process occurs in a relatively natural way without the need for intervention or direction. On the other hand, children with autism spectrum disorders require our help to facilitate this process. In so doing, we allow children to begin where they are developmentally rather than attempting to push them to where they "should" be chronologically.

Sensorimotor activity is children's introduction to play and the basis for all future play-based experiences. In infancy and early childhood, we begin to play and explore through sensation—through sound and touch. For the child with ASD this is typically where we must begin. This type of play is especially relevant for the child who is just beginning to explore and experiment with toys and objects but has not yet developed the skills to play symbolically (Cattanach, 1994). Sensory play involves exploring the world through sound (i.e., music, rhythm), and through touch (i.e., slime, water, sand, clay, marbles, rocks, shells). For the child with autism, this play often becomes the road to connection as child and therapist share the sensory experience. We bury our hands in the sand, experiencing the idea of here and not here—a rudimentary hide-and-seek.

As children begin to master sensory and sensorimotor play, the next goal is to assist them toward exploring symbolic play. In the evolution from sensory to symbolic play, we first may witness symbols used to depict events or experiences—real or imagined. For example, a truck delivers mail, blocks are lined up to represent a road, a pile of sand is transformed into a volcano. We can move any sensory experience toward a symbolic experience by giving meaning—to voice, movement, inanimate objects. When children begin to understand that toys and objects can be transformed and used to represent and symbolize other things, whether real or imagined, symbolic play has begun (Cattanac, 1994).

As this predramatic play deepens, children move toward the projection of personal feeling and experiences that involve emotion. Through projective play, feelings, emotions and other human qualities are projected onto the toys and objects. The truck excitedly delivers mail to or from Daddy, the bus hurriedly races the children to school, people run in fear from the erupting volcano. Projective play infuses thoughts, emotions, and experiences into the play, moving the play and the social connection to another level.

From projective play there is a natural progression to sociodramatic play. Through sociodramatic play, we witness the first true movement of the child with ASD from monologue to dialogue. It is through sociodramatic play that play becomes a truly shared experience—where others are allowed in and true joining occurs. The entire room becomes the play space. Various environments are created as play develops: house, store, post office, school. Roles are established, costumes are donned, and props are used to enhance the improvisational experience. Voices and bodies are used to establish characters. Self is distinguished from other. Feelings and emotions are explored. Problem solving and empathy skills begin to develop.

Involving Parents in Dramatic Play

Involving parents in the drama therapy sessions of children with ASD enhances the child's ability to develop and maintain new play skills. Coaching parents both in and out of session can assist them in establishing an environment for dramatic play at home, to engage in play with their child on a regular basis, and to support the continuity of interventions used in the drama therapy sessions within children's natural environments. Greenspan and Wieder (2006) encourage parents to get involved in their children's dramatic play by taking on a role in their play and actively engaging in the drama. Parents are encouraged to prioritize dramatic play time at home. A list of recommended toys and materials is offered to parents. The more children engage in dramatic play the greater the chance that these behaviors will generalize to other environments and situations—specifically with peers. Parents are encouraged to schedule play dates with peers on a regular basis, gradually increasing the frequency and length of the play dates. Parents are advised to allow the play to naturally evolve from parallel play to interactive play and on to dramatic play and to avoid the urge to force or expect their child to play at a developmental level that they haven't yet reached. The National Research Council report, as cited by Rogers and Vismara (2008), maintains that parent involvement in treatment of children with ASD is especially important. Parent involvement should include both training in effective ways of helping and interacting with their children and instruction in ways to support their child's newly learned skills at home and within the community (Kasari et al., 2006).

Case Presentation: Max

Max is a 4-year, 3-month-old child diagnosed with PDD-NOS, whose parents had received the results of their son's comprehensive evaluation just a week before their first meeting with me. Max had been referred to me for play and drama therapy, and both parents expressed an appreciation of the importance of this type of intervention. Max's parents reported that they were devastated by their son's diagnosis but on some level were not surprised. They had sensed that something was wrong with Max from the time he was an infant. He had not developed as had their two older children, particularly in the areas of socialization, social and emotional connectedness, and play skills. They described Max as "inflexible, unyielding, and rigid." They worried that he isolated himself from others, especially his peers, and showed little interest in interacting with others. Though his parents believed that Max was obviously bonded with them, they complained that his hugs always seemed superficial and that he had habits that they found quite strange. He opened and closed doors incessantly, paced the house listing or naming things, and though his older siblings tried they could not engage Max in play. Max had great difficulty dealing with transition times, unexpected changes, and large social events. Such situations would often lead to anxious pacing, rocking, screaming, and at times full-blown "meltdowns" as they described them. Max had a large vocabulary but used language primarily to name objects or to recite scripts from his favorite videos or television shows rather than to communicate with others. His parents and teachers expressed concern that Max would sometimes look as though he wanted to play and interact with other children but didn't seem to know how to initiate interaction or even how to respond to another child's invitation to play. Max would often totally ignore both peers and adults who attempted to engage him in conversation, and, of particular annoyance to his parents, he would often completely ignore their requests. He had a passion for maps, airplanes, cars, street signs, and anything mechanical.

During the initial parent session, I explained the importance of parent involvement in the therapy sessions, and both parents made a commitment that at least one of them would participate in each of Max's sessions. I explained that during the sessions with Max I would model responses and interventions and encourage them to engage directly with Max to increase their comfort with the approach and increase the likelihood that they will follow through at home. I informed Max's parents that it would be essential for them to establish an environment at home that would foster dramatic play and that it would be important for them to engage in dramatic play with Max daily to support the new play skills Max would be learning during his sessions. We discussed the types of toys and play materials that they might want to make available to Max at home, including a variety of dramatic play materials that would support Max's newly developing play skills. At the end of my initial session with Max's parents, I asked them to identify their greatest wish for their son. Max's mother stated "that he learn to play and have fun and interact more with others." Max's father stated only "that he have friends."

When I observed Max at his preschool prior to my first session with him, I saw a child who isolated himself on the playground, staring blankly through the fence or picking up and dropping random items he would find on the ground. He did not engage his classmates, nor did they engage him. During circle time in the classroom Max was fixated by fibers on the carpet, the pattern on the sweater of the girl sitting in front of him, and the tiny string hanging from the hem of his jeans. At snack time, while the other children laughed and talked, Max counted his crackers as he popped them into his mouth. Fortunately the school was willing to work with me and with Max's parents, and together we developed a list of guidelines for the teachers and school personnel that would support the goal of helping Max to play, interact, and communicate more effectively with his peers.

Max attended his first therapy session in my office with both parents present. He reluctantly held his parents hands as he walked into the building but darted away from them before they could get him through the door of my first-floor office. Instead, Max ran up and down the steps leading to the second-floor offices, counting steps, naming things he saw—"banister," "skylight," "doors." Max's parents finally coaxed him down the steps and led him into my office waiting room.

When I walked out to the waiting room to meet Max and his parents, I found him crouched over the floor register that covered the air conditioning vent. He stared into and put his hand over the vent, feeling the cool air. He laughed as the air blew on his face. The disturbance in texture of the grate on the smooth wood floor and the cool air were likely what attracted Max (and several other children I have worked with diagnosed with ASD) to the vent on the floor. Max remained transfixed by the physical sensations and did not respond as I called his name several times. I grabbed a tissue, sat on the floor next to Max, and put the tissue over the vent. Max continued to ignore me but laughed as the breeze blew the tissue off the vent. I caught the tissue and covered the vent a second time. This time, Max and I both laughed when the tissue was blown from the vent. I held the tissue behind my back. Max watched the vent for a few seconds, waiting to see the tissue trick again. Finally Max looked in my direction, and I smiled and said, "Hi, Max." Max responded "Hi," and then looked behind me for the tissue. When Max found the tissue, he grabbed it from my hand, dropped it in my lap, and shouted, "Do it again." I put the tissue over the vent, and when it blew off I handed it to Max and said, "Your turn." Max took the tissue and placed it over the vent. When it blew off Max looked at me and we both laughed. Max handed the tissue to me and said, "Your turn." We continued the tissue game for the next few minutes. Each time Max looked at me as we laughed together. We had made our first connection and shared our first playful experience. Max's parents reported that Max was eager to return for his next session.

The air vent game involved the physical sensations of sensory play. As in play with an infant, feeling the air on his face allowed Max to connect first with the physical sensations and then with the source of the sensations—which included me. During the next several sessions we continued to engage in sensory play. I introduced Max to the sand tray, and together we explored the soft, cool texture of the sand. I dug my hands into the sand and playfully poked one finger at a time up out of the sand. Max smiled and remained engaged and after a few minutes joined me in this game of peek-a-boo. We played with sand toys, allowing sand to stream onto our hands from increasingly larger funnels. We used a spray bottle to spray water onto our hands and then into the sand, changing the texture from soft and smooth to wet and lumpy. As we played, I began to hide objects in the sand—rocks, shells, marbles—as Max excitedly searched for them in our basic game of hide-and-seek. I began to add animal figures into the sand, and we continued to bury and forage for the figures. Max's continued rigidity and need for repetition were evident as he methodically lined up the animals and other objects that found their way into the sand tray. As the objects were covered with sand, Max began to use the spray bottle to wash each object clean. As the objects were sprayed I began to give them voice shouting, "Oh I'm all wet!" Max laughed each time I did this and sprayed some more. Max then raised the spray bottle higher and sprayed water all over the sand tray. He then looked at me and at his mom and stated, "It's raining!" Max had made the jump to symbolic play—giving the spray bottle a new identity as the rain.

Despite Max's foray into the world of symbolic play, he continued to engage in a fair amount of rigid and repetitive play with toys and objects. He would often stare at the wheels of the toy cars and trucks, spinning the wheels, opening and closing the doors, lining them on the floor or in the sand tray. He brought an ambulance close to his face and in a high-pitched sing-song voice repeatedly named the parts: "wheels," "doors," "lights," "bumper," "siren." Max rolled the wheels with his fingers and opened and closed the ambulance doors. At this point in Max's therapy my attempts to engage him in more imaginary and symbolic play with the ambulance did not typically garner much success.

One activity that seemed to especially grab Max's interest involved a small dollhouse with a garage door that could be raised and lowered. Max would lie on the floor with his face as close to the garage door as possible, repeatedly moving the door up and down as he stared incessantly. Like much of the repetitive play often seen in children with ASD, this activity appeared to have no apparent purpose. I decided to intervene and engage Max and the door in a drama. At the back of the garage was an opening meant to symbolize a door. As Max closed the garage door I put my finger through the back door. When Max raised the garage door he saw my finger and laughed. From this point on the raising and lowering of the garage door took on a purpose (i.e., seeing my finger) and a connection (i.e., attending to and laughing at my action). During the next session when Max again played with the garage door, I moved people figures through the back door and eventually gave them voices. "Open the garage door; I want to get out!" I shouted. Max opened the garage door, and as I tried to push the figures through he quickly closed the garage door, looking at me and smiling as he did so. As we continued this drama, Max began to respond to my figure's pleas with statements such as, "No you can't come out." At times he would actually tease saying, "OK!" and then quickly close the garage door as he laughed heartily. When I added to the conversation with lines such as, "But I have to go to work!" Max opened the garage door and let the person out. I asked, "Where's my car?" Max quickly grabbed a car and pushed it into the garage. I put the person into the car and pushed the car through the garage door. Max rolled the car around the room voicing the figure in the car. "I have to go to work." I added other figures into our drama engaging Max's figure in conversation and activity. This game continued throughout much of Max's therapy, with the drama expanding in each session. The person in the car eventually became people, who traveled to school, work, home, the supermarket, usually starting out from behind the garage door.

Over time, Max was able to add more drama into all of his play. The ambulance picked up sick or injured people and transported them to the hospital where a doctor would tend to them and family members would express worry and concern. His repetitive play with other vehicles such as the mail truck evolved into an elaborate game of mail delivery as we created a mailbox, the post office, and pieces of mail to be delivered to real and imaginary recipients. In the sand tray, roads were created as cars traveled to Grandma's house or to Aunt Annie's in Tennessee. Volcanoes spewed lava and dinosaurs battled. For many months, most of this play relied on the distance afforded by the use of objects and toys as opposed to the use of role play and improvisation that is the basis of sociodramatic play—the ultimate goal of the many months of drama and play. But Max was obviously moving ever closer to this goal.

Sociodramatic play for Max began with the use of a cash register and a couple of phones. Max had played with the toy cash register before, but his play was for the most part repetitive as he pushed buttons and listened to the sounds. The play had little purpose and was for the most part a solitary activity. During this session, I moved a box of pretend food and two telephones next to where Max was playing. Max began to use the cash register to scan the food items. I began to dial on one of the phones and asked Max's mom to answer with the other phone. I told her I was calling the supermarket to see what time they opened so that I could do some shopping. Mom handed the phone to Max telling him that a customer was calling to ask what time the store opened. Max excitedly grabbed the phone and yelled, "Two o'clock!" I then pretended to drive to the store and shopped for groceries as Max played the cashier. Over the next few weeks as we continued the store theme, the whole room evolved into a mall with signs identifying the various kinds of shops. In addition to Max's supermarket there was an ice cream shop, a toy store, a tool store, and several others. Max and I, along with whichever of his parents was present, would don different hats, costume pieces, and props and take turns playing the roles of customers and store keepers. Through our roles, we engaged in reciprocal conversation, responded to requests, and engaged in a variety of interactive tasks and activities. Our sociodramatic play expanded from week to week as we enacted scenes in places such as restaurants, hospitals, and school.

Max always took on the role of teacher, which is typical for most children. However, in the initial weeks of dramatic play Max's teacher role was limited to listing the day's activities, classroom rules, vocabulary words, or homework assignments on the dry erase board. Although his parents and I attempted to engage Max by taking on the roles of students Max did not interact with us and often would completely ignore our attempts to engage him. But as we became more playful and intrusive in our student roles, Max began to respond to our behavior. I especially liked to play a rambunctious, noncompliant student, who called out, interrupted my teacher, and bothered my classmates. Max would scold me for my misbehavior, and I would often be sent to "time-out" until I could follow the rules. School continues to be a favorite scenario for Max. He still prefers to play the teacher while his parents and I are assigned the roles of students, establishing different names, identities, and personalities. Max's mom will often get a star for following directions while I typically get my name on the board for unruly behavior. On a good day my behavior might even warrant a phone call home to my parents.

Today there are few monologues in Max's play—and his ability to dialogue and connect increases steadily both in and out of the playroom. His parents continue to engage in dramatic play with him at home and to arrange play dates on a regular basis. In his kindergarten class, Max has begun to spontaneously engage with other children on the playground and to interact verbally during snack time. He has identified several of his classmates as his friends and has had successful play dates with two children from his class. In his classroom, dramatic play has become Max's favorite activity as he engages with other children in both fantasy and real-life play scenes. Now when Max comes in for his weekly drama therapy session, we set the stage by moving furniture and fashioning fabric, props, and other materials to create our sense of place. Our dramas continue to develop, and new themes emerge as we battle with swords, shop at the mall, and fly off to distant lands—together.

Dramatic Play Dyads and Groups

Once children such as Max have journeyed through the dramatic play continuum and can engage comfortably in symbolic, projective, and sociodramatic play, the next developmental step should involve peer group drama therapy experiences. Participation in such a group offers children with ASD the opportunity to continue to strengthen their emerging play and social skills, provides a supportive and safe environment to experiment with new interactive skills and behaviors, and enhances feelings of social connectedness and competency. For children not yet ready for a group experience, dyads—involving two children appropriately paired based on characteristics such as common interests, social/developmental level, or communication skills—affords children the opportunity to practice their skills in a therapeutic setting with only one other child at a time. As with dyads, groups can be formed for general dramatic play, bringing together children of similar ages and social skill levels. Alternatively, groups can be formed around a specific theme. A popular group theme is that of superheroes. Many children and teens with ASD identify with superhero characters for a variety of reasons and are able to use these characters to explore significant issues of their own. Self-identity and bullying are consistent themes, for as Rubin (2007) notes, "Superheroes rarely fit in" (p. 17). Tony Attwood (2007) extols the benefits of role play involving super heroes with children with Asperger's disorder. "Often the super-hero is someone who has two identities, a timid and often meek and unsuccessful person who is able to transform himself into someone with special abilities, able to conquer adversity" (p.187). The common superhero themes of power and transformation (Attwood, 2007; Rubin, 2007; Scanlon, 2007) resonate with many boys including those with autism spectrum disorders.

The Super Friends Group
Jeremy, Alex, David, and Tim are four boys ages 8 through 10 who participated in a weekly drama therapy group over a period of 6 months. Jeremy, the youngest of the group, was diagnosed with Asperger's disorder. His verbal interaction with others tended to be perseverative and repetitive. He often bluntly criticized both adults and peers and attempted to control any social situation. Alex and David, both diagnosed with autism, had language and articulation delays, adding to their already pronounced deficits in social interaction skills. Tim was the oldest of the boys, and though he was quite verbal his social vocabulary was generally limited to talking about or scripting lines from his favorite cartoons. All four of the boys had a great deal of difficulty understanding and interpreting social cues, which lead to conflict and hurt feelings in typical play or social settings. And all four of the boys had a passion for comic books and superheroes, which were the common threads that motivated them to come together and enabled them to ultimately connect. By the third group session they had named their group "The Super Friends Group," a symbol of their deepening connection. Goals for the boys included enhanced feelings of social competence, increased use of spontaneous reciprocal conversation, and improvement in peer interaction, perspective taking, emotional flexibility, collaboration, and compromise. Each week over the 6-month period the boys came together and created and enacted stories involving super heroes. During the first weeks the stories closely mimicked comic book stories they had read or cartoons or movies they had seen. Characters engaged primarily in monologue or soliloquy as opposed to dialogue or reciprocal conversation. When conversation did take place it rarely involved listening

or an exchange of ideas but rather was limited to each boy waiting for the other to finish speaking so he could have his turn. Even in those weeks, however, the boys began to learn how to compromise and negotiate to turn four ideas into one story that they could enact. The boys used fabric, furniture, props, hand-drawn scenery, and costumes to enact the stories they had created. As the weeks went on I encouraged them to create characters and stories of their own and the boys worked together to develop their own superheroes and villains. Some of the characters persisted and over time the stories became episodes, with themes developing and evolving from week to week. As the characters interacted, the level of spontaneous reciprocal communication among characters—and among the boys— increased. The characters and the boys began working together to solve problems, listened to each other, and regularly engaged in conversation.

The boys looked forward to their time together and often excitedly arrived for their group with lists of ideas for stories and enactments. Through their stories they explored themes related to a variety of issues including friendship, good versus evil, and family relationships. The boys' typical rigidity softened as they became more obviously flexible and willing to compromise. They were able to more readily recognize the value of someone else's ideas and perspective and to find ways to compromise and merge their ideas into a cohesive whole. They clearly demonstrated an understanding of symbolic, projective, and sociodramatic play and were able to use these skills when involved in peer play outside of the therapeutic environment. All four of the boys expressed less resistance to engaging in peer play experiences both at school and within the community, advancing their play journeys into more natural settings and affording them the opportunity to establish and maintain friendships.

Conclusion

Though anecdotal information such as the cases of Max and the Super Friends Group presented in this chapter appears to provide a foundation for the theory that drama therapy has long-term positive implications for children with ASD, there is an obvious need for scientific investigation and study to provide evidence-based support for this type of intervention. The little research that is currently available can at least be viewed as a stepping stone to the work that needs to be accomplished here. Chasen (2011) focuses on neurobiology and drama therapy. He points to recent research in the field of neuroscience that indicates that imitation and reenactment are the basis "for understanding self and other" (p. 66). Chasen maintains that the "inherently dramatic functions of imitation and reenactment" (p. 64) support the idea that dramatic enactment promotes a stronger social connection and clearer sense of self-identity.

Corbett et al. (2011) report on a brief study into the effectiveness of a program that involves theater as therapy for children with autism spectrum disorders. They report that participants evidenced a "modest" enhancement in skills related to theory of mind and social perception (p. 508).

The protocol presented in this chapter has been shown through observation as well as through parent and school report to enable participants to enhance their capacity for social connectedness, social communication, perspective taking, and shared positive experiences. Such qualities have the ability to gently guide children with ASD from a solitary existence to a life filled with purposeful and joyful interaction and heartfelt, meaningful relationships.

References

Attwood, T. (2007). *The complete guide to Asperger's syndrome*. London: Jessica Kingsley Publishers.

Baron-Cohen, S. (2008). *Autism and Asperger syndrome*. New York: Oxford University Press.

Cattanach, A. (1994). *Play therapy: Where the sky meets the underworld*. London: Jessica Kingsley Publishers.

Centers for Disease Control and Prevention. (CDC). (2009). Prevalence of autism spectrum disorders. Autism and developmental disabilities monitoring network, US 2006. *MMWR, 58*,1–20.

Chasen, L.R. (2011). *Social skills, emotional growth and drama therapy*. London: Jessica Kingsley Publishers.

Corbett, B. A., Gunther, J. R., Comins, D., Price, J., Ryan, N., Simon, D., et al. (2011). Brief report: Theatre as therapy for children with autism spectrum disorder. *Journal of Autism and Developmental Disabilities, 41*, 505–511.

Courtney, R. (1974). *Play, drama and thought*. New York: Drama Book Specialists.

Densmore, A. E. (2007). *Helping children with autism become more social: 76 ways to use narrative play*. Westport, CT: Praeger.

Gallo-Lopez, L. (2005). Drama therapy with adolescents. In L. Gallo-Lopez & C. E. Schaefer (Eds.), *Play therapy with adolescents* (pp. 81–95). New York: Jason Aronson.

Gray, C. (1994). *The original social story book*. Arlinton, TX: Future Horizons.

Greenspan, S. I., & Wieder, S. (2006). *Engaging autism*. Cambridge, MA: Da Capo Press.

Irwin, E. C. (2005). Facilitating play with non-players: A developmental perspective. In A. M. Weber & C. Haen (Eds.), *Clinical applications of drama therapy in child and adolescent treatment* (pp. 3–23). New York: Brunner-Routledge.

Jennings, S. (1993). *Playtherapy with children: A practitioner's guide*. Oxford: Blackwell Scientific.

Jennings, S. (1995). Introduction. In S. Jennings (Ed.), *Drama therapy with children and adolescents* (pp. 1–3). London: Routledge.

Jordan, R. (2003). Social play and autistic spectrum disorders: A perspective on theory, implications and educational approaches. *Autism, 7*(4), 347–360.

Kasari, C., Freeman, S., & Paparella, T. (2006). Joint attention and symbolic play in young children with autism: A randomized controlled intervention study. *Journal of Child Psychology and Psychiatry, 47*(6), 611–620.

Landy, R. (1986). *Drama therapy concepts and practices.* Springfield, IL: Charles C. Thomas.

Lewis, V. (2003). Play and language in children with autism. *Autism, 7*(4), 391–399.

Page, T. (2009). *Parallel play.* New York: Random House.

Rogers, S. J., & Vismara, L. A. (2008). Evidence-based comprehensive treatments for early autism. *Journal of Clinical Child & Adolescent Psychology, 37*(1), 8–38.

Rubin, L. C. (2007). Introduction: Look, up in the sky! An introduction to the use of superheroes in psychotherapy. In L. C. Rubin (Ed.), *Using superheroes in counseling and play therapy.* New York: Springer.

Sandberg, B. (1981). A descriptive scale for drama. In G. Schattner & R. Courtney (Eds.), *Drama in therapy* (pp. 29–50). New York: Drama Book Specialists.

Scanlon, P. (2007). Superheroes are super friends: Developing social skills and emotional reciprocity with autism spectrum clients. In L. C. Rubin (Ed.), *Using superheroes in counseling and play therapy* (pp. 169–191). New York: Springer.

Schuler, A., & Wolfberg, P. (2000). Promoting peer play and socialization: The art of scaffolding. In A. M. Wetherby & B. M. Prizant (Eds.), *Autism spectrum disorders: A transactional developmental perspective* (vol. 9, Communication and Language Intervention Series). Baltimore: Brookes.

Stahmer, A. C., Ingersoll, B., & Carter, C. (2003). Behavioral approaches to promoting play. *Autism: International Journal of Research and Practice, 7*(4), 401–413.

Wolfberg, P. J. (2009). *Play and imagination in children with autism* (2nd ed.). New York: Teachers College Press.

CHAPTER 6

LEGO-Based Play Therapy for Improving Social Competence in Children and Adolescents With Autism Spectrum Disorders

DANIEL B. LEGOFF, G. W. KRAUSS, AND SARAH LEVIN ALLEN

Introduction

Children with autism and related conditions, by definition, are often diffi-cult to engage in play, especially interactive play. This is not a trivial aspect of their condition. Play is at the core of childhood development in all its dimensions. Language, social competence, problem solving, motor skills, technology, identity, moral reasoning—all important aspects of learning—are apparent in the self-directed practice evident in various forms of play, from stacking blocks to blasting aliens. At the core of autistic pathology is the absence or deficiency of adaptively relevant play. The LEGO®-based approach has much in common with many play therapy approaches that focus on using whatever elements or approximations of adaptive play are evident and then engage with and expand that core. Fortunately, for many children with autism spectrum disorders (ASD), there is not only an inter-est and an island of efficacy with regard to constructional play, and espe-cially LEGO play, but also a shared interest.

This is not exclusive to LEGO, of course, so the natural question is, "Why LEGO?" To some extent this was arbitrary or accidental—the result of finding a common interest among a number of children with autism and taking advantage of that motivation to increase willingness to participate in a group activity. On the other hand, the sustained interest and growth of the LEGO therapy approach has not been accidental. Currently, LEGO-based therapy is being used with children with autism and other disabilities throughout North America as well as in the United Kingdom (Owens, Granader, Humphrey, & Baron-Cohen, 2008), Asia, Australia, South America, and Africa. There is definitely something relevant with regard to this population about the use of LEGO materials and the resulting therapeutic benefit.

Children play with LEGO bricks all the time—LEGO has been consistently in the top ranks of toy manufacturers since the 1970s (Hansen, 1982; Wiencek, 1987). What is it about this common play toy composed of little more than simple snap-together primary-colored plastic blocks and the process of constructing things with them that can make it therapeutic? Over the years, my colleagues and I have formally and informally deconstructed this approach and have identified some key therapeutic features:

- Likely first and foremost is the high level of motivation that many children with autistic spectrum conditions have for this particular activity and play materials—motivated participation is obviously going to be key to any therapeutic intervention, especially a child-led approach based on play.
- An often overlooked aspect of LEGO materials is the high rate and frequency of discrete actions, and repetition. A typical LEGO activity will involve hundreds of actions and objects and at least that many opportunities for interaction and communication in less than an hour. Clearly, this is a fundamental aspect of learning. Social competence is not something that children with autism learn through insight; they learn through practice and repetition—slow approximations, similar to learning to play a musical instrument.
- As Golan et al. (2009) pointed out, LEGO play is very systematic, and this play activity capitalizes on the strong systematic reasoning abilities of individuals with autism. The system of LEGO then can lead directly to acquisition of a system for interacting with others: accessing the underlying norms and rules of social interaction that have been previously invisible to them.
- LEGO Corporation expends an enormous amount of effort and ingenuity on an ongoing basis in product development. The range and diversity of LEGO materials lends itself to both the idiosyncratic interests of the population of children with autistic conditions as well as to their typically developing peers. There is virtually no idiosyncratic interest that could not be accommodated by the ever-expanding range of LEGO materials.

- Finally, LEGO toys are simple and sensorily appealing, elements that are attractive to children who have difficulty managing complex and changing visual stimuli and patterns.

Theoretical and Empirical Rationale

The use of LEGO bricks as a therapeutic medium to enhance the social and communication skills of children with autism spectrum disorders was initially developed in the mid-1990s and was introduced to the research literature about 10 years later (LeGoff, 2004; LeGoff & Sherman, 2006). This approach did not evolve strategically from a given methodology or intervention and was not based on a preexisting theoretical framework. Rather, a number of coincidental findings led me (LeGoff) to consider the potential use of LEGO bricks as a therapy tool—I had been exposed to them as a play material as a child but had not seen them used in any of my training as a child psychologist. Of course, I'm sure many of my colleagues would agree that there is a considerable overlap between LEGO-based constructional play and that of other materials, such as clay, sand tray figures, blocks, and K'Nex. Nonetheless, there also seemed to be something unique and powerful about the LEGO play system, particularly for the emerging population of children—mostly boys—identified as autistic.

One key aspect of this particular approach is, of course, the LEGO materials themselves. This is not by accident. LEGO Corporation, based in Billund, Denmark, has conducted its own research on the nature of play and utility of play activities for cognitive and social development for decades (Papert, 1999; Weckstrom, 2010). Obviously, for reasons of corporate competition, LEGO Corporation does not typically share its research and development findings publicly. There may be a number of reasons for the popularity of LEGO materials with this particular population, such as their systematic nature (Baron-Cohen, 2003) or the ever-changing themes that capture the interests of the autistic population (e.g., Star Wars, comic-book superheroes, robots, trains). Of course, LEGO toys are equally popular with typically developing children, especially boys—although there has not been any evidence of a gender difference in response to LEGO bricks as an educational or therapy tool (LeGoff, 2004; Papert, 1999).

As has been previously reported (LeGoff, 2004), the initial advent of the therapeutic use of LEGO resulted from the observation of spontaneous social interest and social interaction between two boys, both diagnosed with mild autism spectrum disorders. After noticing that each of them had brought LEGO creations to share with me, they took it upon themselves to begin meeting in the waiting room of my clinic to discuss their shared interest. Taking the advice of Attwood (1998), I decided to capitalize on this interest. Attwood's approach capitalizes on the cognitive-behavioral theory of self-efficacy (Bandura, 1977, 1997)—that is, the use of intrinsic motivation and the experience of a sense of mastery to help enhance motivation for social engagement and interaction.

Without additional structuring, the LEGO therapy approach would have likely been limited to primarily individual play intervention. Many years of experience with this population has taught me that most children with autistic disorders will withdraw quickly from social interaction if they are allowed to pursue a solo activity. A key aspect of LEGO therapy is the enhancement of motivation for social interaction and social self-efficacy (Bandura, 1997) through the experience of a potential intrinsically rewarding group activity. This is achieved through the use of a technique I refer to as *horizontal task analysis.* Most professionals who work with children with developmental disabilities are familiar with traditional task analysis, which is vertical in the sense that it breaks down more complex sequences of actions into linear, sequential steps (Jonassen, Tessmer, & Hannum, 1999). A horizontal task analysis involves breaking down a task into interdependent components that can be engaged in simultaneously or that at least can occur in parallel.

The ideal social learning context involves three key components: (1) a positive and meaningful experience (i.e., personally relevant); (2) a high frequency of rewarding social interaction (i.e., the experience of others as helpful and collaborative and the experience of self as efficacious); and (3) an experience of joint accomplishment (i.e., successful interdependence). The LEGO structured group play activity emphasizes all three of these. At the same time, a critical aspect of the LEGO approach is the high frequency of opportunities for positive interaction. This is an inherent aspect of the LEGO building process itself: Each LEGO activity—whether it is a simple set-building project or something as elaborate as a stop-motion film project—involves many steps, each requiring joint attention, joint decision making, and reciprocal communication (verbal and nonverbal). The following provides a review of the previously published outcome research as well as further detail regarding implementation of this particular method of structured group play intervention.

Level One—Building Skills

Collaborative set building can be initiated once children show independent abilities to identify pieces and then sort and select them based on either the instructions or their own basic imitation. Medium-level sets (50–150 pieces) can be introduced. The LEGO age guidelines provided on sets can be very useful in determining the next level for a given child. Parents should be encouraged to attempt sets at home that are at the next level of difficulty above the one most recently mastered. Often, at this level, the child will need adult prompting and help, especially with parts that are more difficult to assemble (e.g., wheels, smaller parts). Once able to consistently collaborate with an adult and stay focused on task appropriately without requiring external reinforcement for each step (i.e., rewards can be delayed to final completion), children are ready for collaborative building with a peer.

Level Two—Collaborative Building With One Peer
Level-two activities involve collaborative building with one peer and often require close adult supervision. It is often helpful, especially initially, to have a typically developing or at least more advanced peer mentor as a helper. In this regard, we have often found it useful to match a child who is working on prosocial and helping behaviors with a learner (i.e., a LEGO creator or LEGO master with a LEGO builder or helper—see section LEGO Club Groups and Behavior Management and Rewards). Initially, paired collaborative LEGO projects can be an important precursor to larger LEGO group participation. This involves working on collaborative projects with half a dozen or so peers, often with assigned interdependent roles, that emphasize cooperation, communication, and joint accomplishment as opposed to individual projects and achievements. Although peer mentoring continues at all levels of the LEGO Club groups, at times such as this it is more explicitly the focus of the intervention.

Collaborative Set Building   With pairs, it is often helpful to start off with sets that are within reach of the child who is being helped. As the pair demonstrates reciprocal building (i.e. they are able to complete a small set independently, with minimal adult intervention), the level of complexity of sets can be increased. The helping child may need to be given additional support and rewards for being patient and supportive at this stage, with access to preferred sets or magazines or by earning new sets or desired pieces. Typically, helpers have difficulty allowing the less skilled builder to fully participate and will tend to take over the task completely. For this reason, the adult should strictly regulate the activity by assigning specific tasks as follows.

The child just starting level two will be the parts supplier. His job is to find the correct LEGO pieces and give them to the child with whom he is working. The more advanced member of the pair will be the builder. The builder's job is to put the pieces together according to the instructions. The parts supplier should be encouraged and prompted primarily by the builder, not the adult supervisor. For example, the builder should prompt the parts supplier when they have finished one step and need the next piece.

The builder should be instructed to follow a hierarchy of requests or prompts. First, the builder will ask for specific parts needed to complete the set by verbally describing the pieces (e.g., "Please can I have a black 2 by 2 brick?"). Second, if the parts supplier gives the wrong piece or doesn't respond, the builder should point to the item in the instructions, again giving the verbal label. Finally, if the parts supplier has not yet given the correct piece, the builder should point to the actual piece and again verbally label it. The builder should not take pieces from the parts supplier or take the parts supplier's hand to guide a response. Only when there is a clear failure of verbal and nonverbal requests should the adult give direct assistance by pointing or hand-over-hand prompting. The adult should also repeat the verbal prompt and, if necessary, should place the piece in the parts supplier's hand and then prompt him to give the piece to the builder.

This process of collaborative building with a peer is at the core of the LEGO therapy process and should be learned and perfected as a central skill-building strategy. All higher-level LEGO therapy activities are dependent on mastery of this initial collaborative task.

Once a parts supplier has shown some mastery of this task (i.e., the child spontaneously gives parts and needs fewer nonverbal prompts), then turn taking should be introduced. In this situation, the set is divided according to either number of steps (e.g., one child is builder for the first 20 of 40 steps and the second child is builder for the final 20 steps) or functional design characteristics of the set (e.g., building different parts or sections of a set). On larger sets, with pairs collaborating, it may be necessary to switch more than once during the completion (e.g., switching every 10 steps). Alternatively, turn taking can be determined by time, such as swapping roles every 10 minutes.

Collaborative Freestyle   Once children are able to sustain consistent turn taking and collaboration with a peer on set building, they can be introduced to paired freestyle building. Freestyle building involves designing and building their own creations from nonset-specific LEGO pieces rather than following printed instructions to build a particular model. The adult can help steer the pair toward possible projects, which have good potential for success.

Freestyle building involves an increased demand for communication, sharing of ideas, joint attention, and collaboration. The pair should initially be led by the more advanced child. His role is now the engineer, who is in charge of designing the freestyle creation. The less skilled child, who is working at level two, combines the roles of parts supplier and builder.

The emphasis in freestyle building should be on both effective communication and collaboration. Problem solving, compromise, and turn taking may need to be encouraged, modeled, and supported by the adult. If there is little success initially (e.g., the engineer just takes over and the builder winds up watching or making suggestions, which are ignored) the adult should take a more active role. In this situation, the adult should join in a subservient role (parts supplier or assistant builder) rather than as engineer.

Once the pair has demonstrated some proficiency at independently designing and completing freestyle creations, the less experienced child is ready to take over the role of engineer. Again, the adult may need to be more involved initially and, again, should assist rather than direct the project. Typically, at this stage LEGO helpers will be given a mock diploma recognizing their achievement of the LEGO Club status of LEGO Builder and are eligible for inclusion in larger group settings with age/developmentally similar peers (LeGoff, Krauss, & Allen, 2009).

Level Three—Collaborative Building With Two Peers

Set Building   Group set building within LEGO Club groups usually involves small subgroups. With some of the larger projects undertaken by the older groups, there are often five or six participants working on a project, but with younger groups (age 12 and under), there are usually no more than three participants working on a given project. In the dyads and triads, the members are assigned different building tasks.

The engineer describes which parts are required and where to put them according to the instructions. Bricks can be described according to their color, shape, and size. A good place to find appropriate names for bricks that are quite complicated in shape is either the LEGO Factory website on the pick-a-brick pages (factory.lego.com/pab/) or the private online website Bricklink.com.

Once the engineer has described the bricks, the parts supplier searches through the bricks to find the piece that the engineer has specified and passes the pieces one at a time to the builder. Typically, all the bricks are tipped out onto a tray rather than out onto a table so that pieces are less likely to fall onto the floor and get lost. The parts supplier may have additional tasks during building, such as cleaning parts for reassembly for restoration projects or sorting parts for preassembly on larger projects. The parts supplier may also be assigned some preassembly, when there are a large number of simple units needed (e.g., preassembling wheels, axles, and tires). The builder is given the pieces by the parts supplier and constructs the LEGO set according to the printed instructions and directions from the engineer. Participants then take turns playing each of the different roles (e.g., swap every 10 steps of the instructions). Here is a useful opportunity to practice turn taking in a fair way. It is useful to ask children to generate fair strategies to decide who gets to be builder first (usually everyone wants this job).

With most groups of five or more participants, there are at least two adults in the room to facilitate and supervise. As noted already with single-peer collaborations, it is important not to take a leading role in the set building but to defer most conflicts or problems to the members themselves. Children often seek out the adults for help but should be redirected to the other children in the group as appropriate resources. In some situations (e.g., a critical missing LEGO piece), the entire group may be solicited to provide help. "Search parties" are common during groups in which larger projects are under way.

In younger groups (8 and under) there are more dyads than triads, and there is a need for closer adult supervision. Off-task behavior is more frequent and is tolerated as long as the participants can return to the group, often with peer-mediated prompting, such as, "Hey, I still need your help!" Set building can be very technical and demands considerable attention and close interpersonal contact. Younger group members can rarely tolerate this for more than about 20 minutes at a time. Although some older group members can spend a full hour or 90 minutes building sets, the younger ones will need to have breaks during which they can play with the sets or do some relaxed freestyle building. One way of organizing a 1-hour session would be to have 20–30 minutes of set building followed by a 10-minute break (e.g., for a drink outside the LEGO space) and then another 20 minutes of freestyle building and finally 10 minutes to clean up.

Freestyle Building   In a larger group, it is difficult to maintain close supervision during freestyle building. There is a greater need for movement around the materials, and typically there is more noise and off-task behavior as well. When one participant has an idea for a freestyle design, he is encouraged to share the idea with the group, and other group members are recruited to help. This typically results in two or three small groups working with the engineer who had the idea and two builders or suppliers who assist. The duration of interaction during freestyle building tends to be shorter, as diverging interests draw group members in different directions. Participants are often cued or prompted to recruit helpers, especially when they seek advice or assistance from the adults. For example, consider the following exchange:

Phillip: Hey Dr. Dan, I need another black wheel like this one.
Dr. Dan: I know we have one somewhere, not sure. Who's helping you?
Phillip: No one. I'm building this by myself.
Dr. Dan: Can't do that, Phil, buddy. You'll need help. Find a helper.
Phillip: Hey, who wants to help me find this wheel? Curt? Help me.

Freestyle building in small groups can often take the form of competitions. For example, two triads may be challenged to create the best space ship, monster truck, or fire station. The group members and the group leaders later judge the results. Or there may be some objective assessment procedure, such as a race, completion of a stunt or trick, or a *drop test* (LEGO creations are tested for engineering quality by being dropped from a certain height—the creation that loses the fewest pieces wins).

Other more complex issues can also be worked on, including active listening and expressing empathy, social problem solving and conflict resolution, and assertiveness. For these skills, it is important to use examples and situations that occurred in the group context rather than hypothetical situations, which tend to be ineffective in eliciting the appropriate behavior in natural settings. During individual sessions, participants are asked to review events that occurred during groups, sometimes with videotaped evidence to help. Following this, the participant is encouraged to role play alternative responses or to practice skills:

Dr. Dan: Tony, remember when Burt came to group last week? He was late.
Tony: Yeah, he was late.
Dr. Dan: What was he doing when he came in?
Tony: He was being late.
Dr. Dan: Yes, but what else?
Tony: [Laughing] He was crying.
Dr. Dan: Right, he was upset about being late. It bothered him. What did you do when you saw him?
Tony: I teased him ... Oh, I said, "Cry baby, did you poop your diaper?"
Dr. Dan: Yeah. Then what happened?
Tony: Burt threw the train and broke it. He ran out there, and he was knocking things in the waiting room!
Dr. Dan: Do you think you made him more upset?
Tony: Yeah, I think so. I shouldn't have teased him.
Dr. Dan: OK. So what could you have said to him instead of teasing?
Tony: I should have said it's OK, don't worry.
Dr. Dan: How about this—I'll pretend to be Burt, and you practice saying something that will help me feel better.

In general, the format in a group session moves from a higher degree of structure and control by the leaders to more self-directed and less structured activity toward the end. The first part of the session sets the tone for the rest of the time so it is important to have a strong presence and a clear agenda at the outset. Following the usual chaos of bringing members in from the waiting room and talking briefly with parents there should be a clear set of options or an established procedure to get the group engaged in a productive and semistructured activity. Allowing free play at the beginning of a session, as opposed to the end, essentially guarantees that the rest of the group time will be spent in semichaotic individual activities.

Group-Based Semistructured Activities

This is the core of the group session and the time during which the group members are actively engaged in an activity. During this time, the group leader may need to be very active with members, or less so, depending on the skills and developmental level of the group. It also depends on the novelty of the task. For newer, less familiar tasks, there is a need for much more input from the leader. Younger group members or inexperienced builders also tend to require more input. If the group activity is chosen appropriately, the leader can focus more on the social and communication coaching and less on helping get the project done on time.

It is best to try to limit the group to an achievable number and complexity of tasks at the beginning. This can take some experience to know how long a given building task may take. For set building, a rule-of-thumb formula for gauging time requirements is

Number of LEGO pieces involved/Developmental age
of group members (years) = time (minutes)

For example, a group of children with the building skills of average 10-year-olds can put together a LEGO set with 600 pieces in 60 minutes. Keep in mind that that is an uninterrupted and intensive 60 minutes. Alternatively, a group of children with the developmental age of 4 years would accomplish the same task in about 150 minutes.

Less Structured, Creative Time

Following the main structured activity, there is often some time remaining, and this is a good time to allow a relaxation of structure and allow the members to pursue their own interests and projects. As much as possible, during this time it is useful to try to link members up in pairs to work on joint projects or match together members who may be engaging in play activities with similar themes.

Cleanup Time

Start giving cleanup time warnings about 5 to 10 minutes ahead of time, depending on how involved and complex the ongoing projects are and the extent of the mess in the room. Give at least two or three warnings before announcing cleanup time. Following the first warning, make sure no new projects are started and no new play themes or LEGO sets are taken down from the shelf: "Don't start anything new; it's almost cleanup time, and you have 3 minutes to finish up what you're doing." Announce cleanup time at roughly 15 minutes prior to the group ending—don't be flexible about this, or the group leader will spend an inordinate amount of time ordering and cleaning the materials. Be sure to indicate that all materials must be returned to their original locations, and all members should help each other put all materials away, not just the pieces they were personally using. This is a good team-building exercise. Remind the group members that any pieces left on the floor will go into the vacuum cleaner. We have routinely offered *LEGO points* to younger members for gathering up stray LEGO's under tables.

Farewell and Parent Review

Once the room is put back in order and everything is off the floor, cue group members to give age-appropriate farewells, including use of members' names. While group members are rotating through their farewells, I usually head out to the waiting room to give a brief feedback to parents about the group session, progress, problems, and concerns. There are inevitably a second set of farewells in the waiting room and often a continuation of this process out the door. At times, parents may be late in getting their child following a group. This elicits a wide range of reactions from the members, few of which are positive. A couple of times parents have neglected to return to pick up their child following a group. It is a good idea to remind parents ahead of time that this is not acceptable and that they need to be on time to get their child after the group. Of course, this is not a problem for school-based or other groups in which parent transportation is not an issue.

LEGO Club Rules

Parents as well as teachers and other therapists who are not familiar with this treatment approach often ask about discipline or behavior control procedures. It turns out that problem behavior is quite rare using this approach, especially when the participants are highly motivated and have been properly prepared during the initial interview.

A key to LEGO therapy is establishing self-regulation and using peer-mediated corrective feedback. These skills are aided by the use of posted rules, the LEGO Club rules. During the initial interview, potential participants are told, "If you want to come to the LEGO Club, you have to be able to follow the rules." For nonverbal or preverbal children, this message is usually conveyed by correcting their behavior during individual therapy sessions. Children without verbal communication skills are not included in groups until they are proficient at the required skill set, which includes behavioral compliance. The LEGO rules were developed by the original participants in the first LEGO-based social skills groups and reflect the consensus regarding a necessary and sufficient set of rules for peer-mediated regulation of the group process (LeGoff et al., 2009):

LEGO Club Rules

> If you break it, you have to fix it.
> If you can't fix it, ask for help.
> If someone else is using it, don't take it, ask first.
> No yelling. Use indoor voices.
> No climbing or jumping on furniture.
> No teasing, name calling, or bad words.
> No hitting or wrestling—keeps hands and feet to yourself.
> Clean up—put things back where they came from.

The rules are printed in large print so they can be easily read and are posted on the poster board in the LEGO therapy room. Whenever a new member is introduced to a group, one or more of the group members are asked to review the rules with the new member, and we often then have a group discussion about how each of the members has occasionally needed to be corrected about a rule violation.

An important aspect of using the rules is implementing them consistently and without negativity. The leader should typically not offer direct feedback regarding inappropriate behavior. Instead, whenever possible, the leader will request that the other children in the group remind each other about the rules. Using indirect and ambiguous terms enhances the participants' abilities to identify inappropriate behaviors in others and in themselves. For example, when a child climbs onto a chair to retrieve something from a high shelf:

Dr. Dan: Hey guys, is someone in here breaking a rule?
David: Uh, yeah, Peter is hogging the big truck wheels.
Dr. Dan: Anything else?
Peter: Yes! Sam is climbing on furniture. Get down, Sam; that's rule number 5.
Dr. Dan: Good point, Peter. Sam?
Sam: Sorry, Dr. Dan, I just wanted to get R2-D2 for my X-wing.
Dr. Dan: Well, what should you do?
Sam: I couldn't reach it without getting up ...
Dr. Dan: LEGO Club, what should Sam do?
Group (together): He should ask for help!

Rules of Cool   Unlike the proscriptive LEGO Club rules, the *Rules of Cool* are implicit, prescriptive rules that are not overtly written or otherwise indicated. These implicit rules are actually defined by the group members as part of an ongoing discussion that takes place informally during sessions. The topic is introduced to members in situations in which there may be socially inappropriate or stigmatizing behaviors evident but that do not necessarily violate one of the LEGO Club rules. Positive or prosocial behaviors exhibited by group members should be noted and pointed out by the therapists or instructors: for example, "Hey, Matt, thanks for sharing with Nick. That was cool. Wasn't that cool guys?" Also encourage group members to comment on other's behaviors, both positive and negative: for example, "Hey, John, did you see Sean just grab that out of David's hand? Was that cool? What should he have done—tell him."

The LEGO Club Level System   Similar to many aspects of the LEGO approach, the level system evolved over time and was used as a strategy to support social development based on direct clinical evidence. The LEGO Club levels are in place to reward children and to motivate children to improve. There are five LEGO Club levels that are outlined next. Once the skills for a particular level are demonstrated, children are given a LEGO Club certificate or diploma (which many group members have kept and cherished for years). Rather than the group leader awarding a certificate, it is the peers in the group who review whether a child's project meets the specific criteria for a given level.

In general, there is a clear and persistent interest by group members in attaining higher levels within the system, and this often leads to improved motivation, task persistence, and willingness to undertake difficult tasks (LeGoff et al., 2009).

LEGO Levels

1. LEGO Helper   Participants are considered to be at the helper level when they first join a group. At this level, they are encouraged to "help out" the group activities by presorting pieces when set building (e.g., all the gray pieces together), sorting freestyle pieces, checking sets for integrity against directions when completed, ordering and cleaning the LEGO room. This level serves different functions for children depending on their skills: For children who are not yet proficient at set building or who do not have the ability to sustain attention on a task long enough, this allows for participation and provides the context for peer approval and appreciation of input. For children with more advanced skills, these activities motivate them to demonstrate their proficiency at higher-level skills needed to move up to the next level, including gaining peer approval and building peer alliances.

2. LEGO Builder   Once a LEGO helper has demonstrated that he can construct LEGO sets of a moderate size (100 pieces and above) and can take the role of builder in a group set-building activity, the group members will be asked if the participant warrants graduating up to LEGO builder status. If the group agrees, the participant is then awarded a diploma, which is signed by the therapist and all other group members.

3. LEGO Creator   The challenge for a LEGO builder who wants to move up to being a LEGO creator is to construct a freestyle creation. This has to be an original idea, with a certain degree of complexity and Gestalt integrity that makes it appealing to the other members. The other group members again make a group decision regarding the creation, and if they are agreed the participant is given a second diploma.

4. LEGO Master   The challenge at this level is to lead a group project. The participant must have either initiated the purchase of a large LEGO set (over 300 pieces) for which he then coordinates the construction or the presentation to the group of a desirable group freestyle project (e.g., build a complex building, a small town, an airport, or a zoo, or construct a series of creations such as a set of vehicles, robots, or other craft). The important point here is that the group members are assigned tasks and roles by the leader, and he effectively directs the project, enlisting support and input from other members, resulting in a project that all group members are agreed was challenging and worthwhile.

5. LEGO Genius   This level was actually created to appease a few LEGO masters who requested a new challenge against which to pitch their LEGO leadership skills. The criteria for achievement at this level include writing a movie script or story that they present to the group (they can choose a reader for this). The script must be critiqued by other members and edited as necessary. The final script is then analyzed in terms of how the project can be translated into a LEGO-based stop-action animated short film. This is a new development in LEGO Club, and the details of LEGO stop-action film making are beyond the scope of this manual but may be covered in more detail later. The LEGO master must lead the group in the project, including assigning building tasks for the set and characters; assigning action, voice, and sound-effects roles; controlling or assigning control of the camera and computer (a digital video camera and laptop with editing software are used); and then directing the film itself.

The project can take numerous sessions to complete and requires considerable leadership skill to get all members to sustain focus on the task for the required length of time. The resulting animated short film is then edited by the producing member and is shown to the group and other groups, and the group members and participant discuss whether the work qualifies as worthy of the LEGO genius diploma. This level has been attained by only four members to date. They have ranged in age from 9 to 12, and all four had different developmental levels and diagnoses.

Guidelines for Using This Approach

There are three ways to set up and implement LEGO therapy:

1. Permanent LEGO room: This requires setting up a designated LEGO therapy room where all the materials are to be kept and where all therapy sessions take place.
2. Temporary setup: This approach uses a specific site, but the materials are not permanently installed or displayed so that they can be moved or stored separately.
3. Portable materials: This involves using a portable set of materials that are transported to different sites (e.g., schools, community settings, libraries).

Choosing Materials   The choice of materials is a key issue in implementing LEGO-based interventions, for obvious reasons. Unlike many other approaches, however, the process of choosing the materials is an integral part of the therapy itself. Participant selection of LEGO materials can be a part of both individual and group therapy sessions and should be both structured and facilitated by the therapist.

When you are starting a program, it is useful to begin with several LEGO sets. Bear in mind that an important element of LEGO therapy is allowing the children to choose models themselves and to discuss as a group which models to get. However, as this is not always possible when setting up a group, leaders should speak with children individually to find out what sort of LEGO they enjoy and find motivating. This can be done by showing children LEGO magazines or LEGO catalogs or by looking at the LEGO website.

Choosing Materials: Freestyle LEGO   Freestyle LEGO materials can be acquired either directly from LEGO or informally as the remnants of defunct sets, donated shoeboxes full of abandoned bits, or large bins or sets that have multiple possible uses. As much as possible, the freestyle materials should be kept organized in plastic, see-through bins. A large supply of freestyle materials is needed to facilitate the wide range of interests and the tendency for group members to reify freestyle creations. Although members can be encouraged to "recycle" freestyle pieces, certain groundbreaking masterpieces tend to take on particular importance for all concerned. A large supply of freestyle materials can be acquired via donations, although these often require extensive sorting and cleaning, which is time-consuming. LEGO Educational Division also offers a large range at reduced cost to educational and nonprofit organizations.

Assessment Procedures

A key component of any intervention is a thorough assessment. The assessment process allows the leader to determine areas of need and strength as well as to establish objective baseline data for assessing progress in the future. The assessment process has two elements: the initial assessment and the progress assessment. Although there will be considerable variability across leaders and individual participants, the following general guidelines have been established as core features of LEGO-based therapies through both clinical experience and research.

Initial Interview   The assessment process should begin with an introductory interview of the participant and family, typically lasting 1 hour. This interview is designed both to provide information regarding the methodology and procedures to participants and parents and to collect information about participants that will help with further assessment and treatment planning. If the leader will be using a permanent LEGO room site, then the interview should be conducted in that room and should begin with an orientation to the room. If the site is a temporary one (multipurpose room), then the LEGO materials should be present. If the participant will be attending a portable site, the interview can be conducted at the site or at the leader's clinic or office. In any case, it is helpful for information sharing, as well as for establishing rapport, to have LEGO materials available at the initial interview.

The interview should be conducted in a relatively informal and unstructured manner. References to the mental health aspects of LEGO intervention should be minimized (e.g., therapy, interventions, diagnoses, social skills), with an emphasis instead on the activities, requirements for participation, and the social nature of the group.

Most of this information is conveyed directly to parents during the interview. It is also helpful to have written information, in the form of a brochure or single-page description, which may be shared with parents and educators either at the initial interview or beforehand. Many parents find this helpful as there is often too much information to absorb in one interview. Participants should be directly involved in the discussion of the LEGO Club Rules and asked if they understand and can comply with the rules as a condition of participation.

Case Example

Background

Colin was 10 years old when I first met him. He was referred initially by his parents at the recommendation of his school counselor. Colin had been previously diagnosed with oppositional defiant disorder (ODD) and attention-deficit/hyperactivity disorder (ADHD) and was taking a psychostimulant medication. He lived with his parents and two younger brothers, both of whom were noted to be doing well academically and socially. Colin's father was a successful architect, and his mother had a bachelor's in education but was working at home. It was clear from the time I met the family in the waiting room at a large outpatient clinic that they were exasperated with Colin. They described him as "rude" and "annoying" and noted that he was unable to make friends and was more or less constantly in trouble at school. He had been referred to the principal for discipline multiple times and to the school counselor, who didn't know what to make of him.

Colin's mother described him as " . . . a pain from birth on." She had difficulty breastfeeding him as an infant, and he did not snuggle with her. He kept his body rigid and had a harsh, persistent cry, which his mother felt helpless to stop. He was her first child, however, and she often blamed herself for being inept as a mother. As a toddler, Colin seemed aloof and liked to play with his father's tools and drafting table. He began reading almost before he could talk. His early language acquisition was rapid, but he often repeated phrases from TV or other media. While in his car seat, at the age of 3, Colin would read out the road signs and other printed advertising they passed. That year he also spent a lot of time watching TV and, on his own, learned how to turn on the subtitle text for the hearing impaired and would turn off the sound and read the text rather than listen to the TV. He preferred news and informational shows and liked to watch Japanese soap operas that his grandparents watched.

When Colin attended preschool, his teacher was impressed with his reading skills but noted that he did not want to participate in group activities. He refused to sit on the carpet for circle and did not want to join the group for snack or naptime. At times, he would wander out of the classroom and would go out to the playground to look for insects in the shrubs or in the grass. He had a fascination with insects and would pick them up and put them in his pockets. Colin had a precocious vocabulary and often spoke in a rapid half-whisper, often talking to himself or carrying on long monologues, much of which was repeated from the news or weather announcements. Colin refused to wear what most of his peers did—T-shirts, shorts, and flip-flops ("slippers"). He insisted on wearing long pants, golf shirts or Aloha shirts, and penny-loafers, like his father and grandfather wore.

Initial Interview

Colin presented as a small Asian–Caucasian boy, neatly dressed in adult-like clothing, and indifferently groomed, with a mussed mange of straight black hair, dark brown eyes, and glasses, seated on the edge of a waiting room chair, still wearing his bulky backpack. His parents were seated across the room from him. He did not make eye contact or respond in any way to my greeting. When I came over to him and crouched down, he stared at the floor.

I interviewed Colin's parents first, getting a developmental history, and we completed the Vineland Adaptive Behavior Scales. I then went back out to the waiting room for Colin. He had taken a marker from the reception-ist's desk and was writing on the wall, recreating a spelling test he had taken earlier that day. His parents were upset and loudly chastised him for this, but Colin just shrugged, "I was bored." When I asked him to come with me, he refused and looked to his parents: "Do you have permission to abduct me this way?" Colin's parents told him it was okay, and he eventually agreed.

Colin kept his jacket and backpack on in my office. He sat on a chair near the door and looked like he was ready to bolt. "What are you going to do with me?" he asked. He remained anxious and guarded throughout an hour, during which I tried to engage with him. He got up at one point, took a ceramic mug from the top of a filing cabinet, and dropped it to the floor, smashing it. He looked at me, apparently anticipating my reaction. He opened the filing cabinet drawers, exploring them, and then came over to the desk, where he pushed me out of the way while he rummaged through the drawers. In one drawer, he found some mints and helped himself to a handful. When the interview was over, Colin ran down the hall to the waiting room, jostled by his heavy backpack.

Therapy Process

Based on my review of Colin's history and initial interview, I informed his parents that I strongly suspected that he had Asperger's disorder, not ODD or ADHD. I asked to observe him at school and subsequently got permission from his school administrator to observe him there. I watched him in his classroom, where he was isolated from the other students at a single desk in the corner, next to his teacher's desk. He seemed to enjoy the learning assignments but often talked loudly to his teacher or to himself, as if there were only the two of them in the room. On the playground at recess, Colin explored the bushes, looking for insects. Later he told me he had seen a gecko there before and was hoping to find it and adopt it as a pet. At one point, he went over and stood next to the school janitor, who was out looking at a broken window. He discussed the window and the repair process with the janitor.

At the initial therapy visit, Colin met me at my private office—different from the state health department office where we had initially met. He seemed confused by this, and was pacing and complaining in the waiting room: "I thought I was here to see Dr. Dan. Why am I here? This is not Dr.

Dan's office." He was not reassured by seeing me. "Why are we here?" He did come in though and immediately went over to the toy shelf where there was a bin of LEGO bricks. "Can I use these?" he asked. He took the bin to a table, dumped it out, and then began sorting the pieces by shape and color. He asked me to keep them sorted like this: "Don't touch anything. I want to work on this some more when I come back."

Colin was very annoyed when he came back and noticed that the LEGO bricks had been moved. "Who did this? Why didn't you keep them the way they were? You promised." I helped him resort the bricks, and then he started building a structure. "I need more roof pieces, more shingles. Can you get those for next week?" I agreed and did buy more. The next week he came in with a drawing of the building he wanted to make, which was a complexly designed home, with many windows and doors and a gabled roof. He also noted that another client of mine, a boy about his age, had started building a LEGO set, a pirate ship. He asked who was building it and then asked the boy's name and age.

One week, Colin and the other boy, Juan, met in the waiting room. Juan had brought a small LEGO creation—a spaceship—and Colin approached him. They chatted about LEGO sets and freestyle building and surprised both of their parents with their animated and amicable interaction. I later asked the parents' permission to work with the two of them together, and they agreed. Colin and Juan were clearly excited to be together and quickly began sharing ideas about new projects. I had some LEGO catalogs in the waiting room, and they had agreed that they would ask me to purchase a pirate castle that they could build together.

The pirate castle project took a few weeks to build (1 hour per week). Colin and Juan agreed to take turns building or giving each other pieces. As the project developed, other clients of mine noticed the progress and commented on it. Eventually, other students asked if they could join in with Colin and Juan, and they agreed "as long as they can build." Colin and Juan continued as leaders in the growing group of clients, all of whom had been diagnosed with Asperger's disorder or high-functioning autism. They reviewed the latest catalogs and had lengthy debates about what to choose next for the growing LEGO collection. They also shared ideas about freestyle projects and brought sketches to help guide the team. The LEGO creations eventually eclipsed all the other materials in the playroom (e.g., drawing materials, puppet theater, sand table, dolls, stuffed animals, plastic dinosaurs, Play-Doh), and became an impressive display.

Colin's parents reported that he was now very enthusiastic about his new "LEGO Club." He made a sign for the door of the playroom, "Dr. Dan's LEGO Club," on his computer at home. He told his classmates at school about it and invited them and his younger brothers to come by and see it. Colin became much more interested in interacting and collaborating with his peers at school, including non-LEGO projects. Colin's occupational therapist reported that he had made significant improvements in fine motor skills since starting the LEGO play at my office and also that he was much more cooperative and willing to try difficult tasks. At an Individualized Education Program (IEP) meeting, his teacher reported that Colin had improved dramatically in his willingness to participate in group activities and in spontaneous interactions with peers during lunch and recess.

Outcome

Colin had been participating in individual therapy with me for about 3 months and in group therapy for another 3 months. To further assess the reported improvements in Colin's behavior at school and at home, his parents were interviewed and completed the Vineland Scales again, and Colin was observed at school, during both class time and lunch and recess. Colin's Vineland results were significantly improved, with gains on the Communication and Socialization domains of over 1 standard deviation within 6 months of therapy. His parents reported that he was much less oppositional at home, was much more willing to help out with his younger brothers, and was much less "...rigid and self-centered." At school, Colin was observed to have developed a few peer relationships—primarily other students who were interested in LEGO blocks or Star Wars, which was an emerging interest of Colin's. He sat with peers during lunch and initiated conversations and was able to sustain conversations for more than a few minutes. He played at recess with other students—although his "play" was mostly talking to peers about his own interests—but they were apparently shared by others enough that they were willing to sustain the interaction. Colin had his first playdates with typical peers—focused on LEGO play, of course—and his parents were pleased with the outcome.

Colin continued to attend LEGO Club groups on and off for the next 7 years. He often adopted a leadership role and identified himself as "... one of the founding members." He did very well academically, and his Vineland scores rose to above age level. He had many creative ideas about LEGO Club creations. During high school, Colin came to the group with the idea of making a stop-motion animated film about the NASA Apollo 13 mission using LEGO blocks as a history project for school. This idea was well received, and the others helped him make the film using a combination of LEGO, fabric backdrops, and a handheld video camera. Colin got an A on the project, and he shared his teacher's positive feedback with the group. Other group members subsequently shared stop-motion film ideas and scripts, and LEGO-mation projects became the main focus of group activity.

Colin graduated from a large public high school on the honors list. He had decided not to go to college, as his parents had wanted, but enlisted in the U.S. Marine Corps hoping to eventually get his education through the military. Colin had to stop taking his medication and then worked hard on paying attention to commands and collaborating with his fellow induct-ees. He emailed me daily during his induction and training and seemed very proud of himself. The structure and discipline of the Marine Corps suited him well. Colin was subsequently deployed into active duty in Iraq. He sent an excited email the morning before he left for the Middle East. Sadly, he was subsequently killed in action during a brave standoff with rebels at a U.S. checkpoint. His parents were initially very angry—they felt the military should not have accepted him—but a year later, his father emailed me that they had finally accepted this, and both of them were very proud of their son.

Conclusion

The LEGO therapy approach is a mixed form of intervention, combining individual and group approaches with adult-directed, child-led, and peer-mediated approaches (NRC, 2001). The interventions capitalize on the natural interests of many of these children in a construction toy system and emphasize the enhancement of peer identification and development of social identity. The methodology is flexible enough to allow for both highly structured and adult-led methods (Level 1), leading to increased child-initi-ated and peer-mediated activities. To date, two outcome studies have shown clinically significant positive gains in social development for children with autism spectrum disorders who participated. Methods for using this toy system as a remedial tool with this and other populations of children are continuing to be explored and expanded. A replication study using a ran-domly assigned comparison group design was completed by Dr. Gomez de la Cuesta at the Autism Research Center at Cambridge University, under the direction of Simon Baron-Cohen (cf. Owens et al., 2008).

While many current social intervention strategies focus on improv-ing social reasoning (Gray, 1998) or on selecting specific behaviors using behavior analytic techniques (Koegel & Koegel, 1995), the LEGO therapy approach attempts to improve abilities as well as skills and performance characteristics. That is, the method seeks to fundamentally change social development, leading to sustained and generalizable gains in social func-tioning. It is the authors' belief that the benefits of an intervention are more likely to be meaningful if they are based on improvements in core social abilities and social identity rather than reflecting more superficial changes in specific social behaviors. With regard to this belief, clearly there is a need for continued research on social development.

References

Attwood, T. (1998). *Asperger's syndrome: A guide for parents and professionals.* London: Jessica Kingsley Publishers.

Bandura, A. (1977). Self-efficacy: Toward a unifying theory of behavioral change. *Psychological Review, 84*(2), 191–215.

Bandura, A. (1997). *Self-efficacy: The exercise of control.* New York: Worth Publishers.

Baron-Cohen, S. (2003). *The essential difference: Men, women and the extreme male brain.* Penguin/Basic Books.

Gray, C.A. (1998). Social stories and comic strip conversations with students with Asperger syndrome and high-functioning autism. In E. Schopler, G. B. Mesibov, & L. Kunce (Eds.), *Asperger syndrome or high functioning autism?* (pp. 167–198). New York: Plenum Press.

Hansen, W. H. (1982). *50 years of play.* Billund, Denmark: The LEGO Group.

Jonassen, D. H., Tessmer, M., & Hannum, W. H. (1999). *Task analysis methods for instructional design.* Mahwah, NJ: Lawrence Erlbaum Associates.

Koegel, R. L., & Koegel, L. (1995). *Teaching children with autism.* New York: Paul H. Brookes Publishing.

LeGoff, D. B. (2004). Use of LEGO© as a therapeutic medium for improving social competence. *Journal of Autism and Developmental Disorders, 34*(5), 557–571.

LeGoff, D. B., & Sherman, M. (2006). Long-term outcome of social skills intervention based on interactive LEGO play. *Autism, 10*(4), 1–31.

LeGoff, D. B., Krauss, G. W., & Allen, S. L. (2009). LEGO-based play therapy for autistic spectrum children. In A. Drewes & C. Schaefer (Eds.), *School-based play therapy* (2d ed.). New York: John Wiley & Sons.

National Research Council. (NRC). (2001). *Educating children with autism.* Washington, DC: NRC Press.

Owens, G., Granader, Y., Humphrey, A., & Baron-Cohen, S. (2008). LEGO therapy and the Social Use of Language Programme: An evaluation of two social skills interventions for children with high functioning autism and Asperger syndrome. *Journal of Autism and Developmental Disorders, 38*(10), 1944–1957.

Papert, S. (1999). *Study of educational impact of the LEGO dacta materials.* Boston, MA: MIT Press.

Weckstrom, C. (2010). *LEGO Corporation's education and innovations contributions.* Personal communication.

Wiencek, H. (1987). *The world of LEGO toys.* New York: Harry Abrams Publishing.

CHAPTER 7

Touching Autism Through Developmental Play Therapy

JANET A. COURTNEY

I think it's very important to desensitize autistic children to touch, because all children need to be touched. (Temple Grandin, *Animals in Translation*)

Introduction

Over the past several years, mental health practitioners, medical personnel, policy makers, and parents have witnessed a dramatic increase in the diagnosis of autism spectrum disorders (ASD). According to the Centers for Disease Control and Prevention (CDC, 2011) an average of 1 in 110 children in the United States has ASD with the incidence predicted to rise. Inherent with this rise in autism is an increasing quandary about how to effectively assess and treat children with autism (Baker, McIntyre, Blacher, Crnic, Edelbrock, & Low, 2003; Bromfield, 2010; Gray, 2011). One approach called developmental play therapy (DPT), as formulated by Viola Brody in the 1960s, has long been recognized as an effective therapeutic approach used in the treatment of autism (Brody, 1993, 1997b).

DPT shares its roots with Theraplay (Booth & Jernberg, 2010; Jernberg, 1983; Jernberg & Booth, 2001; Koller & Booth, 1997; Munns, 2003) and therefore may be considered a "close cousin" (Myrow, 2000) in approach. Although Viola Brody, who died in 2003, was the major contributor to the literature, research, and training in DPT, the DPT model continues to be taught, practiced, researched, and evolved by her students (e.g., Bailey, 2000b; Clarke, 2003; Courtney, 2004, 2005, 2006, 2010; Courtney & Gray, 2011; Fauerbach & Wibbe, 2003; Schwartzenberger, 2004a, 2004b; Short, 2008). In addition to the effectiveness of DPT in the treatment of ASD, it is also widely recognized as an effective modality in the treatment of children identified as having an attachment disorder or attention-deficit disorder and those suffering from severe emotional and psychological trauma (Brody, 1963, 1978, 1987, 1992, 1993, 1994, 1996, 1997a, 1997b; Brody, Fenderson, & Stephenson, 1976; Burt & Myrick, 1980; Courtney, 2006; Mitchum, 1987; Short, 2008).

Theories Supporting DPT

The underlying theory base of DPT (Brody, 1976, 1993, 1997a, 1997b, 1999) is an alchemy of several different theorists and researchers including Ainsworth (1969), Ainsworth, Blehar, Waters, and Wall (1978), Bowlby (1969, 1979), Barnard and Brazelton (1990), Buber (1958), Des Lauriers (1962), Harlow (1958), Montagu (1986), and Spitz (1946). The overriding theme common to these authors is the emphasis on early infancy and childhood physical and emotional relationships and their impact on later development.

DPT also draws on the writings of Martin Buber (1958) who described the intimate relationship in terms of the "I–thou" relationship. Buber's main thesis is that an individual develops a sense of "I" only in the interactions with another person ("Thou").

Brody (1993, 1997b) identified this "I" as the *core self* that emerges from the experience of touch in a caring relationship. It is the sensation of touch that ultimately produces the condition for a child to develop a *core self,* a basic human need for growth (Barnard & Brazelton, 1990; Brody, 1993, 1997b; Des Lauriers, 1962; Harlow, 1958; Montagu, 1986; Spitz, 1946). Anthropologist Ashley Montagu (1986) determined that "the skin as the sensory receptor organ which responds to contact with the sensation of touch, a sensation to which basic human meanings become attached almost from birth, is fundamental in the development of human behavior" (p. 401). Psychologist Des Lauriers (1962), an early mentor and supervisor of Brody, maintained that the development of the self began with the appreciation of the body. He called this early consciousness of body the *bodily self.* Des Lauriers believed the bodily self had to emerge before there could be the further development of the emotional self. Harlow's monkey experiments in 1969 indicated that maternal touch and comfort were essential for normal development in animals and, presumably, humans too. Brody (personal communication, September, 19, 2002) cited the research of Tiffany Field at the Touch Research Institute at the University of Miami as supporting validation to the emphasis of touch in the DPT model (Field, 1995, 2001; See Touch Research Institute website for further information: http://www.miami.edu/touchresearch/).

Treatment

The DPT format can vary from individual sessions with a child to parents observing and participating along with the practitioner to group therapy where each child is paired with a DPT practitioner. DPT uses "first play" activities initiated by the therapist including touch and "seeing" games that one might observe between a mother and a young child as in singing games, patty-cake, or hide-and-seek. The therapy focuses on the reciprocal nature of a relationship and is dependent on the interactions between what is transpiring in the here-and-now moment. Therapeutic interactions may stimulate regression that assists children to pick up what they missed from an earlier stage of development (Brody, 1993, 1997b; Center for Play Therapy, 1995; Jernberg & Booth, 2001). Thus, interventions are aimed at meeting children at their developmental age level and not necessarily their chronological age (Brody, 1993, 1997b; Koller & Booth, 1997).

It is important that the type of touch given should be pleasurable or fun. Brody (1997a) addresses the significance of touch:

It is the pleasure element in this touching relationship [between adult and child] that enables the child to feel his body. Through his felt body the child becomes aware of himself.... Out of the repeated felt experiences of one's body comes the ability to talk, to image, to fantasize, and to think abstractly. A child who has experienced this repeated body contact with an adult who is fully present with him will always have a solid sense of his body—a "home" or "centering place" within himself.... The basics include experiencing the awareness of the body when touched. This awareness creates an inner self that enables the child to deal with the world from the inside out. (p. 161)

Training

In addition to teaching the theoretical foundations of DPT, training encompasses a series of exercises that gives practitioners an opportunity to practice a "new awareness of themselves" (Brody, 1993, 1997b, p. 341). There is a presumption that the practitioner may better be able to assist children through DPT interventions if they have also experienced what that intervention feels like. Brody (1976) postulated, "It is just as important to help the adults experience and define their own feelings....In fact, many times, the adult cannot understand the child's feelings until he becomes more aware of his own feelings" (p. 39).

Autism Spectrum Disorders

According to Temple Grandin, made famous for her introduction of the Squeeze Machine (a two-sided padded panel that works with compressed air to give a deep pressured squeeze that can produce a calming effect on children with ASD), most children with autism do not like to be touched. However, she writes, "I think it's very important to desensitize autistic children to touch, because all children need to be touched. It's not that autistic children don't want to be touched; it's that their nervous systems can't handle it" (Grandin & Johnson, 2005, p. 118; see Perry & Szalavitz, 2006, pp. 140–142 for a touch desensitization case example). Individuals with autism can overcome their aversion to touch, such as the "real" Rain Man, Kim Peek. Note that according to Kim's father, Fran Peek (2008), Kim's official diagnosis is prodigious memory savant with autistic characteristics. After the movie *Rain Man* was released and Kim began to receive a tremendous amount of positive affection and attention, he had a "near-miraculous transformation" (p. 70). Fran Peek observed that Kim, who was once described as having no social skills, introverted, shying away from others, lacking any sense of humor, and avoiding eye contact with anyone, suddenly after the movie became quite the opposite. His miraculous change included an ability to make eye contact and to initiate hugs and handshakes when meeting new people. Consequently, what Kim was not able to differentiate was an ability to pick up on social cues, and he therefore wanted to hug everyone he came in contact with—a problem Kim's father was deftly able to manage.

Behavioral therapy has been the primary focus of intervention for children diagnosed with autism spectrum disorders (Bromfield, 2010; Grandin & Johnson, 2005; Perry & Szalavitz, 2006) with experiential play therapy interventions slowly gaining acceptance as a viable treatment modality (Bromfield, 2005, 2010; Hess, 2005; Kenny & Winick, 2000; Lanyado, 2005; Solomon, 2008; Yonge, 2004). Additionally, any touch types of interventions are more commonly included as part of the work done by pediatric occupational therapists or massage therapists (Field, Lasko, Mundy, Henteleff, Talpins, & Dowling, 1986; Grandin, 1992; Grandin & Johnson, 2005). Few psychotherapeutic modalities have approached the treatment of autism with an emphasis on touch considered as the key change agent.

Brody (1993, 1997b) perceived that as children with autism are often withdrawn and difficult to engage, and parents may experience "heartbreaking frustration, anger, and increasing alarm as their autistic child continues to live at a far psychological distance from them" (Brody, 1997b, p. 44). Consequently, bonding between a parent and a child with autism can be compromised, resulting in a disconnected parent–child relationship. Brody noted:

Bonding begins immediately after birth and forms as parents touch and feed the child and continues to be cemented by the quality of the interactions necessary between the very young and the parent. Such bonding is the essential soil for nourishing the growth of the child's self. Without it, the child is bereft of the center that chooses, directs, and evaluates her individual life. (p. 45)

The DPT model works to bridge this impeded bond. With children with autism, Brody advocated for a treatment plan that included the parent as part of the session. In that way Brody would promote the parent–child bond by teaching the parents through modeling how to touch and connect with their children.

Touch Considerations

Our current day society is highly sensitized to the issues of touching children. The apprehension over touching and the potential consequences associated with it has infused itself into the playroom. However, in spite of any misgivings a practitioner might have, touch is an essential component to the treatment of the child with autism (Brody, 1993, 1997b, 2000; Grandin, 1992; Grandin & Johnson, 2005; Perry & Szalavitz, 2006; Thomas & Jephcott, 2011). Brody (2000) writes pointedly, "Regardless of the 'Don't touch' warnings, it does not make sense to deprive these children of this life-giving sustenance-caring touch from a caring adult" (p. 1). The Association for Play Therapy (APT) provides a list of clinical, professional, and ethical recommendations regarding touch contributed by play therapists Trudy Post Sprunk, JoAnne Mitchell, David Myrow, and Kevin O'Connor (n.d.) in "Paper on Touch" (pp. 1–2) and summarized as follows:

1. Provide caretakers with an informed consent to obtain a written release for physical contact.
2. Touch should be considered only if it meets the treatment goals and individual needs of the child.
3. Seek supervision.
4. Ethically practitioners should never touch a child if they are uncomfortable with the touch, sexually aroused, or angry.
5. Practitioners need to be more vigilant regarding touching if the child has been physically abused.
6. Some children may need to be physically restrained to maintain safety, which requires training.

Regarding the DPT model and its emphasis on touch, some clinical recommendations were made by Brody (1993, 1997b, 2000) and further contributions expounded upon by this author:

7. A practitioner must receive specialized training in touch prior to implementing touch-based therapeutic interventions.
8. The practitioner must set appropriate physical boundaries in regards to touch. For example, Brody (1987) tells a child not to touch her "bumps!" as she moves a child's hand away from her breast during a video demonstration. Conversely, if children ask to be touched in their genitals, state, "That is something I am not going to do. That part of your body belongs to you. No one should touch it but you" (Brody, 1993, 1997b, p. 361).
9. When touching legs, never touch above the knee.
10. A child can feel seen and "touched" by practitioners without ever physically touching them.
11. Touch can be done through the use of an object such as a puppet (e.g., puppets that have movable mouths can count fingers).
12. Never tickle a child. (Even a light touch stroke can feel like a tickle.)
13. Touch should be gentle and firm enough for a child to sense the touch but never enough to hurt or cause pain.
14. Never reject a child's reach or desire for a hug or appropriate touch.
15. Never force touch.
16. The therapist's "first task" is to find the "right" touch for each individual child. For example, when children say, "Do it again," they are confirming that the therapist has found the right touch.
17. Brody (1993, 1997b) emphasized that before a practitioner is able to give loving and caring touch, a practitioner must first learn and practice *how* to be loving (see also Erich Fromm, 1956, *The Art of Loving*, Chapter 4, "The Practice of Love").
18. Be aware of the cultural differences related to touching.

Case Presentation

Case Background and Presenting Problem

A referral was made from the school counselor recommending play therapy for Dallas, age 6 years, due to severe behavioral problems. He was recently enrolled in the first grade during the middle of the school year after his custody was transferred from his mother, Alena, to his father, John. Alena was diagnosed with bipolar disorder and had a history of hospitalizations due to psychosis, depression, and suicide attempts. Dallas came to live with John after Alena called in a panic shouting, "Come and get Dallas." She believed Dallas was the Antichrist, was physically attacking her, and wished she was dead. He had missed several weeks of school and was failing first grade. Additionally, Alena's current boyfriend was physically abusive to Dallas.

Dallas's parents divorced when he was 1 year old, and he remained in primary custody with Alena who refused visitation with John despite court orders. Alena would tell Dallas that his father did not love him and did not want to see him. Furthermore, Dallas had a history of multiple babysitters and day-care settings. After Dallas moved in with his father, Alena ceased contact with him and was unavailable for an interview.

Diagnosis

John stated that Dallas was "different" even from birth and was described as a difficult baby: "not like the other kids I knew." When in preschool, Dallas was diagnosed by a psychiatrist with attention-deficit/hyperactivity disorder. In kindergarten, he was also diagnosed by several different practitioners as having oppositional defiant disorder, posttraumatic stress syndrome, reactive attachment disorder, and sensory integration dysfunction. By first grade, he had been diagnosed by a psychologist as having Asperger's. Brody (1993, 1997b) and others (Perry & Szalavitz, 2006; Webb, Amend, Webb, Goerss, Beljan, & Olenchak, 2005) observed that many children with autism often have an early childhood history of differing and uncertain diagnoses.

A collateral contact with Dallas's teacher revealed several behavioral problems within the school environment including an inability to get along with his peers, inappropriate touching or hugging of others, pushing and punching other children even without provocation, teasing peers, throwing sand, poor physical boundaries, ignoring directions, belligerent behavior, inappropriate comments in the classroom, displaying anger at trivial things, destroying items in the classroom, refusal to participate in classroom activities, and problems staying in his seat.

Preparation of DPT With Father

John's plea: "I just want to have a good relationship with my son. I love him and will do anything I can to help him, but it's so frustrating. I have tried very hard to be in my son's life, and I am thankful that we can finally be together." In addition to a lack of secure attachment between John and Dallas, several problem areas were identified including Dallas's refusal to wear his school uniform as it was too "itchy," a refusal to eat anything but macaroni and cheese, a refusal to go to bed on time or to take a bath, hiding when it was time to leave the house, and no peer friendships. DPT was determined to be the best treatment of choice as it seeks to enhance the parent–child bond through touch and pleasurable activities—a core problem lacking in the relationship between John and Dallas. Increased adult and child attachment naturally leads to greater child cooperation (Bailey, 2000a).

Since DPT is a different type of therapeutic intervention from other child therapies, caregivers need to be educated about what to expect. John was prepared in the following ways. First, he was enlightened regarding the DPT model and the theories related to attachment and to the importance of touch and pleasure to the therapeutic process. Next, he was given a videotape (Brody, 1998) to watch so he could observe DPT interventions in action. John was also advised to expect daily "home-play" activities to practice with Dallas.

Observations of Dallas and Process of Therapy

Unlike many children with Asperger's that do not like to be touched, Dallas desperately wanted to make contact through touch; however, he did not know how. His behavior was indicated as, on one hand, hugging even "strangers" to the extreme of impulsive hitting and punching. From a DPT standpoint, he lacked any sense of a core self that flowed from a sound sense of his body and its relationship to others. His history of abuse and neglect while living with his mother coupled with his early disrupted relationship with his father created a lack of secure attachment that was compounded by the characteristics of the Asperger's diagnosis. Bromfield (2010) writes, "Having Asperger's as a primary diagnosis does not grant children immunity from other problems such as trauma, abuse, loss, neglectful parenting, family dysfunction not related to Asperger's, alcoholism and substance abuse, delinquency, and antisocial behavior, and on and on" (p. 118).

Dallas was seen for six sessions because John moved out of the area at the end of the school year. This case example was chosen for several reasons. Foremost, it is an example of the implementation of DPT with a child diagnosed with Asperger's. Next, this case demonstrates the modeling and bridging of DPT interventions with a parent. It also highlights the intensity of DPT and the changes that can occur even over a few sessions. Finally, the process recordings are intended to provide the reader with a better understanding of what is meant by reaching children through DPT touch interventions.

Treatment Plan

The initial treatment plan revolved around several factors including the building of a therapeutic relationship with Dallas through DPT interventions and the setting of limits. Next was to model DPT interventions with John and then to transfer and support DPT parent–child interactions within the session and at home. Parenting issues were discussed with John regarding boundaries, limits, and structure at home. A collateral contact was arranged with Dallas's teacher, and a referral was provided for continued therapy upon John's relocation. The following process transactions are abridged excerpts from DPT sessions with Dallas.

Session 1

DPT: Hello. (I greet Dallas in the waiting room. He glances at me and with head down he races forward, ramming his head into my stomach.)

Dallas: Hi! (wrapping his arms tightly around my waist)

DPT: Hey, hey, wait a minute. Do you know me? (I take Dallas's hands and step back for Dallas to look at me and place one hand on his shoulder.) What do you do when you meet someone for the first time? How do you say hello?

Dallas: (Stares blankly at me.)

DPT: How about if we shake hands to say hello?

Dallas: Yes. (shaking his head up and down)

DPT: (I hold out my right hand). Hello, my name is Miss Janet.

Dallas: (He squeezes my hand tightly yanking my arm strongly up and down.) Hello.

DPT: I can see how strong you are, but that is too strong for me. Let's try that again. Let me show you how I like to shake hands. (I take control of his hand so he can feel a gentler shake.) Now let's try saying hello with your other hand.

Dallas: (Smiling, he lifts his left hand and gives a gentler grip).

DPT: I like the feel of that handshake.

Dallas: (Runs into the office and crouches behind a chair.)

DPT: Where is Dallas? Where did he go? (I act like I am searching around the room.)

Dallas: (Pops up from behind the chair) Here.

DPT: There you are. I see you. (He gets excited but makes no facial or eye contact. I repeat, "There you are," every time he looks at me.)

Dallas: (Looking down at the floor.)

DPT: Where is Dallas? Where is he? (Stated in a happy sing-song voice.)

Dallas: (Looks up at me and then away.)

DPT: (Game is repeated, and John is observing from the couch.) What type of games do you and Dallas play together?

Father: Well, I pick him up and roll him over my shoulder.

DPT: That must be fun. Dallas, can you show me what you do?

Dallas: (Sits on John's lap.)

Father: (Flips Dallas over from one side of this arm to the other.)

Dallas: (Giggling.) Do it again.

Father: (Repeats activity.)

DPT: Wow, that looks fun; what else can you both do?

Father: Umm, well we do this... (picks Dallas up and flips him over his arm.)

Dallas: Dad, do that again. (Jumping up and down anxiously)

Father: (Smiling and holding onto Dallas he repeats the activity.)

DPT: Dallas, it's fun when you get to play with Dad.

Dallas: (Giggling) Yes, I like this.

DPT: It's getting time for us to say good-bye. Dallas, when you come here we will always end the session with Dad holding you. Dad can you show me how you cradle Dallas?

Father: (He places Dallas across his lap with one arm under his head and the other under his knees.)

Dallas: (Dallas squirms in his father's arms but then relaxes.)

DPT: (I am sitting in a chair close to the couch.) It's nice when you and Dad can have some special time together. Dad what do you see when you look at Dallas?

Father: I see his eyes.

DPT: What color are they?

Father: Brown.

DPT: Yes, I see they are brown. Dallas, what color are your dad's eyes?

Dallas: Uh, brown.

DPT: Yes, I see. You both have brown eyes. And Dad is looking at you, and you are looking at him. It would be good if you both can have some cradling time together every day—maybe before bedtime. Dallas, you will be coming back next week. How about if you and Dad make up some new tricks and show them to me next week. Dallas, how would you like to say good-bye to me today?

Dallas: Shake. (Holds out hand.)

DPT: Great, let's shake. (His grip is easier.)

Comments   The waiting room meeting with Dallas illustrates how the DP therapist sets limits and takes immediate control. As well, Brody (1993, 1997b, p. 53) notes that some children with autism need to touch "hard" just to be able to feel the sensation of touch. The "There you are" game represents an important early childhood developmental stage. The modeling of DP by the therapist is then transferred to the father through the initiation of "tricks." Dallas's statement of "Do that again" is an indication of the right kind of touch. Cradling was introduced to Dallas as part of the ritual for ending each therapy session.

Session 2

Dallas: (Runs toward me and gives a tight squeeze around my waist.)

DPT: That's a hard hug that squeezes me. I like to have gentle hugs. How about if we practice giving gentle hugs?

Dallas: Okay.

DPT: (Squatting down at his level, I put my arms gently around Dallas's shoulders and give a hug.) How did that feel for you? Now you try.

Dallas: (Reaches out and imitates the hug by softly putting his arms around me.)

DPT: Wow, I really like that. That feels good. (The hug practicing is repeated and also practiced with John.)

DPT: (Dallas and I then sit on the floor across from each other. John is sitting on the couch. I begin to look down at Dallas's hands.)

Dallas: (Unexpectedly, Dallas draws his arm back and punches me hard in the nose.)

Father: Dallas, NO!

DPT: No hitting, Dallas. (Stated firmly. I take his hand in mine and hold it up at eye level.) Do you know you have a hand?

Dallas: (Stares at me blankly.)

DPT: Look, Dallas, look at your hand. Do you know you have a hand? (I start to move his hand and arm to bring his attention to his hand.)

Dallas: (His eyes then shift to looking at his hand.)

Father: Say you're sorry, Dallas. (Stated in a firm voice). Are you okay?

DPT: (I indicate yes toward John but focus on Dallas.) Dallas, I see your hand. Let's look at it. (I begin to open up his fist.) You have fingers here and fingernails. See them? (I touch and point at each finger and fingernail.)

Dallas: (Dallas starts to show some awareness of what happened and begins to look scared.) I'm sorry. (Slumps his body and looks at his father.)

Father: (Nods his approval.)

DPT: I can see you are sorry, and I know you will never do that again. (Focusing back on his hands.) Let's count your fingers to see if they are all still there.

Dallas: (Dallas looks down at his hands.)

DPT: (I start at the base of his thumb and move to the top of each finger counting with a light squeeze.) One, this is your thumb; two, this is your pointer finger; three, this is your big boy finger; four, this is your ring finger; SIX! this is your little boy finger, pinky. (I wiggle his pinky and deliberately miscount.)

Dallas: (Looks up.) Six?

DPT: Oh, did I miscount? Let me try that again. One, two, three, four, five. Five fingers on this one. Is that right?

Dallas: Yes. (He lifts his other hand to give to me.)

DPT: Look, this hand wants to be counted too. (I count his other hand and then bridge the therapy to John.) Dad, would you like to count Dallas's hands too?

Father: Sure.

Dallas: (Moves over to the couch and puts his hands on John's legs.) Okay.

DPT: (I sit close to guide the interaction.)

Father: (John quickly slides up Dallas's middle finger.) One.

DPT: Okay John let's go a little slower and put a little pressure on his finger from the bottom to the top. Dallas, can I show Dad? (I demonstrate the technique again.)

Father: This is your thumb. (Counts fingers on one hand.)

Dallas: (Giggles and gives John his other hand.)

DPT: (I count along and when finished I transition to cradling.) Okay, it is getting time for us to say good-bye. Dallas, what do we do here before it's time to leave?

Dallas: (Moves up to his father's lap.)

DPT: That's right, we have cradle time. Dad, do you have any songs that you sing to Dallas?

Father: Not really. (Shrugs shoulders.)

DPT: How about if we sing "Row, Row, Row Your Boat"? (I begin to sing keeping the pace slow and soft. Father sings along.)

> Row, row, row, your boat,
> Gently down the stream,
> Merrily, merrily, merrily, merrily,
> Life is but a dream.

Dallas: (Dallas is quiet. Looking up, he reaches out and touches his father's face.)

DPT: Let's practice the cradling and hand counting this week. I would also like to see some of the new tricks you do together next week.

Comments   The blow to the nose took the DP therapist by surprise and came without warning; however, she immediately set limits and took control. Since Dallas lacked an awareness of his bodily self, the DP therapist kept bringing the focus of attention directed back toward his body. The transfer of the hand touching to John led to Dallas receiving an intimate touching experience with his father. Dallas's touching of his father's face while cradling is an indication of regression to an earlier developmental stage.

Session 3

Dallas: I brought my hands with me today. (He is excitedly running down the hallway holding his arms up in the air shaking his hands.)

DPT: Yes, you did. Should we count them to make sure they are all still there? (He holds out his hands, and I count his fingers.)

Dallas: (Smiling and looking at his hands while I count.) I had a good day today at school, and this week I got all "green lights."

DPT: That's great. I can hear that you are really trying.

Father: That's right; I have been getting good reports. (Smiling.)

DPT: What did you do this week? Can you show me any new tricks?

Father: Yes, we call this airplane. (John lies on his back with his knees bent. He takes Dallas's hands and placing his feet on his stomach pulls him up.)

Dallas: (Laughing, Dallas puts his arms out in the air as his father moves back and forth.)

DPT: Wow, look at you two. It's fun to play with Dad. I want to show you another game you can play with Dad. (Dallas sits across from me on the floor.) Do you know your face is like a house? Your brown eyes are like windows and your mouth is like a door.

> *Knock at the door* (I take my knuckles and lightly knock on his forehead)
> *Peek in* (I touch below his brows with my fingers and look in his eyes.)
> *Lift the latch* (touch his nose.)
> *And, walk in . . .* (I "walk" with two fingers and find his mouth shut.)

> *Oh, the door is closed. No one is home. I better walk around the house and try again. With two fingers I go around his face and start at the top again. (I repeat the activity. This time he opens his mouth.) Look at all those teeth in there. I bet you take good care of those teeth. Right, Dad? I see a tongue in there. (He moves his tongue.) Oh, and the tongue moves. Look at it go up and down, back and forth.*

Dallas: (Starting to laugh in a regressed baby voice.) Do that again.

DPT: How about we have Dad try this time?

Dallas: Okay.

Father: (Sits in front of Dallas on the floor. I sing as I direct John with the hand motions. When John gets to his mouth it is closed.)

DPT: Dad, what are we going to do now?

Father: Walk around the house?

DPT: Yes, we are going to walk around the house to see if the door will open.

Dallas: (Gives a big belly laugh, when his father comes to the "closed door.") Do that again. (Stated in a regressed baby voice.)

Father: (Repeats activity.)

Dallas: (Opens mouth quickly and then closes it. Opens again and then closes.)

DPT: (Father is repeating activity, and I am commenting.) Your mouth is open. Now it's closed. Oh look it just opened again. I see inside. Dad, can you see? Now it's closed again. (Repeat activity until it is exhausted.) It's getting time for . . . what, Dallas?

Dallas: Uh . . . cuddle time.

DPT: Oh is that what you call it now? I like that. Yes, it's time for cuddle time.

Father: (Sitting on the couch, he holds Dallas in his arms.)

Dallas: (His body is less stiff more relaxed.)

Comments Activities completed at home were bridged to the office for demonstration. A new activity was modeled and transferred for John to practice. Regressed behaviors are observed in the interactions between John and Dallas when Dallas giggles and speaks in a baby voice. The ending ritual of cradling between Dallas and John is revealed as an accepted part of the therapy routine.

Session 4
DPT: Have I shown you the Rainbow Weather Massage yet?
Dallas: No. (Sits with his back to me on the floor.)
DPT: This is how it goes. First "wipe the slate clean" (Move hand to brush
off his back). There once was a little boy who was outside playing. (Draw a stick figure outline.) It was a beautiful day and the
sun was shining bright. (With palm make a circle.) The rays of
the sun shone out in all different directions. (Draw long "rays"
to all sides.) The little boy was having fun laughing, running,
skipping, and jumping around. As he was playing he looked up
in the sky and saw some dark clouds rolling in. (Draw clouds).
Then the little boy saw a beautiful castle. Dallas, what color do
you think the castle is?
Dallas: Purple!
DPT: The castle is purple. He runs into the castle, and he is all *safe* and *protected* inside. Then the wind comes and it blows harder... and
harder... and harder... (I move my hand across his back first
with the flat palm and then with the back of my hand.) Then it
begins to rain. (I stroke down with my finger pads.) It rains so
hard that it turns into hail. (I play with my fingertips all over his
back.) Then the lightning starts. (With fists I make long zigzag
motions.) Then it begins to thunder. (I pound lightly with fists.)
Then the tornado begins. (I start at the base of his spine and
make swirling motions upwards.) All of a sudden a strong wind
comes and blows all those dark clouds away. (I sweep across his
back from right to left.) The sun shines again, and the boy comes
out of the castle. He looks up in the sky and sees a beautiful
rainbow. The rainbow has all different colors. It has a blue color.
(With my fist I sweep half-circles across his back for each color.)
Dallas, what other colors do you think are in this rainbow?
Dallas: Red! (Shouts out.)
DPT: Okay, red. What else?
Dallas: Green.
DPT: Good, what else?

Dallas: Purple.

DPT: Okay, purple. What else?

Dallas: Brown.

DPT: Brown. Now something very special happens. The little boy looks up toward the sky, opens his mouth, and swallows the rainbow. All those colors move to every part of his body. The blue color goes where?

Dallas: Uh, to his head.

DPT: To his head. (I touch the top of his head.) Where does the red color go?

Dallas: Here. (Points to his hand.)

DPT: Okay, it goes to his hand. (I continue the activity by touching his forehead, throat, stomach, shoulders, arms, knees, and feet until the colors are exhausted. When finished, I bridged the activity to John to practice with Dallas.)

Comments Dallas enjoyed this activity and when John practiced Dallas corrected him if he missed something. The Rainbow Weather Massage evolved from the *Weather Massage* shared with this author from Xenia, Lady Bowlby, wife of Sir Richard Bowlby (personal communication, June 16, 2004).

Session 5 John picked Dallas up from school and arrived at the session carrying Dallas, who clearly was not feeling well, lethargic, and warm to touch. Dallas's head was resting on his father's shoulder. Dallas drank some water, and we wrapped him snuggly in a blanket. Cradled now in his father's arms he fell asleep as I sang a lullaby:

> Rock-a-bye Dallas
> In the treetop
> When the wind blows
> The cradle will rock
> When the bough breaks
> The cradle will fall
> And down will come Dallas
> And Dad will catch you.

Comments As the school year end was emerging, John advised that they would be moving to a town closer to his parents. The next session was thus planned for termination of treatment and a referral of services. I called Dallas the next day to see how he was feeling and for him to sense my care and concern. I stated to Dallas that as he and Dad were moving, our next appointment was planned to be our time to say good-bye.

Termination

In many cases, therapy can end abruptly for many different reasons, and the therapist needs to be prepared to figure out how best to address the child's needs in the last session. Ideally, in the DPT model three sessions are allotted for termination with the last session entailing a review of all that occurred throughout the course of therapy (Brody, 1997). In this last session the review of therapy was done through a made-up song. The drawing of hands was meant to signify our connectedness and to provide a transitional reminder of our time together.

Session 6

Dallas: I brought a flower for you. (He holds it out for me to view.)

DPT: I see, Dallas, how beautiful. Thank you so much. Today is our day to say good-bye. Do you remember on the first day that we measured you on the wall? Let's do it again to see how much you have grown.

Dallas: (Leans head against the wall standing straight.)

DPT: (I mark his new height and compare. Indeed he had grown!) Dallas, look you have grown! You're growing, Dallas!

Dallas: Dad, see.

Dad: I see, Dallas, you're getting bigger.

DPT: (Dallas is sitting in his dad's lap on the floor with me). How about if we make up a song about our time together? Let's call it "Dallas's song." (I make up a tune and begin to sing making hand motions for all the different activities we did together. John and Dallas add to the song. When finished, we move to the children's table where I have paper and markers.)

DPT: Dallas, I am going to draw your hand and fingers. (I name and outline his fingers while he holds his hand flat on the paper.) How about if we have Dad draw your other hand?

Father: (Picks up markers and outlines Dallas's hand.)

DPT: Dallas, how about your Dad's hands?

Dallas: Yeah, Dad.

DPT: Dallas, where would you like to draw Dad's hands on the paper?

Dallas: Here. (Outlines Dad's hands next to his and names the fingers). Now you.

DPT: Me too? Where do you want my hands to go?

Dallas: Here. (Pointing above his hands).

DPT: (He places his hand on top of mine and while tracing he calls out the finger names. We all sign our names, and I write down some of the activities we did together.) Let's call this Dallas's graduation good-bye picture.

Dallas: (Starts to look worried.) So I won't see you again?

DPT: No, Dallas probably not, but I will always remember our time together. Do you know where? It will always stay here. (I point to my heart.) How should we say good-bye to each other?

Dallas: Hug. (Gives a tender hug.)

DPT: That's a great hug. That feels good.

Discussion

This case example demonstrates the intimacy and intensity of DPT and the changes that can occur with a child diagnosed with Asperger's even over a few sessions. Although the course of Asperger's disorder is known to be "continuous" and "lifelong" (APA, 2000, p. 82), problems of attachment and behavior experienced by a child with Asperger's can improve. At the time of discharge, John reported that the indiscriminate touching and hugging of strangers by Dallas had stopped, and his teacher reported a decrease in the aggressive acts toward his peers. John stated that the enjoyment in their relationship had increased and that Dallas was listening better at home. Like a sponge, Dallas seemed to "soak up" all the touching and affection given to him by his father and the DP therapist, and by the end of therapy he was better able to make eye contact and his ability to show affection was less aggressive and more genuine.

Practitioners must keep in mind that children with autism have different tolerance levels for touch. DPT interventions should therefore be adjusted to meet the individual needs of the child. As an example, Brody (1993, 1997b; see Chapter 3 for the full case study) describes a child with autism who stiffened his body during an attempt at cradling. For him to feel a cradling experience Brody instead swung him, with the help of his mother, in a sheet. In the case example of Dallas presented in this chapter, as with many other children with ASD, DPT has proven to be an effective therapeutic treatment approach.

References

Ainsworth, M. (1969). Object relations, dependency and attachment: A theoretical review of the infant–mother relationship. *Child Development, 40,* 969–1025.

Ainsworth, M. D., Blehar, M. C., Waters, E., & Wall, S. (1978). *Patterns of attachment.* Hillsdale, NJ: Erlbaum.

American Psychiatric Association. (APA). (2000). *Diagnostic and statistical manual of mental disorders* (4th ed., text rev.). Washington, DC: Author.

Bailey, B. (2000a). *Easy to love, difficult to discipline.* New York: HarperCollins.

Bailey, B. (2000b). *I love you rituals.* New York: HarperCollins.

Baker, B. L., McIntyre, L. L., Blacher, J., Crnic, K., Edelbrock C., & Low, C. (2003). Pre-school children with and without developmental delay: Behaviour problems and parenting stress over time. *Journal of Intellectual Disability, 47*(4–5), 217–230.

Barnard, K. E., & Brazelton, T. B. (1990). *Touch: The foundation of experience.* Madison, CT: International Universities Press.

Booth, P. A., & Jernberg, A. M. (2010). *Theraplay: Helping parents and children build better relationships through attachment based play* (3rd ed.). San Francisco: Jossey-Bass.

Bowlby, J. (1969). *Attachment and loss: Vol. 1, Attachment.* New York: Basic Books.

Bowlby, J. (1979). *The making and breaking of affectional bonds.* New York: Methuen.

Brody, V. A. (1963). Treatment of a prepubertal twin girl with psychogenic megacolon. *American Journal of Orthopsychiatry, 33,* 3.

Brody, V. A. (1976). *Results from one developmental play program for first grade children in the Pinellas County schools of Florida.* Unpublished manuscript, copy in possession of author.

Brody, V.A. (1978). Developmental play: A relationship-focused program for children. *Child Welfare, 57*(9), November.

Brody, V. A. (Producer). (1987). *Developmental play: The intimate relationship* [Video no longer available]. Copy in possession of author.

Brody, V. A. (1992). The dialogue of touch: Developmental play therapy. *International Journal of Play Therapy, 1*(1), 21–30.

Brody, V. A. (1993). *The dialogue of touch.* Treasure Island, FL: Developmental Play Therapy Associates.

Brody, V. A. (1994). Developmental play therapy. In B. James (Ed.), *Handbook for treatment of attachment-trauma problems in children* (pp. 234–239). New York: Free Press.

Brody, V. A. (1996). Play therapy as an intervention for acting-out children. In G. L. Landreth, L. E. Homeyer, G. Glover, & D. S. Sweeney (Eds.), *Play therapy Interventions with children's problems* (pp. 22–24). Northvale, NJ: Jason Aronson Inc.

Brody, V. A. (1997a). Developmental play therapy. In K. J. O'Connor & L. M. Braverman (Eds.), *Play therapy theory and practice: A comparative casebook* (pp. 160–183). New York: John Wiley & Sons.

Brody, V. A. (1997b). *The dialogue of touch: Developmental play therapy* (2nd ed.). Northvale, NJ: Jason Aronson.

Brody, V. A. (Producer). (1998). Developmental play therapy with attachment problem four year olds. [Video no longer available]. Copy in possession of author.

Brody, V. A. (1999). Circle time in developmental play therapy. In D. S. Sweeney & L. E. Homeyer (Eds.), *Group play therapy: How to do it, how it works, whom it's best for* (pp. 139–161). San Francisco: Jossey-Bass Publishers.

Brody, V. A. (2000). *The role of touch in child play therapy.* [Handout from workshop.] Copy in possession of author.

Brody, V. A., Fenderson, C., & Stephenson, S. (1976). *Sourcebook for developmental play.* Tallahassee: State of Florida Department of Education.

Bromfield, R. (2005). Psychodynamic play therapy with a high-functioning autistic child. In G. L. Landreth, D. S. Sweeney, D. C. Ray, L. E. Homeyer, & G. Glover (Eds.), *Play therapy interventions with children's problems: Case studies with DSM-IV-R diagnoses* (pp. 51–53). Lanham, MD: Rowman & Littlefield Publishing Group.

Bromfield, R. (2010). *Doing therapy with children and adolescents with Asperger syndrome.* Hoboken, NJ: John Wiley & Sons.

Buber, M. (1958). *I and Thou.* New York: Scribner.

Burt, M., & Myrick, R. D. (1980). Developmental play: What is it all about? *Elementary School Guidance & Counseling, 15,* 14–21.

Center for Play Therapy. (Producer). (1995). *Developmental play therapy: A clinical session and Interview with Viola Brody.* [Video tape]. (Available from Center for Play Therapy website: http://cpt.unt.edu/)

Centers for Disease Control and Prevention. (CDC). (2011). *How many children have autism?* Retrieved on March 25, 2011 from http://www.cdc.gov/ncbddd/features/counting- autism.html

Clarke, A. (2003, Summer). Viola Brody and developmental play. *Play for Life,* Newsletter of Play Therapy International. East Sussex, England.

Courtney, J. A. (2004, October). *Tribute to Viola Brody.* Paper presented at the General Assembly of the 21st annual Association for Play Therapy, Denver, CO.

Courtney, J. A. (2005, October). *Developmental play therapy: Theory, practice and research.* Association for Play Therapy International Conference, Nashville, TN.

Courtney, J. A. (2006). *Assessing practitioner experiences of developmental play therapy* (Unpublished doctoral dissertation). Barry University, Miami Shores, FL.

Courtney, J. A. (2010, May). *Research analysis of child psychotherapists and play therapist's experiences of developmental play therapy training.* Paper presented at the 2010 International Play Therapy World Congress, Marrakech, Morocco.

Courtney, J. A., & Gray, S. W. (2011). Perspectives of a child therapist as revealed through an image illustrated by the therapist. *Art Therapy: Journal of the American Art Therapy Association, 28*(3), 132–139.

Des Lauriers, A. (1962). *The experience of reality in childhood schizophrenia.* Madison, CT: International Universities Press.

Fauerbach, P. J., & Wibbe, K. (2003, September). *Our time: A group process utilizing Developmental play therapy to promote attachment and bonding in a child protection system* [Lecture handouts]. Workshop presented, St. Petersburg, FL.

Field, T. M. (Ed.). (1995). *Touch in early development.* Mahwah, NJ: Erlbaum.

Field, T. (2001). *Touch.* Cambridge, MA: MIT Press.

Field, T., Lasko, D., Mundy, P., Henteleff, T., Talpins, S., & Dowling, M. (1986). Autistic children's attentiveness and responsivity improved after touch therapy. *Journal of Autism and Developmental Disorders, 27,* 329–334.

Fromm, E. (1956). *The art of loving.* New York: Harper & Row.

Grandin, T. (1992). Calming effects of deep touch pressure in parents with autistic disorder, college students, and animals. *Journal of Child and Adolescent Psychopharmacology, 2*(1). Retrieved from http://www.grandin.com/inc/squeeze.html

Grandin, T., & Johnson, C. (2005). *Animals in translation.* Orlando: Harcourt, Inc.

Gray, S. W. (2011). *Competency-based assessments in mental health practice: Cases and practical applications.* Hoboken, NJ: Wiley.

Harlow, H. (1958). The nature of love. *American Psychologist, 3*, 673–685.

Hess, E. (2005). Floor time: A play intervention for children with autism. *Association for Play Therapy Newsletter, 24*(3), 17–18.

Jernberg, A. (1983). Therapeutic use of sensory-motor play. In C. E. Schaefer & K. J. O'Connor (Eds.), *Handbook of play therapy* (pp. 128–147). New York: John Wiley & Sons.

Jernberg, A., & Booth, P. (2001*). Theraplay: Helping parents and children build better relationships through attachment based play* (2nd ed.). San Francisco: Wiley.

Kenny, M. C., & Winick, C. B. (2000). An integrative approach to play therapy with an autistic girl. *International Journal of Play Therapy, 9*(1), 11–33.

Koller, T. J., & Booth, P. (1997). Fostering attachment through family Theraplay. In K. J. O'Connor & L. M. Braverman (Eds.), *Play therapy theory and practice: A comparative presentation* (pp. 204–233). New York: John Wiley & Sons.

Lanyado, M. (2005). Treating autism with psychoanalytic play therapy. In G. L. Landreth, D. S. Sweeney, D. C. Ray, L. E. Homeyer, & G. Glover (Eds.), *Play therapy interventions with children's problems: Case studies with DSM-IV-R diagnoses* (pp. 54–56). Lanham, MD: Rowman & Littlefield Publishing Group.

Mitchum, N. T. (1987). Developmental play therapy: A treatment approach for child victims of sexual molestation. *Journal of Counseling and Development, 65*, 320–321.

Montagu, A. (1986). *Touching: The human significance of the skin* (3rd ed.). New York: Harper & Row.

Munns, E. (2003). Theraplay: Attachment-enhancing play therapy. In C. E. Schaefer (Ed.), *Foundations of play therapy* (pp. 156–174). Hoboken, NJ: Wiley.

Myrow, D. L. (2000). Theraplay: The early years. In E. Munns (Ed.), *Theraplay: Innovations in attachment-enhancing play therapy* (pp. 2–8). Northvale, NJ: Jason Aronson.

Peek, F. (with Hanson, L.). (2008). *The life and message of the real rain man: The journey of a mega-savant.* Port Chester, NY: Dude Publishing.

Perry, B. D., & Szalavitz, M. (2006). *The boy who was raised as a dog and other stories from a child psychiatrist's notebook: What traumatized children can teach us about loss, love, and healing.* New York: Basic Books.

Schwartzenberger, K. (2004a, January). *Developmental play therapy.* Retrieved from http://playtherapyseminars.com/Article.aspx?articleID=10000

Schwartzenberger, K. (2004b, October). *Developmental play therapy.* Paper presented at the 21st annual Association for Play Therapy International Conference, Denver, CO.

Short, G. F. L. (2008). Developmental play therapy for very young children. In C. E. Schaefer, S. Kelly-Zion, & J. McCormack (Eds.), *Play therapy for very young children* (pp. 367–378). Lanham, MD: Rowman & Littlefield Publishers.

Spitz, R. (1946). Hospitalism: A follow-up report. *Psychoanalytic Study of the Child* (Vol. 2). New York: International Universities Press.

Sprunk, T. P., Mitchell, J., Myrow, D., & O'Connor, K. (n.d.). *Paper on touch: Clinical, professional & ethical issues.* Retrieved from Association for Play Therapy website: http://www.a4pt.org

Solomon, R. (2008). Play-based intervention for very young children with autism: The play project. In C. E. Schaefer, S. Kelly-Zion, & J. McCormack (Eds.), *Play therapy for very young children* (pp. 379–402). Lanham, MD: Rowman & Littlefield Publishers.

Thomas, J., & Jephcott, M. (2011, Winter). Touch is a "hot topic." *Journal of the International and UK Societies of Play and Creative Arts Therapies*, p. 5.

Yonge, C. (2004). An investigation into the application of the principles of emotional literacy through the arts: A case study on autistic spectrum disorder. Unpublished manuscript, School of Emotional Literacy, Southhampton, UK.

Webb, J. T., Amend, E. R., Webb, N. E., Goerss, J., Beljan, P., & Olenchak, F. R. (2005). *Misdiagnosis and dual diagnosis of gifted children and adults: ADHD, bipolar, OCD, Asperger's, depression, and other disorders.* Scottsdale, AZ: Great Potential Press.

CHAPTER 8

Relational Intervention

Child-Centered Play Therapy With
Children on the Autism Spectrum

DEE C. RAY, JEFFREY M. SULLIVAN, AND SARAH E. CARLSON

A six-year-old boy named Andrew bursts into the playroom with his therapist just behind him. He is excited and out of breath but manages to gasp, "I just...just...I unlocked...You just earned a new spell." As Andrew is talking, he is swinging a toy snake vigorously around and around. Andrew suddenly yells out with unbridled enthusiasm, "The snake is Timmy!!!" The therapist replies, "You have a new spell."

Andrew has received a diagnosis of Asperger's disorder, which lies on the autistic spectrum of disorders, meaning that he is delayed in his social understanding and communication and displays rigid or ritualistic behaviors. The room he has entered is a play therapy room, and it is filled with toys that he can play with in lots of the ways he wants. Andrew's therapist is a play therapist, and, unlike other therapists with whom he has worked, she is not there to teach him social skills or instruct him on how to engage in particular styles of play. She is there to understand and accept Andrew fully and without condition and enter into a relationship with Andrew through his natural language of play.

Introduction to Child-Centered Play Therapy

Child-Centered Play Therapy Definition and Background

Child-centered play therapy (CCPT) is a mental health intervention that recognizes the relationship between therapist and child as the primary healing factor for children facing many types of challenges. CCPT therapists use a playroom with carefully selected toys to match the developmentally appropriate communication style of children, which is play, thereby supporting the message that the therapist seeks to understand the whole child in the context of his or her world. By understanding and accepting children's world, the therapist offers them an environment that unleashes their potential to move toward self-enhancing ways of being. The growth that children experience through CCPT typically results in reducing their relationally or physically harmful ways of interacting as well as increasing their sense of self-responsibility toward behavior.

CCPT was developed in the 1940s, distinguishing it as one of the longest-standing mental health interventions used today. Based on Rogers's (1951) person-centered theory, Virginia Axline (1947) presented the first structure of CCPT by operationalizing the philosophy of person-centered therapy, so aptly described for adults, into a coherent working method for children. Axline referred to this approach as nondirective play therapy, which was later termed child-centered play therapy. In the years since the introduction of CCPT, 62 outcome studies have explored its effectiveness and have summarily concluded that CCPT offers a viable and effective intervention for children (Ray, 2011). Currently, CCPT is recognized as the most widely practiced approach to play therapy in the United States (Lambert et al., 2005), and the approach has earned a strong international reputation (see West, 1996; Wilson, Kendrick, & Ryan, 1992).

Theoretical Rationale for CCPT

In developing person-centered theory, Rogers (1951) introduced 19 propositions to explain personality development and behavior. The 19 propositions provide a framework for human development and explain in great detail how maladjustment in the human condition occurs. These propositions also provide the rationale for CCPT intervention and serve as a guide for play therapists in understanding and facilitating the change process. According to Rogers, the human response to experience is organic and holistic, forward moving, and striving for enhancement of the organism (organism is the term invoked by Rogers to describe the individual person). The essential concept for growth and change is that personality development lies in the phenomenological experience of the organism. The propositions emphasize that persons are the center of their own perceived phenomenological field, meaning that their perception of experience represents reality for them. Individuals' phenomenological experience, which encompasses the perception and integration of experiences from the phenomenological field into perceptions of self, guides the growth and development of the self.

The self develops through interactions with significant others throughout development. The development of the self is separate from the phenomenological field but is also highly influenced by it. One eventually comes to evaluate self-worth based on the perceived expectations and acceptance of others (termed *conditions of worth*). Conditions of worth eventually integrate into the developing self, so that subsequent experiences represent individuals' internalized representations of how they are valued. Thus, people's valuing process may or may not contribute to optimal growth based on how internalized representations of being valued relate to the self-construct.

The propositions further delineate the roles of behavior and emotion in the development of the self. Behavior, described as one's interactions with the phenomenological field, is directly consistent with the view of self and valuing process, whether it is within the awareness of the person. Behavior is seen as an attempt to maintain the organism and have one's needs met depending on the perceived expectations of the environment, whereas the emotion accompanying behavior is seen as dependent on the perceived need for behavior. Hence, a person will behave and emotionally respond in a way that is consistent with the view of self, even if the view of self does not facilitate the optimal growth of the individual.

A person's ability or inability to integrate experiences into a personal self-construct greatly influences how adjustment or maladjustment may develop. Experiences that are not integrated can be perceived as threats to self, even if those experiences are potentially enhancing to the organism. For instance, if I do not feel worthy of receiving love from others based on internalized conditions of worth that I am unlovable unless I am perfect, then love experienced from others may be seen as a threat to self and rejected. This internalized condition is counterproductive to growth and interferes with the development of meaningful relationships. Rogers proposed a path to which the person, when given a nonthreatening environment, can examine experiences in a nonjudgmental way and integrate them into a self-structure that is respectful of the intrinsic direction of the organism, thereby enhancing relationships with others.

In more simplistic terms, specifically regarding children, a child is born into the world viewing interactions in a unique and personal way that is apart from reality or others' perceptions. However, the child will move holistically toward what is most enhancing for the self-organism. A sense of self is established through interactions with significant others and the child's perceptions of those interactions. A child's interactions result in an attitude of self-worth that is influenced by a perceived sense of acceptance by and expectations of others. If a child feels unworthy or unaccepted for certain aspects of self, this sets up barriers for self-acceptance. Because the organism is holistic in movement, a child's feelings and behaviors will be consistent. More concretely, if a child feels unaccepting of self or unaccepted by others, feelings and behaviors will be more negative and less self-enhancing.

Based on these basic beliefs about human nature, CCPT therapists seek to establish environments in which a child will feel fully accepted by another (the therapist) and will learn to develop self-acceptance. The given theoretical outcome of self-acceptance is the resulting movement toward more positive feelings and behaviors. Hence, therapeutic movement is dependent on several factors including the person of the therapist, the person of the child, the level of acceptance established in the therapeutic relationship, and the therapist's trust in the child to move naturally toward self-enhancing ways of being.

Conditions for Therapeutic Change in CCPT

Because CCPT is based on person-centered theory, principles underlying the change process identified by Rogers (1957) apply to the provision of CCPT. Six postulated conditions must exist for the therapeutic process to work effectively. All six conditions are based on the primacy of the relationship between therapist and child:

1. Two persons are in psychological contact.
2. The first person (client) is in a state of incongruence.
3. The second person (therapist) is congruent in the relationship.
4. The therapist experiences unconditional positive regard for the client.
5. The therapist experiences an empathic understanding of the client's internal frame of reference and attempts to communicate this experience to the client.
6. Communication to the client of the therapist's empathic understanding and unconditional positive regard is to a minimal degree achieved.

In the first condition, the therapist and child must be in psychological contact or, in simpler terms, a relationship. In this relationship, both the therapist and child must be in each other's awareness, allowing the other to enter the phenomenological field. Secondly, the child must be in a state of incongruence, which may be demonstrated through anxiety or vulnerability. Conditions 3, 4, and 5 are typically considered the core conditions provided by the therapist, more accurately referred to as attitudes (Bozarth, 1998) and traditionally labeled as congruence, unconditional positive regard (or acceptance), and empathy. These attitudinal therapist conditions provide an environment that promotes the actualizing tendency accessible within all persons, including children.

Congruence is described by Rogers (1957) as the ability to feel free to be self within the therapeutic relationship and to be able to experience congruence between experience and awareness of self. Congruence involves a combination of the therapist's self-awareness, acceptance of such awareness, and appropriate expression of awareness to the client. Congruence of the therapist is a prerequisite to the expression of empathy and unconditional positive regard. Hence, if the play therapist is not authentic, the child will not be able to fully accept the therapist's provision of unconditional positive regard or empathy.

Unconditional positive regard is a warm acceptance of all aspects of the client's experience, without judgment or evaluation (Rogers, 1957). Additionally, unconditional positive regard is a therapist-felt condition in which the therapist experiences a feeling of trust in the child's ability to move toward actualization of the organism. Unconditional positive regard serves as the curative factor in CCPT, a natural antidote to the conditions of worth taken on by the child during development (Bozarth, 1998).

The final therapist attitudinal condition is the provision of empathic understanding, entering the child's world as if it were one's own without losing a sense of self as the therapist. A play therapist typically communicates empathy through reflective responses to the child. Empathic understanding is intertwined with the concept of unconditional positive regard, as empathy may be considered a vehicle for the expression of unconditional positive regard (Bozarth, 2001). When a therapist enters the world of the client, there is an underlying message that the client's world is a valuable world, one in which the therapist has the utmost respect for the client's experience and abilities.

The final condition states that the client must be open to receiving empathy and unconditional positive regard from the therapist, representing an element of therapy over which the therapist has little control. All previous conditions may be met, but if the child is unable to receive some level of unconditional positive regard or empathy from the therapist then therapy will be minimally effective or not at all. Generally, if a therapist is able to achieve the prior conditions, a child will perceive such conditions and engage in the therapeutic process of change.

CCPT Process Structure

CCPT is characterized by a nondirective attitude toward the child. Nondirectivity is not a set of passive behaviors but is an attitude that promotes the client's self-sufficiency by not guiding the client's goals or therapeutic content (Ray, 2011). The child leads what is said and done in a play session. Axline (1947) offered guidelines to enact the philosophy of nondirectivity in the context of the CCPT structure. They are referred to as the 8 Basic Principles, paraphrased as follows (pp. 73–74):

1. The therapist develops a warm, friendly relationship with the child as soon as possible.
2. The therapist accepts the child exactly as is, not wishing the child were different in some way.
3. The therapist establishes a feeling of permissiveness in the relationship so that the child can fully express thoughts and feelings.
4. The therapist is attuned to the child's feelings and reflects those back to the child to help gain insight into behavior.
5. The therapist respects the child's ability to solve problems, leaving the responsibility to make choices to the child.
6. The therapist does not direct the child's behavior or conversation. The therapist follows the child.
7. The therapist does not attempt to rush therapy, recognizing the gradual nature of the therapeutic process.
8. The therapist sets only those limits that anchor the child to reality or make the child aware of responsibilities in the relationship.

These principles provide the structure for play therapy, encouraging the therapist to accept, trust, and follow the child. Using the principles to operationalize play therapy, specific types of responses guide the therapist's enactment of the nondirective philosophy. They include reflecting feelings (you feel angry), reflecting content (your mom was fighting with your dad), tracking behavior (you're moving to over there), facilitating decision making (you can decide), facilitating creativity (that can be whatever you want), encouraging (you're trying hard on that), facilitating relationship (you want to make me feel better), and limit setting (Axline, 1947; Ginott, 1961; Landreth, 2002; Ray, 2004).

Limit setting is used as necessary when the child might be a threat to self, others, or the room. For limit setting, Landreth (2002) offers a three-step approach titled ACT: Acknowledge the feeling, Communicate the limit, Target an alternative. In ACT, the therapist first and foremost seeks to understand and communicate understanding of the child's intent by acknowledging the child's feeling (you're really angry with me). Second, the therapist sets a clear and definitive limit (but I'm not for pushing). Finally, the therapist provides an alternative to allow the child appropriate expression of the feeling (you can push the bear). Limit setting allows the child to perceive the playroom as a safe environment. Although CCPT therapists have provided specific types of responses to help concretely structure CCPT, it should be remembered that the attitudinal conditions provided by the therapist always take precedence over a rigid approach to responding to a child.

Playroom and Materials

CCPT is conducted in a playroom stocked with toys that encourage the expression of all feelings by a child. The playroom sends the message that all parts of the child are accepted in this environment. Although Landreth (2002) recommended that play therapy be conducted in a room measuring 12 feet by 15 feet, smaller or larger rooms can be used. Smaller rooms should ensure that there is enough space for the toys and open space for the child to move. Larger rooms can be sectioned off with curtains or shelves to limit the size of playroom so that it is not overwhelming to the child. Materials for the playroom include toys, craft materials, paints, easel, puppet theater, sand box, and child furniture. Kottman (2003) provided categorization of materials in five general areas: family/nurturing, scary toys, aggressive toys, expressive toys, and pretend/fantasy toys. In selecting toys, the most fundamental criterion is that the toy serves a purpose in the playroom. Ray (2011) suggested that each therapist should ask the following questions regarding toy selection: (1) What therapeutic purpose will this serve for children who use this room? (2) How will this help children express themselves? (3) How will this help me build a relationship with children? When toys meet a therapeutic purpose, help children express themselves, and help build the relationship between therapist and child, they can be considered valuable to the playroom.

CCPT With Children on the Autism Spectrum

CCPT is a way of working with children that emphasizes relationship and communication. In CCPT, the primary healing therapeutic factor is the relationship between therapist and child. The playroom offers a venue for communication that is developmentally appropriate for a child. Hence, CCPT is philosophically positioned to address the salient characteristics of children on the autism spectrum.

To understand the effectiveness of CCPT with children diagnosed with autistic spectrum disorders (ASD), including autistic disorder, Asperger's disorder, and pervasive developmental disorder—not otherwise specified (PDD-NOS), it becomes necessary to understand core problems that designate a child as challenged with these disorders. Although much attention is paid to obvious behavioral symptoms associated with autism such as echolalia, stereotypy, or self-stimulation, these are secondary symptoms indicative of the deeper pervasive relationship limitations. Greenspan and Wieder (2006) identified three core problems that must be considered when diagnosing children on the autism spectrum: (1) establishing closeness; (2) exchanging emotional gestures in a continuous way; and (3) using words or symbols with emotional intent.

When children establish closeness with others, they exhibit warmth toward others, seek support from adults with whom they are comfortable, and show enjoyment in their close relationships. When children exchange emotional gestures, they engage in emotional signaling with significant others through smiles, frowns, and other interactive gestures. Finally, when children use symbols with emotional intent, they use words meaningfully and with desire as opposed to the use of words concretely (the difference between "I love my doggy" and "This is doggy"). Because the diagnosis of ASD is often identified on a continuum and not categorically, children's level of effectiveness in these three core areas determines how challenged they are by the disorder.

When conceptualizing ASD according to the three core problems, it can be clearly observed that children who are correctly diagnosed with ASD are challenged in relationships. Within those relationships, communication is a primary concern. All people are on the relationship continuum, but children who are diagnosed with ASD tend to aggregate toward one end. The ability of an individual with ASD to communicate within relationships is often evaluated based on each person's abilities, needs, and characteristics.

As described previously, CCPT is a relationship-based intervention in which the relationship and the ways of communicating within relationships serve as the therapeutic factors for change. Hence, if ASD is conceptualized in part as a relational communication disorder, CCPT is equivocally matched as a relational communication intervention. The goal of CCPT is to provide a relationship for children in which they feel free to move toward self-enhancing processes of growth. The CCPT relationship allows full acceptance of their world, which, for children with ASD, is organized differently from that of typically developing children, so that they determine how much and when they will engage with the therapist. When children engage with the therapist, the self-enhancing behaviors will continue to grow to other external relationships.

The CCPT therapist does not seek to "fix" the secondary symptoms of children with ASD, such as eye contact, verbal responsiveness, or rigidity. CCPT actively addresses the primary core areas of ASD by providing relationship and communication to counter their challenges in this area. CCPT does use behavioral techniques to train children to do something that is incongruent with their way of being. So then, one might ask how can CCPT be helpful in improving problems of children with ASD? Several essential elements of CCPT result in the improvement of behaviors related to autism.

First, the full acceptance of the child by the therapist in CCPT is a condition that is often unavailable to the child diagnosed with ASD. Because of the high level of parental stress related to parenting a child with ASD and because of prevalent intervention methods to change the child's behavior on a daily basis, children with ASD rarely experience understanding and acceptance of them as they are. In addition, children with ASD are often forced to interact in the adult's version of the world, and few adults enter into the child's world on the child's conditions. CCPT offers the unique experience to the child with ASD that the therapist will enter the child's world on the child's terms and at the child's will. This full acceptance, unconditional positive regard, sends a message of respect and safety to children to enable them to share their world freely. When they feel safe and understood, their motivation to interact with the external world increases.

For children who exhibit symptoms associated with Asperger's syndrome, this acceptance and attention to them is especially salient. A commonly described quality of individuals with Asperger's is a strong desire to connect with the social world but a lack of social understanding to do so effectively (Attwood, 1998). However, when the therapist actively listens and intently reflects within children's long soliloquy on, say, dinosaurs, over time they are able to organically feel that acceptance and engagement of the therapist. As a result, it is typical for these children to begin to try to engage the therapist in a two-way conversation. They are able to transfer this new relationship ability to relationships outside of the playroom.

The nonverbal focus of CCPT is also a beneficial therapeutic factor for children with ASD. In CCPT, they are not forced to talk or interact with the therapist. The therapist is verbally and nonverbally engaged through continual reflections of the children's behaviors or reactions and through following them with eyes and body. The therapist seeks to match the children's tones and movements through not only verbal but also nonverbal reflections. This following of behavior allows the children to communicate in nonverbal ways to increase meaningful interactions through gestures. Because the impairment of meaningful symbolic interaction is a core problem for children with ASD, the nonverbal child–therapist interaction helps to enhance children's communication.

Another positive outcome of CCPT for children with ASD is the decrease of emotionality and behavioral problems associated with the disorder. Parents of children who participate in CCPT typically report a lessening of tantrums, yelling and screaming, and extreme emotionality. Although it is difficult to distinguish between symptoms associated with the disorder and symptoms of comorbid disorders that may develop with these children, CCPT appears to be effective at helping reduce these more emotionally related problems. Children with ASD may also be challenged with depression, anxiety, and attentional problems (Howlin, 2005). CCPT offers a place where children can express self-doubts verbally or through play, which allows them to work through the negative sense of self and emerge with hope.

Finally, one of the most important aspects of CCPT compared with other more behaviorally oriented interventions for children with ASD is that children are creating a sense of self and making changes from an intrinsic need. In CCPT, they are not pressured to be different from what they are. Hence, when children begin to exhibit new behaviors and relational abilities, these are developed from within them. There is no reward that must be provided to them for good behavior. They have established an internal reward for change, and thereby the changes will be integrated into their experience. These changed behaviors will not dissipate when therapy ends or when rewards are withdrawn; they will now be a part of who they are.

Opportunities to play in a nondirective manner allow the child with ASD to choose the pace and focus of change, instilling an intrinsic motivation to engage in the world of others rather than enacting a style of play learned through a set of skills (Josefi & Ryan, 2004). The relationship that is built between therapist and child through CCPT will eventually be transferred to other adults and children in the child's life. Because relationship is a core problem of ASD and relationship is the core focus of CCPT, the effectiveness of therapy serves to help the core issues of the child.

Although CCPT therapists report working with children with ASD quite often, research on CCPT with this population is limited. Josefi and Ryan (2004) presented a case study comparing CCPT and behavioral interventions with a child with severe autism. They concluded that this preliminary case study indicated that nondirective play therapy may enhance and accelerate the emotional/social development of children with severe autism. Beckloff (1998), using an intervention that taught CCPT skills to parents of children with ASD, found an increase in parents' ability to recognize their child's need for autonomy and independence. One could also argue that Virginia Axline's (1986) seminal case study of CCPT, *Dibs: In Search of Self,* presented a detailed account of a successful intervention using CCPT with a child on the autistic spectrum. In addition, CCPT has demonstrated effectiveness with many populations through randomized controlled studies such as Schumann (2010) with children who were aggressive; Ray, Schottelkorb, and Tsai (2007) with children who had attentional difficulties; and Blanco and Ray (2011) with children academically at risk. However, there appear to be no clinical trial studies exploring the effectiveness of CCPT with children on the autistic spectrum. Several difficulties arise in conducting research with children on the spectrum including challenges related to identifying a large enough sample to meet criteria and willingness of participants to commit to 10–16 sessions of CCPT intervention.

Case Example

Andrew was a 6-year, 6-month-old boy enrolled in kindergarten who had been diagnosed with Asperger's disorder. Andrew's teacher referred him for individual play therapy due to his difficulty getting along with other children, difficulty in transition, and low frustration tolerance. According to his teacher, Andrew was at or above grade level in all of his subjects, although his teacher expressed concern about his writing and possible deficiencies in fine motor skills. Andrew lived with his mother and maternal grandparents. Andrew's mother reported no other significant relationships outside of the family and that Andrew focused his energy on video games. Andrew attended individual CCPT once per week for a total of 24 sessions.

Throughout play therapy, Andrew routinely displayed high energy and enthusiasm. He often rocked from side to side in an animated fashion, flailed his arms, and jumped up and down excitedly. Andrew used an extensive array of sounds and noises in his play and communication with the therapist and often experienced shortness of breath due to his excitable and energetic play. Andrew's conversation typically included his sharing knowledge of video games in painstaking detail, although such conversation was typically one-sided and conveyed little awareness of the play therapist's interest in the topic. However, Andrew routinely checked with the therapist to ensure that she understood what he was communicating.

During initial sessions (1–7), Andrew put a lot of physical distance between himself and the play therapist and did not make eye contact. Andrew engaged verbally, but with excessive verbal overflow, often making it difficult for the play therapist to reflect his actions or feelings. His play typically included drawing pictures of Pokémon and Mario Brothers on the easel, which he explained in great detail to the play therapist. He invoked an array of sounds and noises while playing. The following excerpt takes place after attending several sessions of play therapy.

Andrew: A brand new galaxy is born, that is…that means a brand new galaxy and a…and a planet is born. (He is wandering around the room, rocking from side to side as he moves.)

Play therapist: You know when a new galaxy is born.

Andrew: (Andrew hands the wig and the butterfly wings to the play therapist from the side of his body.) A magic wig and these… these…wings and spells.

Play therapist: You want me to have these.

Andrew: (Moves over to the shelf and picks up the ring toss.) Pshew… pshew…sheeh. (Andrew dumps the rings into the sandbox.) These are…magic rings…magic rings, and you can use these spells like this (throws the bottom of the ring toss to the bop bag.)…And you can use these spells…Uh, uh…

Play therapist: You know what to do.

Andrew: This is a trick, you, you, you, can, you, have to, you can, you can, super do it, but you have to watch out for the mean evil plants.

(Andrew is leaning over the sandbox with his hands in the sand, sitting perpendicular to the play therapist.)

Play therapist: You want me to be careful of the mean evil plants.

Andrew: Oh but... oh but... watch out for those mean evil screaming plants.

Play therapist: So, the plants are evil and they scream.

Andrew: No, there is one plant that... that screams like EEEEEEEEEEEE! (Andrew screams a very high-pitched scream.)

Play therapist: Oh, it makes that noise.

Andrew: Vooomp! (Andrew takes all the rings out of his hands and throws them across the room.)

Play therapist: You threw them over there.

Andrew: Whew. (Andrew sighs and moves over to the kitchenette.) But... but... I... I... got some... I'm giving out free food. Cause I'm gonna stand at the free food stand and get me some food. (Andrew sits down.) 1 dollar, 1 dollar, 1 dollar, get some, some, food from our food stand, and, and, bring it to him, OK. (Andrew is out of breath.)

As seen in the transcript, Andrew had very little meaningful interaction with the therapist, mostly focused on speaking his own thoughts from his own world. In the initial sessions of CCPT, the play therapist entered Andrew's world without questions or judgment. Rather than correcting Andrew or trying to focus his attention on one single topic or particular type of play, she followed Andrew through verbal reflections as he explored the playroom and his world, conveying her unconditional acceptance of his experience.

Throughout the middle sessions (8–14), Andrew's experience of feeling understood and accepted began to emerge in his play. He engaged more with the play therapist and started to make eye contact, though it was often out of the corner of his eye. Andrew also began involving the play therapist in his play and offering the play therapist toys from around the playroom, which he did not do in early sessions. The play therapist continued to demonstrate the core conditions of congruence, unconditional positive regard, and empathic understanding and did not shift her approach. She continued to allow Andrew to direct the play sessions as she entered his world and communicated to him her understanding and acceptance of his experience.

Andrew: (Andrew is sitting behind the puppet theater and pops up suddenly.) But how about we play trains also?

Play therapist: You have another idea.

Andrew: OK, OK, OK, pretend, you, OK... I am going to be on a train... and, and, I'm gonna put milk in it. I need to get my milk from over there.

Play therapist: You have a plan.

Andrew: Choo, choo...hmm, hmm, choo, choo. (Child is getting large bricks from the pile again and placing them in a stack.)

Play therapist: You are getting that how you want it.

Andrew: Here's the milk, choo choo, choo choo. (Child gets a pail full of sand and brings it over to the brick structure, but stops.)

Play therapist: You are getting it all set up.

Andrew: (Andrew teeters back and forth until he dumps the sand in the sandbox.) I'll...I guess I just dump it in here.

Play therapist: You've decided where it goes.

Andrew: Oh, but, oh, but...there's something...that's your table. (Child looks at the brick structure.)

Play therapist: You decided it's a table.

Andrew demonstrated increased connection and trust in the play therapist. Throughout much of his time in play therapy, Andrew had kept a physical distance between himself and the play therapist, but the understanding and acceptance conveyed by the play therapist instilled in Andrew a sense of safety, confidence, and trust. As sessions progressed, Andrew increasingly included the play therapist by engaging in more cooperative types of play where the play therapist and child fight "bad" characters together. This level of cooperation and coordination by Andrew was completely absent in early sessions and represented a strength of the relationship that he perceived between him and the play therapist.

Andrew: Now, would you like to play food store?

Play therapist: You can decide.

Andrew: OK, so, I get my food... (Andrew takes the plastic fruit and places it on plates. He then carries the plates to the table, positioned next to the sandbox.) Now you get food.

Play therapist: I need to pick my food out now.

Andrew: Yeah. (Andrew watches the play therapist get her food and watches her sit down in the chair, next to the table.) Is that your food? (Andrew begins singing.)

Play therapist: It sure is.

Andrew: (Andrew begins to put his hands in the sand and pour sand on his legs, all while sitting in the sandbox. Without looking at the play therapist, Andrew asks her a question.) Do you want to get in here?

Play therapist: You want me to sit with you.

Andrew: Mmm, hmm.

Play therapist: (The play therapist moves to sit on the corner of the sandbox and notices that Andrew moves over to make space). You want me to sit next to you in the sandbox. (The play therapist sits in the sandbox next to Andrew, with the therapist and child sitting closely, shoulder to shoulder. This continues uninterrupted for 3 more minutes.)

After attending 24 sessions of child-centered play therapy, Andrew and the play therapist forged a strong relationship built on the therapist's willingness to enter his world with acceptance and understanding. Although many features of his presentation continued to be on the autistic spectrum, his being in proximity, making more frequent eye contact, and engaging in more reciprocal play demonstrating turn taking and cooperative activities reflected Andrew's experience of the relationship. Andrew's increased desire to be in relationship with the play therapist was not the result of being rewarded for staying on task or demonstrating particular play behaviors but because he was open to receiving the acceptance and unconditional positive regard offered by the play therapist, demonstrating his intrinsic motivation. Andrew's increased two-way communication indicated that he might be prepared to transfer those skills outside of the playroom. Andrew began CCPT group therapy with another child where he developed and used appropriate social skills to communicate with both the therapist and child. His teacher additionally commented on his increase in social skills in the classroom and his improved ability to socialize with other children.

Guidelines for Implementation of CCPT With Children With ASD

Although CCPT is nondirective in nature, in keeping with responsible practice, child-centered play therapists should adhere to particular guidelines in their work with children with ASD. Before engaging with a child diagnosed with ASD, a CCPT therapist should be knowledgeable regarding characteristics and symptoms of the diagnosis. Although CCPT is conducted similarly with all children, children with ASD sometimes present with self-harming or destructive behaviors for which the therapist must be prepared. Initially, a CCPT therapist who begins a therapeutic relationship with a child presumed to have ASD is to conduct a proper assessment of the child. As mentioned, ASD is not a dichotomous, all-or-none diagnosis. Children have varying levels of abilities within the spectrum, and some who have been labeled ASD may not even exhibit the core signs of impairment. Children are most likely to demonstrate lower abilities in the presence of strangers and should be assessed in the presence of and interaction with a primary caregiver (Greenspan & Wieder, 2006). Moreover, diagnosis of ASD should not derive from only one source, such as a single assessment or parent report. Assessments should be multifaceted and take into account assessment scores, parent reports and possibly teacher reports, as well as observation of the child in natural, familiar settings, such as when interacting with the parent. CCPT treatment plans for children with ASD may include individual CCPT and consistent parent consultations. Additionally, when the therapist concludes that a child might be ready to transfer relationship skills to another child, group CCPT may be added to the treatment plan.

According to Rogers (1957), making contact is the first condition of effective therapy. When CCPT is conducted with children with ASD, contact may be initially thwarted by the child. In this case, the therapist needs to slowly gain the child's trust by entering the child's world. Using nonthreatening tracking responses such as, "You're moving over there" or "You're playing with that ball" is one way to enter the child's world in an unobtrusive manner. Not overwhelming the child with too much eye contact may also be encouraged with some children. Children with ASD are slow to respond to the relational offerings by the therapist, but this should not discourage the therapist from the process. Additionally, the therapist should not assume that because children are not responding that they are not engaged. Often, children with ASD will be engaged in the relationship, perhaps through listening or silence, long before the therapist is aware.

In play therapy sessions, a CCPT therapist will want to be acutely attuned to the behavioral manifestations of children's neurological functioning, specifically their sensitivity to noise, interaction, and light. Conditions in the playroom may need to be adjusted to help children feel safe, such as lowering the light, ensuring that the facility is not overly busy at their appointment time, and not speaking too loudly or overly animated. As the therapist comes to know these children well, it will be natural to respond to them in the way that is most in contact with their internal system.

Another helpful therapist response to children with ASD, especially those demonstrating symptoms of Asperger's disorder, is to respond in a focused way to them, not following their every verbal lead. As seen with Andrew, children with Asperger's will often jump from subject area to subject area without any apparent connection. Reflections that help close one road of content and introduce a new one can model clear communication and help focus these children. It also helps for the therapist to stay in the moment with them. For example, a therapist might respond, "You were talking about a video game, but now you're talking about the thunderstorm," or, "You liked that movie, but now you want to talk about your bike."

Conclusion

CCPT is a relational intervention that seeks to unlock the potential of all children who are experiencing inner and contextual struggles. Through the relationship with the (CCPT) trained play therapist, a child engages in an environment where a sense of acceptance, warmth, and understanding can be experienced. The therapist offers children understanding based on entering their world, specifically the world of play. These aspects of CCPT are especially salient for children who are diagnosed with ASD. Children with ASD present as unusual based on cultural norms, separated based on lack of adherence to social cues, and alone based on exhibition of "strange" behaviors. In the cases where adults attempt to help children with ASD, children are often sent the message that they are unacceptable and must be changed. CCPT offers children with ASD a place where they can learn and experience their own uniqueness and sense of worth, a place where they are fully valued by another person. Through this experience, they will likely be able to tap into inner resources to develop a sense of self that is forward moving and relationally connected. Often, for children with ASD, this experience leads to an intrinsic motivation to connect and communicate with others. True change occurs, developed from children's inner resources and abilities so that change is substantial and lifelong.

References

Attwood, T. (1998). *Asperger's syndrome.* London: Jessica Kingsley.

Axline, V. (1947). *Play therapy.* New York: Ballantine.

Axline, V. M. (1986). *Dibs: In search of self.* New York: Ballantine Books.

Beckloff, D. (1998). Filial therapy with children with spectrum pervasive development disorders. (Doctoral dissertation, University of North Texas, 1997). *Dissertation Abstracts International*, DAI-B 58/11, 6224.

Blanco, P., & Ray, D. (2011). Play therapy in the schools: A best practice for improving academic achievement. *Journal of Counseling and Development, 89*(2).

Bozarth, J. (1998). *Person-centered therapy: A revolutionary paradigm.* Ross on Wye: PCCS.

Bozarth, J. (2001). An addendum to beyond reflection: Emergent modes of empathy. In S. Haugh & T. Merry (Eds.), *Empathy. Rogers' therapeutic conditions: Evolution, theory and practice* (vol. 2, pp. 144–154). Ross on Wye: PCCS Books.

Ginott, H. (1961). *Group psychotherapy with children.* New York: McGraw-Hill.

Greenspan, S., & Wieder, S. (2006). *Engaging autism: Using the Floortime approach to help children relate, communicate, and think.* Cambridge, MA: Da Capo.

Howlin, P. (2005). Outcomes in autism spectrum disorders. In F. Volkmar, P. Rhea, A. Klin, & D. Cohen (Eds.), *Handbook of autism and pervasive developmental disorders* (vol. 1, pp. 200–220). Hoboken, NJ: John Wiley & Sons.

Josefi, O., & Ryan, V. (2004). Non-directive play therapy for young children with autism: A case study. *Clinical Child Psychology and Psychiatry, 9*(4), 533–551. doi:10.1177/1359104504046158

Kottman, T. (2003). *Partners in play: An Adlerian approach to play therapy* (2nd ed.). Alexandria, VA: American Counseling Association.

Lambert, S., LeBlanc, M., Mullen, J., Ray, D., Baggerly, J., White, J., et al. (2005). Learning more about those who play in session: The national play therapy in counseling practices project. *Journal of Counseling & Development, 85,* 42–46.

Landreth, G. (2002). *Play therapy: The art of the relationship.* New York: Routledge.

Ray, D. (2004). Supervision of basic and advanced skills in play therapy. *Journal of Professional Counseling: Practice, Theory, and Research, 32*(2), 28–41.

Ray, D. (2011). *Advanced play therapy: Essential conditions, knowledge, and skills for child practice.* New York: Routledge.

Ray, D., Schottelkorb, A., & Tsai, M. (2007). Play therapy with children exhibiting symptoms of attention deficit hyperactivity disorder. *International Journal of Play Therapy, 16,* 95–111.

Rogers, C. (1951). *Client-centered therapy: Its current practice, implications and theory.* Boston: Houghton Mifflin.

Rogers, C. (1957). The necessary and sufficient conditions of therapeutic personality change. *Journal of Consulting Psychology, 21*(2), 95–103.

Schumann, B. (2010). Effectiveness of child centered play therapy for children referred for aggression in elementary school. In J. Baggerly, D. Ray, & S. Bratton (Eds.), *Child-centered play therapy research: The evidence base for effective practice* (pp. 193–208). Hoboken, NJ: Wiley.

West, J. (1996). *Child centred play therapy* (2nd ed.). London: Hodder Arnold.

Wilson, K., Kendrick, P., & Ryan, V. (1992). *Play therapy: A nondirective approach for children and adolescents.* London: Bailliere Tindall.

CHAPTER 9

The Narcissus Myth, Resplendent Reflections, and Self-Healing

A Jungian Perspective on Counseling a Child With Asperger's Syndrome

ERIC J. GREEN

Autistics have problems learning things that cannot be thought about in pictures. (Grandin, 2006, p. 14)

Introduction to Jungian Play Therapy

Jungian play therapy (JPT) asserts that children psychologically develop through *introjection* (internalizing beliefs of others) or *identification* (strongly relating to the values and feelings of others) (Green, 2007, 2009, 2011). Feelings, thoughts, and traits of primary caretakers are acquired (or internalized) as well as any associated dysfunction inherent within those significant primary relationships. Jungian play therapists offer children adequate space in an emotionally secure setting so that their personal development (individuation), disparate from the beliefs internalized or identified with, materializes. Individuation characterizes a progress from psychic fragmentation toward wholeness: the acknowledgment and reconciliation of opposites within an individual (Jung, 1951). Jung believed children's psyches contain a transcendent function, or *self-healing archetype* (Allan, 1988), that surfaces through symbol production.

The Jungian approach to psychotherapy depends on the children trusting and allowing the symbols to lead them into healing by *containing* the images. Symbols tell children where they are in the therapeutic journey by pointing to the area of the unconscious that is most neglected. The Jungian counselor accepts that position and supports the children unconditionally along the therapeutic journey. After the self-healing symbol in play appears, the therapist explores children's inner language by reconciling the meaning of the symbol (or archetype) with their assistance (Allan, 1988; Green, 2007, 2010b).

The principal aim of Jungian play therapy is activating the individuation process through a *symbolic attitude* (or sometimes referred to as the *analytic attitude*) where images are honored so that children maintain equilibrium of energy flow between their inner and outer worlds (Allan, 1988; Green, 2007, 2011). A *symbolic attitude* is cultivated when sustained attention allows the symbolic value of an image to be recognized. For example, when children pretend or use the "as if" quality, they are said to have developed a symbolic attitude. The goal of Jungian therapy with children, individuation, is operationalized through the transformation of symbol—the process of their symbols being generated throughout therapy. The symbolic attitude of the therapist permits children to move from impulse or action to the symbolic life, where emotions and images are contained. For example, children may articulate verbally or through symbolic play the phrases, "I do not like" or "I am angry at you," instead of antipathy or physically attacking toys or the therapist.

JPT's treatment plan involves three steps: (1) counseling a child one to two times per week for 50 minutes; (2) conducting one family play therapy session with a child's caretakers every 2–3 weeks; and (3) consulting with a multidisciplinary team of school and community-based professionals to provide holistic care. The Jungian treatment process can be codified into three stages: (1) orientation; (2) working-through; and (3) reparation/termination. During the orientation phase, the therapist builds an alliance with the child by establishing the frame (i.e., consistent time and weekday in specific space), purpose (i.e., playing, talking about worries, sharing dreams), and conditions or limits of therapy. Orientation typically lasts one session to several weeks. Building the therapeutic alliance and creating an atmosphere of permissiveness and safety so that the child's ego may constellate and transfer images unto the toys and therapist involves using empathy, unconditional positive regard, and therapeutic limit setting. In the *working-through phase*, the child's negative behavioral and personality traits appear and transference occurs, in which emotional woundedness, introjections of negative parental imagoes, and rage materialize (De Domenico, 1994; Jung, 1910, 1913). The third stage, reparation (and eventual termination), involves the child reconciling opposites, internalizing a good enough parental image, and developing psychologically healthy mechanisms to cope with anxiety (manageable frustration).

Jungian Play Techniques

Analysis and Interpretation   The aim of child analysis is to provide a facilitative environment where psychological disturbances, which comprise the underpinnings of complex defenses, may be reached. However, analysis, which typically occurs four to five times per week, is not a financially realistic or logistical option for most families today. Therefore, I use the term *therapy*, as in Jungian play therapy, more often to connate the less frequent (usually twice-per-week) therapeutic sessions. One of the inherent difficulties in using analytical play infrequently is the issue of working through resistances. Specifically, if children on the autism spectrum are seen infrequently, they may not sufficiently work through the effects of some of the interpretations because of the expanse of time between play sessions. They build resistances to the interpretations, possibly to ward off anxieties (Fordham, 1944, 1976). Moreover, the value of the analyst's interpretations may become lost between sporadic sessions, thereby creating inherent difficulties when working through complexes. I typically set appointments with children twice per week to meet the realistic demands of families' complicated schedules and still provide adequate support to the needs of the child's ego.

Furthermore, the analysis of children encompasses toys and symbolic play for therapeutic purposes, yet the main component of child analysis is in the therapist's verbalizing and interpreting the action in the playroom and urging the child to do so as well (Allan, 1988; Fordham, 1976; Green, 2008, 2010a). Therefore, analytical play therapy would be appropriate only with sufficiently verbal, high-functioning children on the autism spectrum. The purpose of interpretation is to bring unconscious contents into awareness and to help the child mediate anxiety. The technique of interpretation does not relieve anxiety because the therapist tells children something new about themselves but rather gives them information about their therapist's capacity to (1) hear them, (2) see them, (3) understand them, and (4) ultimately accept them. Interpretation is a key inductive technique when working with children with Asperger's syndrome (AS) as it (1) provides children the abilities to resolve interpersonal deficiencies constellated in the transference and (2) relies on the use of symbols and the theory of archetypes to facilitate their understanding of their fears and fantasies. Through interpretation, Jungian play therapists link symbolic play with personal observations and relevant experiences in children's external world.

One last component of analysis and interpretation specific to working with children with Asperger's syndrome is the reliance on interpretation based on the analyst's own countertransference. Some children with Asperger's syndrome may find interpretations to be persecutory. If a child displays a manageable degree of persecutory tendencies during interpretation, this may be a sign that development is occurring. For example, I had a child client on the autism spectrum who continuously covered his ears when I provided verbalization of play. I gave a voice to the child's transference by stating, "You experience me as bad sometimes." Afterward, the child smiled and nodded his head. There was a sense of mutual understanding that had not occurred before this moment.

When there is repeated failure to get any type of response from a child with Asperger's syndrome during therapeutic interpretations (and the therapist hasn't been overly complicated with language or ill-timed), the therapist should consider stopping and later conducting interpretation. This interpretation is not so much based inductively on the observable evidence in the child but more on the therapist's own countertransference. For example, I once had a 5-year-old client who did not want to leave the play session when it ended. The child charged into the waiting room area and began to harshly scream at and berate his mother, telling her he hated her and that he wished she would die. The mother's eyes began to well with tears. I felt distressed and realized that an interpretation based on observable data may not have been effective. So I used his countertransferential feelings and stated, "Now I feel like crying too because you're hurting your mother's feelings." The child instantly stopped his dysregulated behaviors, calmed himself down, then left without any other protestations. According to Fordham (1976), affective processes activated in the therapist through the countertransference and sensitively verbalized to the child can be highly effective in promoting change in the child's behaviors.

Coloring Mandalas   Jung (2008, 2009) believed the mandala, or an object (perhaps a circle) with an image contained within, represents unity or wholeness. From a Jungian perspective, unity or wholeness is commensurate to psychological healthiness, because Jung believed a reconciliation of opposites has occurred in the individual (*individuation*). In individuation, the child functions outside of the constraints of the ego, operating from the true center of being—the autonomous self.

When coloring mandalas, the Jungian play therapist first asks children to spend a couple of minutes relaxing. With eyes closed in a comfortable seated position, the therapist leads children through a guided imagery technique, assisting them to release any frustrations or anxieties accumulated throughout the school day through deep breathing. Also, therapists may ask them to manipulate Play-Doh or clay as an anxiety-releasing technique while deeply breathing. After a couple of minutes, the therapist asks the children to pick a preconfigured mandala from several choices. These can often be found at no charge by surfing the Internet or in books specific to coloring mandalas (Fincher, 2004). They are then instructed to depict, draw, or color the mandala. Once they finish, the therapist and the child contemplate the images in silence. Then the therapist asks the children to create a color key (similar to a map key) to represent what each color represents. After, the therapists may ask some of the following questions: "Tell me what is the story of this mandala?" "If you could give this mandala a title, what would it be?" and "Write the story of the mandala on the back of the paper. Afterward, let's talk about it."

Sandplay   Kalff's (1980) sandplay was rooted in Jung's premise that the psyche can be activated to move toward healing and that individuation occurs in the sand process through the *temenos*, or free and protected space. *Protected space* refers to the way the therapist listens, observes, and serves nonjudgmentally as a psychological container for the emotional content that becomes activated by the sand therapy process (Green & Gibbs, 2010). The therapist provides the free and protected space in which a creation in the sand may symbolize the inner drama and healing potential of the child's psyche. The therapeutic rationale for sandplay is that children reproduce symbolic scenes of their immediate experience and link opposites from their inner and outer worlds. Through the concretization of unconscious experiences, children's psyches are able to make meaningful links and develop mastery over difficult feelings. Moreover, it is what children experience for themselves that is therapeutic in sandplay, not necessarily the therapist's analysis of the symbols contained within the scene. Kalff (1980) emphasized that the transformative experience of creating a world in the sand contains the healing.

Sandplay typically involves children playing in a sand tray and choosing sand miniatures to create a world, with little to no direction or guidance. Therapists permit children to draw, depict, or create whatever world they choose. The therapist may say, "Create a sand world. There's no right or wrong way to do this. It's completely up to you. After you finish, we may talk a little about your sand world. I'll be quiet while you play unless you ask me a question." After children finish creating their sand worlds, therapists might inquire about the sand world's name or title. Second, therapists may ask, "If you were in this world, what would you feel like?" Third, therapists may probe children further by asking how they felt while forming the world. Sample questions for processing sandplay worlds could include (1) What were you feeling when you placed that castle there? and (2) If this symbol (or object or person) were talking, what would they be saying and to whom? A therapist may use Jungian sandplay techniques to facilitate containment of children's affect in the sand tray (Green, 2010b, 2011).

Theoretical and Empirical Support

At this time, there is a paucity of empirical support for specifically using an analytical child play therapy approach as a part of the multidisciplinary team typically required to treat children with Asperger's syndrome. According to Shunsen (2010), sandplay mediates some of the language barriers of children with autism, stimulates problem solving through simulations in the sand, emphasizes the development of self-reliance and self-control ability via the principles of natural teaching, and improves their imagination and creativeness. In a 10-week school-based action research study with children with autism, Lu, Peterson, Lacroix, and Rousseau (2010) found that sandplay increased verbal expression and symbolic play and improved children's sustained social interaction. The authors concluded that creativity-based interventions, such as Jungian sandplay, provide a complementary approach alongside behavioral models when counseling children with autism. However, substantial research needs to be undertaken before conclusions of efficacy can be made regarding Jungian play's effectiveness with children with Asperger's.

The theoretical support for using Jungian play is that children with Asperger's syndrome have the capacity to communicate verbally, a core requirement for the analytical process. Liu, Shih, and Ma (2011) described how children with Asperger's syndrome scored equal to and often superior to their typically developing peers in areas of creativity and originality. Jungian play therapy incorporates symbol work, which requires children to use creative and original play within the psychotherapy. Therefore, children with Asperger's syndrome may find Jungian play to be appealing and complementary to their attributes and strengths, which may promote self-motivation to resolve psychosocial difficulties.

Temple Grandin (2006) observes that many high-functioning children with AS view the world in pictures or images, and they make sense of external stimuli through visual thinking. This view would be complementary to the analytical premise that symbols and images created in drawings, read about in myths, and enacted in sandplay are integral to a child's psychological growth. Grandin, herself a leading voice and doctoral scholar with autism, comments, "Every problem I've ever solved started with my ability to visualize and see the world in pictures" (p. 4). Her views are substantiated as research demonstrates many high-functioning children with autism score equivalent or superior to their typical developing peers in visuo-perceptual processing (Bertone, Mottron, Jelenic, & Faubert, 2005; Caron, Mottron, Rainville, & Chouinard, 2004).

The term *analysis*, from Jungian *analytical* play therapy, refers to reducing complexes into taut, understandable components through visual means. In play therapy with children, analysis means listening to and observing children to elucidate the complexes that are creating anomalies and need mediation to reduce stress and make meaning out of psychosocial difficulties. Many children with AS rely heavily on the left-brain hemispheric section where analytical processing occurs as opposed to right-brain intuiting and emoting (Rosenn, 2009). So from this viewpoint, Jungian play therapy may be beneficial to children with AS because the therapist may be able to more easily empathize with children's disparate inner world that is sometimes emotionally flat and monotonous, as children with AS may place considerable passion into analytical, rule-based activities (Grandin, 2006). Jungian analyst Michael Fordham (1976) illustrates this concept in his book *The Self and Autism*, as he provides anecdotal support from his various clinical cases when using Jungian child analysis with high-functioning children with autism.

Daniel Rosenn (2009), a medical doctor and expert on Asperger's syndrome, commented on the inherent difficulties but importance of incorporating insight-based psychotherapy (in contrast to cognitive-behavioral therapy) with children with AS:

> After a great deal of tactful and thoughtful effort on the therapist's part, the patient experiences deeply emotional insights or self-revelations, and these presumably lead to internal change and adaptation. These also are very hard to harvest in Asperger's, where most therapy is cognitive behavioral, and relies on patterning of external behaviors and actions. If you are the kind of therapist who searches for these moments of affective transcendency, it can be like panning for gold nuggets in a muddy Sacramento River. So insight-oriented psychotherapy can be very lonely and empty. There are many adults and even older children with Asperger's, with whom one can do satisfying humanistic-relational therapy. (p. 7)

The reader is advised to continue to survey the most current effective treatments and consider incorporating aspects of analytical therapy into their treatment of children with Asperger's syndrome if they deem it may be beneficial to the child and in conjunction with a multidisciplinary team.

Case Example

Background, Presenting Concerns, Assessments

Anthony, a child diagnosed with Asperger's syndrome, was 7 years old when I first met him in the playroom. He had been referred to me by his behavioral analyst. At that time, he was being treated by a multidisciplinary team, including the behaviorist who would visit him at school two times per week for 30 minutes, a school psychologist who had him partaking in group counseling and provided him psychoeducation on Asperger's syndrome, and a pediatric neurologist. A comprehensive assessment for Asperger's syndrome was done a few months before I began counseling him, including a detailed developmental history and review of social, communication, and behavioral development. Specifically, his chart included data from psychometric assessments including the Wechsler Intelligence Scale for Children-Revised (WISC-R) and the Autism Diagnostic Observation Schedule, which was used to observe social behaviors at school necessary for a diagnosis. The Autism Diagnostic Observation Schedule is a semi-structured interview that requires established reliability and conducted by clinicians who specialize in autism spectrum disorders, some of which includes free play (Toth & King, 2008). The results of his assessments indicated a child who scored high in intelligence, had a low frustration tolerance, was socially inhibited, and scored exceptionally high in creativity and imaginative abilities. His history showed that he had intact cognitive ability (absence of mental retardation or intellectual disability) and no delays in early language milestones but was disproportionately anxious. His primary therapy was applied behavioral analysis, and he received social skills competency training from his school psychologist. His comprehensive treatment accentuated his strengths, targeted specific areas of impairment (socialization and academics) as well as comorbid medical or psychiatric disorders, and was implemented across settings to ensure success and generalization of skills. I was brought in as a targeted intervention specialist to augment his more broad-based intervention approaches to assist him in making meaningful connections with peers.

His mother informed me upon our first interview that Anthony needed help with identifying and expressing his feelings and improving his capacity to be comfortable in social situations with peers, especially during the school day. According to his chart and later corroborated by his mother and one of this teachers, there were many incidents at school where teachers reported Anthony would withdraw and refuse to comply with directions and further learning. This seemed to be a product of a distressful social interaction Anthony would have with peers. Fortunately, all of the adults I spoke to and observed interacting with Anthony seemed fond of him and showed him care and respectful treatment. Anthony was fully integrated into a private school in the southern portion of the United States. His grades fluctuated between straight A's and periodic C's in science and reading. I conducted my own extended developmental assessment, including observing him at school, at home interacting with his family (composed of a mother, father, and one younger brother), and in the playroom. I also conducted consultations with his teachers, principal, and close family members (including his grandparents on his mother's side) who provided me input into Anthony's current psychosocial struggles. The consensus was that Anthony was benefiting from the behavioral analysis as he was learning to mediate his anxiety in school and at home. His mother was directly involved with the behavioral treatment and was open and receptive to feedback regarding changes in parenting and discipline to more fully support her son.

As for his presenting problems, some of the children at school were teasing him about being different because he was quiet and often introverted. His mother indicated that a couple of the boys at his school called him "weird." There were a couple of incidents at home that his mother reported where he became intensely angry and violently threw things at her or would try to break whatever was in front of him. She remarked that these hostile occurrences were not frequent and were usually precipitated by her trying to comfort him after a difficult day at school. She also commented that one of his repetitive behaviors was staring at himself in front of the bathroom mirror for lengthy periods of time in silence. She was advised by the behaviorist not to disrupt this activity unless it induced stress in the child.

I worked primarily with Anthony's mother because his father had a demanding work schedule and was often unavailable for consultations. She and I met every 2 weeks for a parent consultation. Anthony's parents were both highly educated and would be classified in the upper-middle-class socioeconomic status. They had tremendous resources and used their financial leverage to assist their child with securing services. Anthony had a primarily positive relationship with both of his parents. He would draw things for them and regularly sit next to either one while watching TV in the living room. They also provided him and his brother lots of positive attention and were seemingly content. There was no indication or admission of trauma, neglect, or abuse in Anthony's childhood history. Anthony also had a significant social support system with his extended family members, who would visit the household multiple times a month. I worked with Anthony twice per week for approximately 5 months.

Implementation of Model

During our first 2 weeks of play therapy, Anthony was relatively quiet. He regularly engaged in symbolic and spontaneous play, especially gravitating toward the sand tray and figurines. He spent most of our time together during this initial *orientation* phase massaging the sand with his hands and creating sand worlds in silence. I attempted to discuss the sand scenes with him afterward, as outlined in a previous section in this chapter, but he did not respond to my questions. He validated my initial clinical impression that he lived primarily in an interior world.

I began using interpretations as he built the sand worlds after the first couple of weeks, and then, interestingly, he began to verbalize. The first verbal communication involved his sand world of chaos and destruction.

It was filled with little green army men and one red dragon and one green dragon with fire coming out of its mouth. The dragons would annihilate all of the army men, and Anthony would make death-cry sounds as the army men perished. I made the interpretation, "Seems like the dragons are really angry at the army men and want to show them how powerful they are." I interpreted he was projecting his inner world of splitting between good and bad objects, possibly similar to what he experienced day after day at school with wanting to be accepted by peers but not knowing how to connect. Therefore, he split and saw others as bad and needing to be destroyed (children sometimes use the death or *thanatos* wish to convey disappearance or removal of). His play began to modify slightly after I began making interpretations while he created his sand worlds of destructive violence and carnage. At one point, he made a laughing noise with the red dragon after he knocked several dead army men out of the sand tray. I responded, "He's happy now that those army men won't hurt him any longer. He's showing them that he's not going to be hurt anymore." His anxious play began to diminish, and he, for the first time, responded, "Yes, the dragon hates these bad guys because they're trying to kill him, and he just wants to live." I analyzed this interaction as Anthony differentiating between good and bad self-objects that were being projected into the sand scene. On one hand, he was feeling omnipotent because he was closely identifying with the symbol of the dragon, which was breathing fire. Jung referred to creating fire as an instinctive behavior related to rhythmic activities from a primitive source. I interpreted Anthony's use of fire to destroy the army men as part of his psyche's *prima materia* being activated in the symbolic play constellation. This provided me with an inference about his unconscious affect, whether defensive or instinctual, that needed to be explored further.

During the next couple of months, Anthony's play could be primarily characterized as the *working-through* phase. He began verbalizing more. He added tremendous narrative content to his sand worlds and seemed to have developed a sense of trust in the analytic relationship. I would make interpretations during his play, and he would sometimes respond and other times continue playing as if he hadn't heard me. As time passed on, some of his sand worlds become anxious and aggressive. I permitted this intense display of aggression since I wanted to uncover the core of his hostility. I needed to ascertain the ideas, fantasies, and beliefs connected with this rage. Some of his violent play included throwing some of the army men at the wall and replying, "Now you're dead, bitch!" I would not stop his affective display of rage but interpreted, "I bet sometimes you wish some of those mean boys at your school would disappear so they can't hurt you anymore." At this point, I interpreted he was living in a terrorized imaginal state. His projections consistently depicted his experience of fantastic ideas and objects as inherently maligning. He exteriorized his conflicts, and I made reflective statements to show him I understood how scary his inner world could be at times. After hearing this comment, he responded acutely, "Yes, they don't like me and I don't know why." His aggression began to sublimate into sadness or despair at this point. It is these feelings that are so important for the therapist to discriminate, as these underlying feelings, which prompt a child's rage, are more important than the rage itself. In this moment, Anthony reached out and began to internalize a good enough father imago within me. I replied, "It sounds like you want to be liked and accepted but don't know how to make friends, and that makes you feel different and strange."

After hearing this last interpretation, he began to cry. He came over to where I was sitting and gave me a hug. This was the first time in our 6 weeks or so of therapy that Anthony physically acknowledged my presence. Before, I was simply another object in the playroom. And he sat there, for a couple of minutes, and cried. I comforted him, and then he sat on a chair across from me and looked down at the floor. I remember his mother telling me that she would offer advice to her son about making friends and sometimes became frustrated when Anthony wouldn't follow her instruction, which would prompt his raging at home. Instead of trying to rescue the child from his despair (which I believe he was anticipating that I would do), I let him sit with the pain. Jung said that to get through the depression we must enter it. And that was an extremely difficult moment for me to get through as clinician as I was experiencing countertransference of wanting to protect him and shield him from the psychogenic pain he was experiencing. The session ended with grounding the child back to his external reality. I asked him to color a mandala. He created an intricate design with dark hues of colors, including black, deep blue, and brown. The mandala he chose was a circle shape with many triangles interlocking. This activity seemed to noticeably calm his affect, as research has found that coloring mandalas can be a soothing activity that decreases anxiety (Henderson, Rosen, & Mascaro, 2007). When the session ended, he gave me a hug and said good-bye.

During the next several weeks of therapy, Anthony remained limited in his verbal interactions with me. His mother began reporting that he appeared less anxious at home and had no meltdowns, and his teachers found him to be less obstinate in class. It seems as though he was indeed aware of his feelings but not overly concerned or even aware of the feelings of others. Sometimes it seemed as though I was doing therapy alone, as he seemed emotionally detached from the play. As the therapy continued, Anthony began to manipulate a small mirror sand figurine. At first, he would include it in his sand scenes by placing it impulsively in the world without much discernable reason. Then he began making it the centerpiece of his play. His mother disclosed to me during our interviews that

Anthony would sometimes stare in the mirror at home for long periods of time. I interpreted his scenes, but I could get no response. His mind was expressing its aptitude for symbolic expression, but I had not yet recognized the myth in which his psyche was unfolding.

During our sessions, I would sometimes read to him fairy tales or myths and ask him to sand a world afterward. During one session, I read the Greek myth of Echo and Narcissus. I explained to him how a mountain nymph (and love-struck admirer) named Echo chased after the beautiful god boy Narcissus who was not all that interested in her. Narcissus had been pursued by many maidens but was excessively proud and wanted nothing to do with them. One day Echo could only use her voice to repeat back the last few words of the other person during a conversation. One day, she attempted to profess her love for him in the forest, and proud Narcissus coldly rejected her. He thought she was a lowly handmaiden, and he wanted nothing to do with her and her repetitive words. One day Narcissus went out hunting and stopped at a fountain to drink. He saw a beautiful image, his reflection. Not knowing it was his him, he admired the reflection. He became enamored by it, so much that he stayed at that fountain staring and talking to his own image. Narcissus withered and turned into a flower after realizing that the image in the fountain was a reflection, like a mirror, and therefore incapable of expressing love. He died lonely and heartbroken. I asked Anthony to sand a world from the story. He made an immediate comparison as he was smoothing the sand: "Me and him both like mirrors." I replied, "Yes, it seems as though you two have something in common."

Anthony then sanded a world with a small blue pool in the middle of the tray. Next to the pool was one male figure and one princess fairy figurine, and a mirror was placed in between the two figures. I asked him to tell me about the scene. "Echo wants to get close to Narcissus. But he doesn't like her because she bothers him. So he told her to leave him alone. But she won't. So he put a mirror between them so she couldn't see him and he could see himself. He liked looking at himself because it was better than looking at Echo." In this projective scene, I interpreted Anthony connecting to the elements inherent within the myth and correlating his subjective experience of feeling socially isolated and alone. Because he did not have the capacity to form social bonds, perhaps it was easier for him and less anxiety-provoking for him to isolate himself behind a façade or mirror. I responded, "What would happen if Narcissus removed the mirror?" Anthony hesitantly looked at me and responded emphatically, "He wouldn't!" So I tried again, "I'm wondering what it would be like if Narcissus felt that Echo wouldn't hurt him. Maybe if he trusted others and himself more? What would it be like then?" Anthony stood quietly for a moment then removed the mirror between them and placed it to the side.

He said, "Narcissus would probably talk to her and tell her he just wants people to like him." So I instructed him to talk through the characters and tell me what it would sound like. He went on to describe Narcissus and Echo having a conversation about taking turns swimming in the pool, but Narcissus told Echo she couldn't ever stare at him too long. Shortly after this scene ended, I asked Anthony to draw a mandala before he left. In his mandala, he depicted a large circle with a blue star in the middle. He also placed some blue star stickers on the mandala as well. I asked him what the title of his mandala was, and he responded with a smile, "Me."

During our next session, he continued sanding a world with the Narcissus and Echo until the mirror finally disappeared and Echo and Narcissus were seemingly friends. He said they enjoyed playing together. I made the interpretation, "Anthony, seems like Narcissus finally let his guard down. Even after being bothered by other nymphs, he finally allowed himself to get close to Echo, and she was nice to him. And he realized he could make friends with Echo and maybe other nymphs if he just trusted in himself. Removing that mirror was a big, scary step." He slightly accepted my interpretation: "Yeah, maybe so." Shortly after this session, the mother reported to me that Anthony asked if he could have a playdate with another boy at his school. This was the first playdate Anthony had ever been on, surprisingly. She asked if I had suggestions to make things go OK so he would want to do it again, and I responded, "Trust yourself and him, and let him be who he is. He needs to play and figure out who is in relation to others. If things don't go well, he'll figure out how to improve. Or maybe he'll ask your help." That playdate went well, fortunately. The mother said the boys played with Anthony's Star Wars LEGO set and built a scene, and there was no tension.

The following week (the reparation/termination stage), Anthony spent most of our play time sanding a world with a castle and many fairies at the top of a mountain he built with moon sand. He placed a gold jewel at the bottom of the mountain. I asked him to tell me about the story of his scene. He said that the fairy princesses had finally found their lost golden egg. One of the princesses had dropped it when she was playing, but they found it and now everyone is happy because it's magical. The psychology of the child archetype here, mainly the "divine child," was activated. Anthony identified in this symbolic play with an omnipotent power that was regained and brought great joy to everyone in the kingdom. He produced the symbols, and he followed them, through carnage and war to magic golden eggs. At this point in therapy, I knew we had gone as far as we could go. Anthony was showing small increments of improvement in his attitude at school and was starting to make new friends. His play at school transformed from scattered, chaotic, and violent to organized, coherent, and even mystical. During this time, he began building trust with others because some of the children who were teasing him stopped. The school psychologist and I worked together to formulate a guidance curriculum on bullying. It seems to have alleviated some of the harassment he and other children were experiencing. Also, though still quiet and seemingly comfortable with being alone, Anthony started to try to use his own unique style of relating to objects to people. As he had worked through conflicts in the sand world, he began to externalize his new found inner reserves. He began to trust in himself and realize that he was worthy to make friend with others and that they wouldn't always hurt him.

Outcome

Anthony's outcome within our psychotherapy was relatively positive. My goals were to enhance his ego-self axis so that he had a strong, valid connection between his rich inner world and sometimes bewildering outer world. Second, I wanted to help him develop a symbolic attitude so that he would follow symbols and allow them to lead to healing. Also, we aimed to help him feel more comfortable with making social bonds. Before this occurred, Anthony needed to internalize that he could trust others and they would not always hurt him. Though Anthony's myth-making may have looked like pure archetypal imagery, there were clear links between his inner and outer realities. He was able to see his *potential future*, as Jung described it (Fordham, 1976), inherent within the symbolic expressions of the self-symbols related to the Narcissus myth. This identification helped compensate his conscious attitude with instinctual root systems of belief, including the potential for wholeness. Once he saw that Narcissus was not happy being alone with only his reflection, he was able to make the affective shift in his own self-alienation. I hypothesized that Anthony's individuating function had already been set in motion before he began working with me based on his material. His strong family and school support systems were working hard to create a cohesive environment for this child. Though I believe some of my interpretations were facilitative, there is clear evidence this child was on his own path to growth. The dialectic was never severed for too long, which undoubtedly helped Anthony, as our biweekly sessions provided a holding effect for his anxieties surrounding socialization. After analyzing this case, I have come to realize that my analysis and play time with him was subsidiary as I did not cure him of his social woes but only provided an environment in which his own therapy was nurtured.

Guidelines for Incorporating Jungian Play With a Child with Asperger's Syndrome

The clinician looking to incorporate analytical play with a child with Asperger's syndrome should do so only in the context of sufficient training with symbol work and in conjunction with a multidisciplinary team of professionals. Furthermore, the clinician will want to have a solid foundation in sandplay and the archetypal imagery inherent throughout. Second, clinicians should be advised that interpretations are extremely important when facilitating change by using analytical play. Therefore, only highly verbal and high-functioning children with autism would be appropriate with this modality. Last, clinicians need to know beforehand that it can at times be a lonely place in the playroom since a hallmark of this population is the difficulty to socially or empathically connect with others. Therefore, clinicians wanting to work with this population by using analytical play should approach it with care and collaborative reliance on the support of other professionals in the field. By reaching out to the inner dimensions of a child with Asperger's syndrome with compassion and dynamic understanding, clinicians are able to help children mitigate psychological obstacles so that they may see their own resplendent reflections, out of which meaningful social bonds may be formulated.

References

Allan, J. (1988). *Inscapes of the Child's World*. Dallas, TX: Spring Publications, Inc.

Bertone, A., Mottron, L., Jelenic, P., & Faubert, J. (2005). Enhanced and diminished visuo-spatial Information processing in autism depends on stimulus activity. *Brain: A Journal of Neurology, 128*(10), 2430–2441.

Caron, M. J., Mottron, L., Rainville, C., & Chouinard, S. (2004). Do high functioning persons with autism present superior spatial abilities? *Neurospsychologia, 42*(4), 467–481.

De Domenico, G. (1994). Jungian play therapy techniques. In K. J. O'Connor & C. E. Schaefer (Eds.), *Handbook of play therapy: Advances and Innovations* (2nd ed., pp. 253–282). New York: John Wiley & Sons.

Fincher, S. (2004). *Coloring mandalas* (2nd ed.). Boston, MA: Shambhala.

Fordham, M. (1944). *The life of childhood*. London: Routledge.

Fordham, M. (1976). *The self and autism*. London: William Heinemann Medical Books.

Grandin, T. (2006). *Thinking in pictures: My life with autism* (2nd ed.). New York: Vintage Books.

Green, E. (2007). The crisis of family separation following traumatic mass destruction: Jungian analytical play therapy in the aftermath of hurricane Katrina. In N. B. Webb (Ed.), *Play therapy with children in crisis: Individual, group, and family treatment* (3rd ed., pp. 368–388). New York: The Guilford Press.

Green, E. J. (2008). Re-envisioning Jungian analytical play therapy with child sexual assault survivors. *International Journal of Play Therapy, 17*(2), 102–121.

Green, E. J. (2009). Jungian analytical play therapy. In K. J. O'Connor & L. D. Braverman (Eds.), *Play therapy theory and practice: Comparing theories and techniques* (2nd ed., pp. 83–122). Hoboken, NJ: John Wiley & Sons.

Green, E. J. (2010a). Jungian play therapy with adolescents. *Play Therapy, 5*(2), 20–23.

Green, E. J. (2010b). Traversing the heroic journey: Jungian play therapy with children. *Counseling Today, 52*(9), 40–43.

Green, E. J. (2011). Jungian analytical play therapy. In C. Schaefer (Ed.), *Foundations of play therapy* (2nd ed., pp. 60–86). Hoboken, NJ: John Wiley & Sons.

Green, E. J., & Gibbs, K. (2010). Jungian sand play for preschool children with disruptive behavioral problems. In C. Schaefer (Ed.), *Play therapy for preschool children* (pp. 223–244). Washington, DC: APA.

Henderson, P., Rosen, D., & Mascaro, N. (2007). Empirical study on the healing nature of mandalas. *Psychology of Aesthetics, Creativity and the Arts, 1*(3), 148–154.

Jung, C. G. (1910). Psychic conflicts in the child. In H. Read, M. Fordham, & G. Adler (Eds.), *The collected works of C. G. Jung (Vol. 17)*. Princeton, NJ: Princeton University Press.

Jung, C. G. (1913). The theory of psychoanalysis. In H. Read, M. Fordham, & G. Adler (Eds.), *The collected works of C. G. Jung (Vol. 4)*. Princeton, NJ: Princeton University Press.

Jung, C. G. (1951). The psychology of the child archetype. In H. Read, M. Fordham, & G. Adler (Eds.), *The collected works of C. G. Jung (Vol. 9)*. Princeton, NJ: Princeton University Press.

Jung, C. G. (2008). *Children's dreams*. Princeton, NJ: Princeton University Press.

Jung, C. G. (2009). *The red book*. New York: W. W. Norton & Company.

Kalff, D. (1980). *Sandplay: A psychotherapeutic approach to the psyche*. Boston: Sigo Press.

Liu, M., Shih, W., & Ma, L. (2011). Are children with Asperger syndrome creative in divergent thinking and feeling? A brief report. *Research in Autism Spectrum Disorders, 5*(1), 294–298.

Lu, L., Petersen, F., Lacroix, L., & Rousseau, C. (2010). Stimulating creative play in children with autism through sandplay. *Arts in Psychotherapy, 37*(1), 56–64.

Rosenn, D. (2009). Asperger connections 2008 keynote speech. *Asperger's Association of New England Journal, 4*, 5–8.

Shunsen, C. (2010). The principles and operations of sand play therapy on children with autism. *Chinese Journal of Special Education, 4*(3), 11–22.

Steinhardt, L. (2000). *Foundation and form in Jungian sandplay*. Philadelphia: Jessica Kingsley.

Toth, K., & King, B. H. (2008). Asperger's syndrome: Diagnosis and treatment. *American Journal of Psychiatry, 165*, 958–963.

CHAPTER 10

Communication and Connection

Filial Therapy With Families of Children With ASD

RISË VANFLEET

Introduction to Filial Therapy

Filial therapy (FT) was the brainchild of Drs. Bernard and Louise Guerney in the late 1950s, and they developed it and the subsequent Relationship Enhancement approach to family therapy throughout their careers. FT is a theoretically integrative psychoeducational model of therapy in which parents serve as the primary change agents for their children. In essence, it is a form of family therapy that uses play therapy methods to enhance parent–child relationships and to resolve a wide range of child and family problems. During FT, therapists teach and supervise parents as they conduct nondirective play sessions with their own children. Parents learn a set of skills that include structuring, empathic attunement, child-centered imaginary play, and limit setting, through which they offer their children a safe and accepting environment with opportunities for the expression of feelings, communication, and resolution of social, emotional, and behavioral problems. With the therapist's guidance, parents also learn to attend to the meanings that play has for their children. The deeper understanding that ensues often shifts parents' negative attitudes and beliefs about their children, helps parents cooperate more effectively with each other, reduces parental stress and frustration, and motivates parents to change some of their own behaviors to create better family relationships.

The theoretical foundations, methods, applications, and research on FT are described in detail elsewhere (Guerney, 1983; VanFleet, 2005, 2006; VanFleet & Guerney, 2003; VanFleet & Sniscak, in press; VanFleet & Topham, 2011). A brief introduction is included here.

Theoretical Foundations

FT represents a comprehensive and thoughtful integration of a number of leading theories: psychodynamic, humanistic, behaviorism and learning theory, interpersonal, cognitive, developmental and attachment, and family systems. Despite significant differences in the underlying assumptions and methods drawn from these theories, their integration is possible because of the psychoeducational nature of FT. Therapists serve as both clinicians and educators, sharing with clients skills and information about child development, parenting, and play while supporting parents as they learn and use these skills with their own children. For example, therapists use empathy and acceptance with parents just as they teach the parents to use the same with their children. Psychodynamic theory offers an understanding of the symbolism and dynamic features of children's play as well as attention to individual, parent, and family dynamics that impact the problems and their resolution. Behaviorism and learning theory contribute the limit-setting process for children and much of the training process for parents, in which parent skill development is accomplished through positive reinforcement, shaping, modeling, and immediate behavioral feedback. Interpersonal psychology and family systems approaches provide a focus on the reciprocal nature of parent–child relationships, and developmental and attachment theories contribute an understanding of child behavior, play themes, the importance of attunement, and the interplay of child exploration and return to a secure base (the parents). Other resources discuss the theoretical components of FT in greater detail (Cavedo & Guerney, 1999; Ginsberg, 2003; VanFleet, 2009, 2011).

Methods

The intervention of FT is deceptively simple. It is straightforward in that the therapist trains parents to conduct the special play sessions with their children, supervises them until they master the skills of doing so, and then helps them transition the play sessions to the home environment where their newfound skills can be generalized. Even so, FT is family therapy, and families are complex and unwieldy at times. Filial therapists must be highly trained as play therapists, have excellent skills for engaging and interacting with parents, and be able to negotiate through the complexities of family relations. Specific methods employed in FT are described briefly here and are available in greater detail elsewhere (Guerney & Ryan, in press; VanFleet, 2005, 2006).

After the assessment and recommendation for FT, the therapist guides parents through several phases of treatment: training, supervised play sessions, home play sessions, and generalization. The entire process typically takes between 15 and 17 1-hour sessions, and it can be applied with families experiencing great distress or as a preventive program. Although it is suited best for children between the ages of 2 and 12 when imaginary play is most active, it has been applied with some types of problems with children as old as 16. This is particularly applicable for traumatized children or children with special needs, where social and emotional development may lag behind that of their peers.

Therapists usually train parents in three to four sessions. First, the therapist conducts a child-centered play session with each child, one at a time, while parents observe. This is followed by a discussion of parent observations and things the therapist wishes to point out. Next, training continues with role played play sessions in which the therapist plays the child role and simultaneously provides encouraging feedback to parents as they practice the skills. In this way, therapists can help parents learn the skills quickly and without pressure.

Parents learn four skills for use during the filial play sessions: (1) structuring; (2) empathic listening; (3) child-centered imaginary play; and (4) limit setting. These are the same skills used by child-centered play therapists (VanFleet, Sywulak, & Sniscak, 2010). *Structuring skill* involves room entry and departure and provides a way to distinguish the special nature of the play sessions from everyday life. Parents learn a room entry statement and give 5- and 1-minute warnings that the session is coming to a close. *Empathic listening* involves watching children closely and briefly rephrasing what they are doing in the play. Parents learn how important it is to reflect children's emotions when present: "Jimmy, you really like that big dragon. He's fierce and powerful." Parents also learn to reflect the feelings of characters in their children's play: "That horse is really sad that the farmer yelled at him." *Child-centered imaginary play* involves the parent engaging in pretend play when children assign a role. They are to play the role as the child wishes, following verbal and nonverbal cues. The parent follows the child's lead but takes on the character role much as an actor or actress would do. One boy, a victim of domestic violence, asked his mother to play a princess and told her to scream. She did as he wished, and he put on a police hat and came to her rescue, clearly enacting issues relating to his trauma. Finally, *limit setting* involves handling situations in which the child is not permitted to engage in certain behaviors, usually because they are destructive or unsafe. Filial therapists teach parents to use a three-step procedure of stating the limit, giving a warning if it happens a second time (including a statement that the session will end if it happens a third time), and enforcing the consequence the third time by ending the session. This procedure helps reestablish parental authority when it is needed.

Next, parents conduct the special play sessions with their children, one on one, while the therapist observes. Filial play sessions at this point range from 15 to 30 minutes. If both parents or more than one caregiver is involved, they sit with the therapist and watch each other's sessions, continuing to learn vicariously. Immediately after the play session, the therapist meets with the parents to provide skill feedback and to discuss the themes of the child's play and the parents' reaction to them. This feedback period focuses heavily on what the parent did well and provides just one or two suggestions for improvement next time. The theme discussions begin to help parents see the possible meanings behind the child's play.

After holding three or four parent–child play sessions with feedback, most parents become quite skillful in conducting them. More emphasis is then placed during postplay discussions on the play themes and how they relate to the child's feelings, perceptions, struggles, and wishes. The therapist's job is to continue to encourage the parents' skillful conduct of the play sessions and to help them gain an accurate understanding from the point of view of each of their children.

After the therapist has directly observed between four and six play sessions for each parent (often with different children), parents usually are quite skillful in conducting them and are able to recognize and interpret play themes quite well. The filial therapist then helps the parents plan to conduct the sessions weekly with each child at home. This requires a special set of toys to keep the sessions special and distinguishable from other forms of everyday play. Planning also includes the location in the home best suited for the play sessions and how to manage interruptions and scheduling so that it least interferes with family life.

During the home session phase of FT, parents conduct weekly filial play sessions at home with each of their children and meet with the therapist weekly or biweekly to discuss them. During these meetings, parents report on the play sessions, their own skills, aspects that went well, and questions that they have. If they are able to make a video, the therapist might review portions of that with them. They also discuss play themes and how they relate to behaviors in daily life. Once this process is moving forward smoothly, the therapist helps parents begin to generalize the use of the skills. In each session, the therapist covers how specific skills are adapted for daily use, gives examples, and asks the parents to practice use of the skills outside the play sessions as well. This is done in a gradual manner to avoid overwhelming the parents. Usually at this point the parents are quite skillful and have seen positive results, and they are motivated to use the skills at other times. Play themes continue to be monitored, as are the real-life behaviors that brought the family to therapy in the beginning.

Once the therapeutic goals have been achieved and parents are competent and confident in conducting the play sessions, a planned conclusion of FT is implemented. Weekly sessions become biweekly; biweekly sessions become triweekly or monthly. Parents continue to hold play sessions at home as long as the children enjoy them and benefit from them, even after formal therapy sessions have ceased.

Research

The efficacy of FT has been supported by nearly 50 years of research. A meta-analysis of play therapy research (Bratton, Ray, Rhine, & Jones, 2005) examined 93 controlled and comparison-group studies of play therapy, including 22 FT studies. The analysis clearly showed the strongest outcomes when parents were involved and highlighted the value of FT. VanFleet, Ryan, and Smith (2005) reviewed the FT research literature, including the historical research as well as 10 more recent controlled studies. In general, the research has shown significant gains in parental empathy and acceptance, parent skills, child behavior, parent stress, and satisfaction with family life. Most recently, Topham, Wampler, Titus, and Rolling (2011) studied a 10-hour FT program following the sequence described here with 27 parent–child dyads. Parents who initially reported higher levels of distress and child behavior problems showed greater reduction in child problems and greater increase in their acceptance, providing preliminary evidence that FT is effective with parents and children with more severe problems, such as poor regulation of emotion, less social support, and more parent distress.

Filial Therapy With Families of Children With ASD

To the author's knowledge, FT has not been widely used with families of children with ASD, nor has any controlled research on FT been conducted with this population. Clinical outcomes and case studies, however, indicate that the potential benefits of FT for these families warrant further consideration and study. Josefi and Ryan (2004) examined the use of nondirective play therapy with a 6-year-old boy with severe ASD, finding preliminary evidence that it appeared to enhance his social and emotional development. Following incorporation of FT with Greenspan's Floortime approach (Wieder & Greenspan, 2005), Duffy (2008) documented positive parent reactions and improved acceptance of FT (Hamilton, personal communication). While there have been ongoing efforts to apply the basic skills, principles, and some features of FT with adolescents and young adults (Pinson, personal communication), this chapter concentrates on its use with younger children, approximately 3 to 12 years of age.

There are a number of reasons FT offers potential benefit to families of children with ASD. First, the nondirective play sessions offer an avenue of expression and communication to children with ASD. While the play of children with ASD differs from that of typically developing children in terms of its reduced flexibility, repetitiveness, and predominance of exploratory play (Jarrold, 2003; Kasari, Freeman, & Paparella, 2006), they nevertheless play. The motivation to play exists when the opportunity is presented, and various forms of play therapy have been applied with good clinical result (Kaduson, 2006). It seems reasonable that when children's ability to express themselves is thwarted, play therapy, which does not rely on verbal or adult forms of communication, might offer an avenue for expression of their feelings, frustrations, and point of view. The nondirective play sessions in FT provide children with play choices that are physically and emotionally safe and comfortable, without pressure to communicate in any given manner. The parents learn to hold back their own questions, ideas, or plans and permit their children to lead the way. By following their children's lead, the parents allow them to explore and express as needed, permit them to work through problems through play, and learn to attune better to their feelings and needs.

Siblings of children with ASD can also benefit from FT. In the full-family therapy form of FT, parents conduct special one-to-one play sessions with all of their children between 3 and 12 years old as well as special child-centered activity times with adolescents (VanFleet, 2005). Siblings of children with ASD appear to be at elevated risk for impairments in social functioning (Yoder, Stone, Walden, & Malesa, 2009), and FT offers the same potential benefits for them to play, express, and be better understood by their parents as with their sibling with ASD. FT gives them the same opportunities for working through problems and testing possible solutions in their play as well. Furthermore, as happens with chronic medical illness in a brother or sister (VanFleet, 1985), siblings of children with ASD may forego some parental attention due to the amount of family energy necessary for coping with the special needs of the child with ASD. A half-hour filial play session per week with each of the other children does not add significant pressure for parents (except in large families) yet helps siblings feel included, special, and cared for. The play sessions also give siblings a chance to express their own feelings, fears, resentments, and hopes through their play and to be heard by their parents. In addition, the filial play sessions have been shown to lead to better problem solving and resolution, even under difficult circumstances. It seems likely that siblings of children with ASD would benefit similarly.

The third area in which FT can be useful to families is in improving how the parents feel about their children and themselves while at the same time giving parents useful skills they can use throughout their children's lives. Studies have suggested that parents of children with ASD can experience depression, anxiety, frustration, fatigue, and significant stress largely based on their children's behavior problems and severity of the ASD (Carter, de L. Martinez-Pedraza, & Gray, 2009; Lyons, Leon, Phelps, & Dunleavy, 2010; Seltzer et al., 2010). Having a child with special needs requires much of parents, and when the child has difficulty communicating and participating fully in relationships, it can be very difficult for parents. Parents often report to therapists that they feel "worn out" by dealing with the child's inflexibility, odd social behaviors, tantrums, and "continuously trying to figure out what's going on." Managing medical, therapy, and special school appointments can also be overwhelming. Although FT adds one more intervention to the mix, it is time limited and provides real coping skills that parents can use at home to help all their children.

FT is an empowering approach, and in the case of children with ASD perhaps it is most empowering of the parents. Competent filial therapists engage the parents as true partners in the therapeutic process, listening to them empathically and considering their input of great importance. Parents receive substantial emotional support while they learn to conduct the play sessions, and therapists help parents understand the possible meanings of their children's play with sensitivity and genuine concern for the impact on the parents. Much as the parents learn to provide a safe and accepting environment for their children through the play sessions, therapists provide a safe and accepting environment where parents can talk about their distress and discover possible solutions to parenting problems. One mother of a child with ASD told the author that the support she received during FT allowed her to voice her long-held fears that there was something wrong with her because she was so frustrated with and disconnected from her son. The empathic conversation that ensued helped her realize that her feelings were normal under the circumstances.

Perhaps of greatest benefit is the potential of FT to open the lines of communication between parents and children with ASD. Reliance on verbal communication can be difficult if not impossible. Using the language of play, parents can gain insight into their child's world without the need of spoken language. While children can and do talk during the filial play sessions, their most important feelings and wishes are gleaned from their play. As therapists help parents understand the potential meanings of children's play, and as patterns in the play confirm these hypotheses, parents become excited by the possibility that they can understand their children in a new way. As one filial therapist experienced in using FT with families of children with ASD stated, "The parents are excited that they now have a way to communicate with their child. They begin to understand things they never did before, and they're excited about what they're learning" (Pinson, personal communication). In the author's experience conducting and supervising FT with children with ASD, it is something akin to the "lightbulb being turned on." The parents begin to see how much more they can and will understand about their child with ASD. The language of play and emotional expression transcends many barriers.

Finally, FT can become a focal point for supportive small groups of parents. While it offers specific strategies through the play sessions and has the flexibility to adapt to each unique child and family, it also gives families an opportunity to meet together to discuss what they have learned and how they are implementing the play sessions. FT can be offered to individual families (VanFleet, 2005, 2006), and it can be offered in a variety of group formats, including the original model (Guerney & Ryan, in press; VanFleet & Sniscak, in press) and in several shorter-term group formats (Caplin & Pernet, in press; Landreth & Bratton, 2006; Wright & Walker, 2003).

In summary, while there is scant research on the use of FT specifically with families of children with ASD, the research surrounding the method and the needs of these families merge in such a way that the use of FT with this population deserves consideration. Clinicians who have used FT with children with ASD, their siblings, and their parents have been universally positive about its helpfulness. Anecdotally, a considerable number of parents have reported greater understanding that helps them establish more realistic expectations of their child with ASD and build more positive and relaxed relationships. Parents have also described feeling relieved that they can offer something beneficial to their typically developing children and that these play sessions have improved their relationships and resolved problems with siblings greatly. Clinically administered pre- and post-tests have supported the idea that FT can meet family needs on multiple levels in satisfying ways.

Case Example

The identifying information in the case example that follows has been changed to protect the privacy of the family.

Sylvia and Red brought their 6-year-old son, Alex, to therapy due to his tantrums at home and in school. He had been diagnosed with high-functioning autism, and he had difficulty transitioning from one activity or location to another. When he was urged by adults with a "hurry up" or "let's go," he shook his head rapidly, threw papers or other items, and shouted loudly. While he had done this from the time he was 3, the frequency had increased since he had begun school. His parents and teachers had established routines surrounding transition times, but this helped only minimally. Sylvia and Red expressed much frustration with this behavior and their inability to know how to help him. They were exhausted from trying to determine how to manage Alex's behavior. They had worked with an in-home behavior therapist a year prior who had helped them use a behavior plan consisting of positive reinforcement and extinction (ignoring) strategies. While this had helped in many ways, they felt no closer to Alex, nor did the plan seem to work with the transition behaviors. His parents were also concerned that Alex was developing some unusual behaviors and had no friends.

Alex had a younger brother, Teddy, who was 4. Teddy was a typically developing child who attended a day care program 3 days a week while Sylvia went to her part-time job. Teddy seemed socially well adjusted with good peer relations, and his parents commented, "Thank goodness he's an easy boy! We don't have any problems with his behavior at all."

After my first meeting with Sylvia and Red when we discussed their situation in detail and went through a developmental history, I asked them to bring both boys the following week for a family play observation. They were to go into my playroom to play while I sat unobtrusively in the corner to observe. Both parents tried to pay attention to both boys. Teddy seemed content to play by himself, but he also enjoyed his parents' attention. Frequently, Alex whined or threw objects, seemingly in frustration, and this drew his parents' attention away from Teddy. This pattern was repeated throughout the 20 minutes of the observation. Sylvia's sister had come with them to watch the boys while I discussed the play observation with Sylvia and Red afterward. When asked what was typical or not of that session, they both remarked that it was common for them to pay much more attention to Alex than Teddy. They expressed regret that this was the case. I commented that Alex had seemed a bit fearful in the playroom, and Sylvia said that was common whenever they took him to new places. He spent most of the session looking at the toys and picking up the puppets.

As I recommended FT to Sylvia and Red, they were surprised that I wanted to include Teddy. When I explained that it would be a way to give him some uninterrupted attention and give him a chance to express his feelings, they agreed. I wanted FT to be a whole-family therapy because the stress involved in parenting Alex impacted all of them.

Considering scheduling and child-care difficulties, we completed the training phase of FT in two 90-minute sessions. Both parents were motivated and learned quickly. After we completed the usual two mock play sessions, we added a third so they could prepare for some of Alex's more difficult behaviors. We practiced accepting Alex's feelings of fear and frustration: "You aren't too sure about being here—it's a little scary for you," and "It's frustrating when things change." We also practiced limit setting for any unsafe or destructive behaviors that Alex or Teddy might exhibit, and we planned what each of us would do if Alex broke a limit three times and the play session had to end. This extra training was needed to help them see how the FT skills would apply with Alex as a child with ASD. We also agreed that we would adjust things that did not work well until we found the approach that suited their family the best.

As we moved on to the supervised play session phase of FT, we planned for each parent to have a 15-minute play session with one of the boys followed by a discussion with both parents alone. Because Alex could not tolerate a stranger for child-care purposes during these discussions, the family brought a relative for the six supervised sessions.

In the first three sessions, Alex mostly explored the room. He picked up different toys, occasionally working them briefly. He said little and showed little emotion. His parents took turns holding the filial play sessions, and both of them did quite well reflecting his actions: "You're checking out that puzzle.... Oh, there's something else that is interesting to you.... Those puppets with the teeth are interesting." During the postplay discussion, I suggested ways for them to pace and vary their comments so they would not feel intrusive to Alex. Teddy did exploratory play for the first two sessions and then settled on creating a birthday party for himself. He put on a hat shaped like a birthday cake, invited many of the stuffed animals and puppets to "attend" (sitting around him on the floor), and told his mother that she had to sing to him. Because no one in the family had a birthday at that time, we discussed the possibility that Teddy's play reflected his need to have some special attention. Sylvia became sad when we talked of this, but I was able to reassure her that she was already providing him with special attention with the play sessions. Nevertheless, both parents began to see how Teddy was reveling in their undivided attention during play sessions.

Because the play sessions had gone well, we extended the length to 20 minutes each for the remaining three supervised sessions, still allowing time for skill feedback and discussion of play themes. Alex started with the exploratory play in his fourth play session, but he eventually sat and played with the bendable dinosaurs. The dinosaurs walked around together and eventually went swimming—Alex had created a pool for them by pouring some water into a bowl. The dinosaurs splashed in the water, bouncing up and down. Abruptly, Alex stopped that play and seemed worried, looking around the playroom. Red, who was playing with him that session, commented throughout this sequence as follows: "Those dinosaurs are bouncing around and splashing. They seem to be having fun. It feels good to splash around in the water." These were all excellent examples of empathic listening. Red also reflected, "Gee, something just happened. You're looking for something. You look a little worried." Alex looked at his father for a moment, looked away, and said, "Towel." Red simply said, "You need a towel." He refrained from helping Alex, as Alex had not requested help. Alex then found the paper towels and dried his hands.

This play sequence generated much discussion with Red and Sylvia. Red was pleased that he had been able to understand Alex's play better. He told me that he realized how much he had been "second-guessing" Alex before and how little he was actually listening. I was able to praise his use of the skills. Red told me that it was actually easier to listen this way than to try to imagine what was going on in Alex's mind. The parents were also surprised that Alex was able to state his need to dry his hands and then take care of it for himself. They had not seen this type of independence in him before. Through my empathic listening about this, they realized that they had always been quick to help Alex when he struggled without giving him much chance to try things for himself.

The dinosaurs figured prominently in the remaining two sessions that I supervised directly in my playroom. Alex did not say much and his face remained relatively expressionless, but the dinosaurs' interactions became livelier and more expressive. Sylvia was able to empathically listen as the dinosaurs had an argument: "Those dinos sure are mad. They are having a big fight. That one seems like a big bully. He's pushing everyone around." Again, as she reflected these feelings that seemed accurate in terms of the dinosaur characters, Alex glanced quickly at her and then back at the toys. Because he rarely made eye contact, this seemed significant. This play was repeated during the sixth observed play session with Red, making us wonder if it was a reflection of something happening at school. Rather than try to talk with Alex about it at that point (as that could shut down the play), Sylvia decided to talk with Alex's teacher and counselor, asking them to be alert for any signs of bullying that might be going on.

During the final supervised play sessions, Teddy's play was quite typical of a well-adjusted 4-year-old. He clearly enjoyed playing with each of his parents, and he readily involved them in his play. He asked them to play various characters with the miniatures and the puppets, which they did quite well. He laughed aloud, clearly delighted. Both Red and Sylvia said they enjoyed these sessions with him immensely. They realized that they, too, were missing something important when Teddy was left to his own amusement so much of the time. Teddy was able to give them social feedback in a way that Alex could not. The parents told me that they actually felt "refreshed" after playing with Teddy—that it replenished their energy for dealing with Alex.

Red and Sylvia both conducted the play sessions very well. They recognized play themes easily and were open to discussing their possible meanings for the boys. They were ready to start their home play sessions. Because of their difficulties finding child care for Alex, we decided to meet every other week. They would hold 30-minute filial play sessions with both boys each week and then discuss them with me during our sessions. They could call in between if needed.

Although Alex still showed little emotion facially, he willingly participated in the play sessions. He continued dinosaur play at home, but the specific dinosaur behaviors changed a little each time. He spoke from time to time but mostly remained quiet. The dinosaurs appeared to be involved in a variety of situations where things did not go as planned. They built a house with some blocks and it fell down. They went for a walk and fell over. They went to sleep and were disturbed by a wolf. Sylvia and Red were able to see how this might reflect Alex's perspective on the world and some of his frustration. We discussed how to continue to reflect the dinosaurs' feelings, based on the context, as they would essentially be empathically responding to Alex's feelings that way. They had noticed that Alex looked at them more often, although still rather quickly. At times they worried that he did not include them in his play as Teddy did, but I urged them to stay the course and let him find his own way. He was already involved in a social interaction program at school, and the play sessions seemed an important way for him to process relationships and feelings, mostly through the dinosaurs. Interestingly, by the time the family began the home sessions, the frequency of Alex's tantrums had reduced.

Teddy continued to enjoy his play sessions and frequently asked when the next one would be. Sylvia and Red thought he seemed more engaged with the family than previously, and they no longer felt so guilty about "ignoring him." Both of them felt more connected to Teddy and, to their surprise, to Alex as well. As Sylvia put it, "It might seem strange to say that we're more connected, but we really are. We understand his world a little better just by letting him play and show us. I think he is responding, too, because he looks at us more, and last week when the dinosaurs went swimming and made a big mess with the water he actually looked toward my face and gave a little hint of a smile. There's a boy in there behind that serious mask! Now we have more of a chance to see that boy and connect, even if it's just a little bit."

During the final phase of FT, we discussed ways to use the empathic listening with both boys outside the play sessions and covered the generalization of the other skills as well. At the time of discharge, Alex still had occasional tantrums, but much less often. Sylvia and Red had learned to reflect his fears, discomfort, and frustration with changes. They also adapted the 5-minute and 1-minute warnings from the play session structuring skill to give Alex some predictability over transitions. They planned to continue the play sessions indefinitely and to check in periodically with me with updates and any problems that might arise.

Guidelines and Adaptations

FT is a process-oriented form of therapy, and, as such, the structure remains much the same with different types of clients. At the same time, it offers flexibility and adaptability because of its collaborative focus and respect for the uniqueness of each individual and family. Although FT apparently has not been used widely with families of children with ASD, it offers some benefits to all family members. Its successful use with other families coping with very challenging and stressful circumstances, such as children with trauma and attachment problems or children with serious medical illnesses, suggests that it might follow a similar trajectory with families of children with ASD.

Because children on the spectrum manifest a vast array of behaviors, strengths, and limitations, it is premature to discuss in any detail where FT would be most useful and how it could be adapted. More clinical experience is needed using FT with this population, and research is vital to provide clearer guidance in its application. Some general observations based on the experiences of a number of filial therapists to date are in order, however.

First, FT seems well suited for high-functioning children with ASD and their families. Adaptations might include additional training for parents to identify feelings from the context of play when the child is not outwardly expressive. Parents might need additional support for their exhaustion or exasperation from dealing with the challenges of ASD. If the child's play becomes excessively repetitive with no variation, the therapist might need to help parents recognize when and how to gently shift rote behaviors back to more flexible play, although this would be done rarely and with caution to avoid interfering with actual play behaviors. For children who talk at length about their chosen area of "expertise" or focus, parents would benefit from knowing how to empathically listen to the feelings behind the words and, in daily life, how to balance the child's interests with greater variety in conversations. FT can easily be used in conjunction with other forms of therapy, and this would likely be needed.

For lower-functioning children with ASD, FT may still offer benefits to the parents and siblings, and it remains to be seen whether it would benefit some children, as the author is aware of only partial application of FT with children with severe deficits to date. One therapist with experience working with all functioning levels of children with ASD suggested that parents could use communication boards during play to point to feelings the child seemed to be expressing. Parents would focus on the child's non-verbal behaviors and expressions as well as the tenor and context of the play scenarios to say and use the communication board to reflect feelings. Because much remains to be learned about the play of children with ASD, especially those with more serious difficulties, further speculation about the use of FT would be misplaced here.

In conclusion, it seems that FT offers a number of potential benefits to families of children with ASD, including a way to communicate that is not primarily dependent on spoken language and a way to connect more fully with the child's feelings. Anecdotal evidence is growing and has been quite positive in terms of parents' stress levels, feelings of competence, awareness and understanding of the child's inner world, ability to communicate and connect, and ability to better meet the needs of siblings. The way forward needs to include further use of FT with families of children with ASD by fully trained filial therapists with experience with these children. Both qualitative and quantitative research are sorely needed and should shed light not only on the efficacy of FT with families of children with ASD but also the circumstances when it is beneficial and when it is not. This chapter has been written with the hope that therapists will more frequently consider the use of FT to help address the social and emotional needs of children with ASD and all members of their families and for the collection of clinical and research data that can refine our understanding of how best to meet the needs of these families.

References

Bratton, S. C., Ray, D., Rhine, T., & Jones, L. (2005). The efficacy of play therapy with children: A meta-analytic review of treatment outcomes. *Professional Psychology: Research and Practice, 36*(4), 376–390.

Caplin, W., & Pernet, K. (in press). *Group filial therapy for at-risk families: A leader's manual for an effective short-term model.* Boiling Springs, PA: Play Therapy Press.

Carter, A. S., de L. Martinez-Pedraza, F., & Gray, S. A. O. (2009). Stability and individual change in depressive symptoms among mothers raising young children with ASD: Maternal and child correlates. *Journal of Clinical Psychology, 65*(12), 1270–1280.

Cavedo, C., & Guerney, B.G. (1999). Relationship Enhancement (RE) enrichment/problem-prevention programs: Therapy-derived, powerful, versatile. In R. Berger & M. T. Hannah (Eds.), *Handbook of preventive approaches in couples therapy* (pp. 73–105). New York: Brunner/Mazel.

Duffy, K. M. (2008). *Filial therapy: A comparison of child-parent relationship therapy and parent-child interaction therapy.* (cardinalscholar.bsu.edu/747/1/kduffy_2008-1_BODY.pdf; DAI: Section B, 2010, 7205)

Ginsberg, B. G. (2003). An integrated holistic model of child-centered family therapy. In R. VanFleet & L. Guerney (Eds.), *Casebook of filial therapy* (pp. 21–48). Boiling Springs, PA: Play Therapy Press.

Guerney, L. F. (1983). Introduction to filial therapy: Training parents as therapists. In P. A. Keller & L. G. Ritt (Eds.), *Innovations in clinical practice: A source book* (Vol. 2, pp. 26–39). Sarasota, FL: Professional Resource Exchange.

Guerney, L., & Ryan, V. (in press). *Group filial therapy: Training parents to conduct special play sessions with their own children.* London: Jessica Kingsley.

Jarrold, C. (2003). A review of research into pretend play in autism. *Autism, 7*(4), 379–390.

Josefi, O., & Ryan, V. (2004). Non-directive play therapy for young children with autism: A case study. *Clinical Child Psychology & Psychiatry, 9*(4), 533–551.

Kaduson, H. (2006). *Play therapy for children with PDD.* [DVD]. Author.

Kasari, C., Freeman, S., & Paparella, T. (2006). Joint attention and symbolic play in young children with autism: A randomized controlled intervention study. *Journal of Child Psychology and Psychiatry and Allied Disciplines*, 47(6), 611–620.

Landreth, G. L., & Bratton, S. C. (2006). *Child parent relationship therapy (CPRT)*. New York: Routledge.

Lyons, A. M., Leon, S. C., Phelps, C. E. R., & Dunleavy, A. M. (2010). The impact of child symptom severity on stress among parents of children with ASD: The moderating role of coping styles. *Journal of Child and Family Studies*, 19(4), 516–524.

Seltzer, M. M., Greenberg, J. S., Hong, J., Smith, L. E., Almeida, D. M., Coe, C., et al. (2010). Maternal cortisol levels and behavior problems in adolescents and adults with ASD. *Journal of Autism and Developmental Disorders*, 40(4), 457–469.

Topham, G. L., Wampler, K. S., Titus, G., & Rolling, E. (2007). Predicting parent and child outcomes of a filial therapy program. *International Journal of Play Therapy*, 20(2), 79–93.

VanFleet, R. (2005). *Filial therapy: Strengthening parent-child relationships through play* (2nd ed.). Sarasota, FL: Professional Resource Press.

VanFleet, R. (2006). *Introduction to filial therapy*. [DVD]. Boiling Springs, PA: Play Therapy Press.

VanFleet, R. (2009). Filial therapy. In K. J. O'Connor & L. D. Braverman (Eds.), *Play therapy theory and practice: Comparing theories and techniques* (2nd ed., pp. 163–201). Hoboken, NJ: John Wiley & Sons.

VanFleet, R. (2011). Filial therapy: What every play therapist should know. *Play therapy: Magazine of the British Association of Play Therapists*, 65, 16–19.

VanFleet, R. J. (1985). *Mothers' perceptions of their families' needs when one of their children has diabetes mellitus: A developmental perspective*. The Pennsylvania State University. (DAI: 47 (1-A), July 1986, 324.).

VanFleet, R., & Guerney, L. (2003). *Casebook of filial therapy*. Boiling Springs, PA: Play Therapy Press.

VanFleet, R., Ryan, S., & Smith, S. (2005). Filial therapy: A critical review. In L. Reddy, T. Files-Hall, & C. Schaefer (Eds.), *Empirically-based play interventions for children* (pp. 241–264). Washington, DC: American Psychological Association.

VanFleet, R., & Sniscak, C. C. (in press). *Filial therapy for child trauma and attachment problems: Leader's manual for family groups*. Boiling Springs, PA: Play Therapy Press.

VanFleet, R., Sywulak, A. E., & Sniscak, C. S. (2010). *Child-centered play therapy*. New York: Guilford.

VanFleet, R., & Topham, G. (2011). Filial therapy for maltreated and neglected children: Integration of family therapy and play therapy. In A. A. Drewes, S. C. Bratton, & C. E. Schaefer (Eds.), *Integrative play therapy* (pp. 165–216). Hoboken, NJ: John Wiley & Sons.

Wieder, S., & Greenspan, S. (2005). Can children with autism master the core deficits and become empathic, creative, and reflective? A ten to fifteen year follow-up of a subgroup of children with autism spectrum disorders (ASD) who received a comprehensive developmental, individual-difference, relationship-based (DIR) approach. *Journal of Developmental and Learning Disorder*, 9, 1–29.

Wright, C., & Walker, J. (2003). Using filial therapy with Head Start families. In R. VanFleet & L. Guerney (Eds.), *Casebook of filial therapy* (pp. 309–330). Boiling Springs, PA: Play Therapy Press.

Yoder, P., Stone, W. L., Walden, T., & Malesa, E. (2009). Predicting social impairment and ASD diagnosis in younger siblings of children with autism spectrum disorder. *Journal of Autism and Developmental Disorders, 39*(10), 1381–1391.

The World of the Sand Tray and the Child on the Autism Spectrum

JANE FERRIS RICHARDSON

The world of the sand tray is a uniquely receptive container within which the emotions, ideas, dreams, and dearly held interests of the child on the autism spectrum can become visible. The holding environment of the sand tray, with its sensory allure, multiplicity of images, and infinite capacity for change and repair, offers a rich opportunity for symbolic and shared play in therapy. Sandtray Worldplay, as developed by Gisela De Domenico (2000) and practiced by the author, is a play therapy approach that builds on the strengths and addresses the challenges of the child and adolescent on the autism spectrum identified by Attwood (2006), Greenspan and Shanker (2004), Greenspan and Wieder (2006), and Wetherby and Prizant (2001); this approach is uniquely suited to meeting these strengths and challenges.

Helping children on the autism spectrum to access and communicate through the language and experience of play demands flexibility, attunement, and acceptance on the part of the therapist. The educators and psychologists of Reggio Emilia, Italy, have constructed an educational model that offers acceptance to all children. Reggio-inspired educators, and therapists, including the author, use the word *languages* (Malaguzzi, 1987) to connote a multiplicity of ways and materials that we can offer children for enriching their experiences of perceiving, expressing, and communicating about the world and with others. They suggest that there are "100 languages" (Malaguzzi, 1987) for apprehending and reaching out toward the world, a concept as valuable for clinicians as it is for educators. No children need this multiplicity of languages to express themselves and be heard and supported more than children on the autism spectrum. These children come to therapy with their own individual mix of the core challenges associated with this spectrum: difficulties with social communication and emotional regulation, sensory challenges, and a high need for supports in understanding and dealing with the world of others (McAfee, 2002; Wetherby & Prizant, 2001). Also, the therapy setting may well be the place where children on the spectrum first fully experience shared play, with its rich symbolic and affective meaning.

Sandtray Worldplay

Sandtray Worldplay is a flexible, multisensory, child-centered way of working with children's growing edge of development (De Domenico, 2000). The growing edge is supported as children explore and express themselves through the play, regardless of presenting condition or "limitations." This attitude of acceptance is crucial to working with children on the spectrum, as any successful interventions must not be targeted solely to remediating deficits (Wetherby, Prizant, & Schuler, 2001), but rather interventions must "create the types of contexts that are more responsive and conducive to communicative intentions" (p. 124). Furthermore, as Greenspan and Wieder (2006) remind us, children "who have motor or processing problems have difficulty imagining the world and thus pretending" (p. 83). These children need extra support to engage in play and explore communication. De Domenico's way of staying with the child playing in the sand is similar to Greenspan and Wieder's description of, "following the child's natural interest" (p. 83) as a way of connecting with the child, grasping every opportunity to "give more purpose or meaning" to any gesture or expression and more fully engage the child's interest. In De Domenico's model, this is translated into the process of amplifying the meaning of the play, through sound, movement, or a shift in the play. The creation of a world in the sand goes beyond words while supporting children's endeavor to find the words that can describe that world and their experience in it. In sharing with the therapist who witnesses the play, verbalization is at the same time important and unimportant to Sandtray Worldplay. Some children may remain silent during play in the sand and may have limited verbal sharing with the therapist. Yet the practice of Sandtray Worldplay is always about "creating living language, living symbols" (G. De Domenico, personal communication, August 5, 2004). For the child with autism, the emotionally charged language of play is particularly important, for it is here children that connect "their own emotions...to their symbols" (Greenspan & Shanker, 2004, p. 215), as Greenspan and Shanker describe the process. This connection is what motivates children to use language in a meaningful and communicative fashion. When a child is actively playing in the world of the sand tray, meaningful communication is encouraged by the sense of self-efficacy the child feels as the builder, by the presence of the therapist, and by the therapist being curious together with the child about what is both emerging and what ultimately emerges. The careful attention to the child playing in the world, and observation of their world building helps to support reciprocity in play and communication.

The therapist may also use other expressive play modalities to engage children and support the play; these other play materials are often chosen by them as they continue their play on the floor or in the dollhouse or through the use of other art materials. Children may play music for the worlds they have built, which often helps them literally warm up to talking and verbally sharing the story of their world. The task of the therapist is always to help children remain connected to play in the world so that they can fully experience and then share their story.

While moving through the stages of Sandtray Worldplay, we as therapists see the construction of the children's world, are introduced to their perspective, and then have the opportunity to experience the world jointly with them, always seeing what we may not always hear. Sharing the world in the sand offers an experience of intersubjectivity that moves at a pace comfortable for the children and a safe space to explore communication, challenges, and emotions. The focus of attention is always in the world they have built, and this is usually a comfort to children on the autism spectrum, who have a preference for looking together over being looked at. There are a number of ways we might either witness or play with children, from moving at their invitation into the sand tray to play alongside them to offering more structured "teaching play" (G. De Domenico, personal communication, August 6, 2004) in which the therapist has the opportunity to offer a new way of looking at or reframing experience.

Moving With the Child Through the Phases of Sandtray Worldplay

During the initial phase of building a world in the sand, the therapist is a silent witness to the child's play. The task of the therapist as the child is building is to fully connect with that emerging world and to record the transformative process taking place in the sand, writing down the child's journey. The child may invite us to actively join in play, in which case the play takes on a shared dimension. There are a number of ways we might witness or play with the child, but we always, as therapists, observe carefully. The child might ask for assistance, which for children on the spectrum may start out as very directive toward the therapist's role and then become more flexible, especially when therapists stay attuned to their own feelings and communicate to the child: "I'm trying to do this just like you want me to." The play may move on to shared sand tray play, in which case the therapist exercises caution not to intrude too much into the play by taking over and playing for the child.

After children have built their world, there is time for a period of silent experiencing and reflection, in which they are encouraged to stay with their creation. The therapist models how to be comfortable with looking at the world. The task of the therapist is to keep children connected to the world they have built so that they may more fully experience and then share this world. This is a time of children being in the world they have created.

The next phase of sharing the world is a time of joint experiencing of the world together. This phase is particularly significant for children on the autism spectrum, as there is joint attention to the world and to all its richness, nuances, and history. The eye contact is with the sand tray at this time and not with the child, which creates comfort for children on the spectrum. When exploring the world and seeking to understand it more fully, we ask for experience, not facts about the world. This may be a challenge for children on the spectrum who are fascinated by the dinosaurs or fossils they have placed in the tray and who are eager to talk about all that they know. Thus, this phase becomes like a dance: acknowledging the children's interest and encouraging sharing affective experience. For example, we might ask, "How is it for the baby dinosaur to be close to his mother?" Such storytelling brings the world to life. Engaging more fully with all the dimensions of the world can be a revelation to children. Here we can learn about the connections to their own life. We explore where and how the world began and what we may take from this world as child and therapist are "joined together, asking questions in the world" (G. De Domenico, personal communication, May 27, 2008).

Sandtray Worldplay as a Support for Children

The need "to play with others, and for others to play with us" (G. De Domenico, personal communication, May 6, 2008) is the same for children on the autism spectrum as for neuro-typical children. Creating the affectively meaningful exchanges so critical to the ability to communicate and form reciprocal relationships (Greenspan & Shanker, 2004) in therapy can offer a bridge to building these meaningful relationships within the family, the school, and the community. Treatment of children and adolescents on the spectrum is complex, as Bromfield (2010) succinctly describes the process, because it must address both the core challenges of autism and the child's emerging feelings and experience. Expressive approaches to play therapy, he feels, provide "alternative options of handling overwhelming events, circumstances, and feelings" (p. 118). Research has found that openness, reciprocity, and the opportunity for shared experiences meaningful to the child are critical elements of play therapy approaches for children and adolescents on the spectrum (Greenspan & Wieder, 2006; Mastrangelo, 2009; Myers, 2009; Prizant, Wetherby, & Rydell, 2000; Schuler & Wolfberg, 2000).

It has certainly been my experience that expressive and shared play allows communicative and relational abilities to blossom. So too does acceptance of children's uniqueness and special interests, allowing them to feel "special" in a positive sense rather than vulnerable to experience the criticism or disinterest from others (Bromfield, 2010, p. 92). In witnessing children's choices of images and themes, the therapist acknowledges the significance of those particular interests, images, and themes to them. The therapist's collection of images for the sand tray is an important ally in this work and must include a broad visual vocabulary. My own collection has grown through the special interests of the children I work with, and this enriched "vocabulary" helps support their communication. Children may also create images to use in the sand, and their creations bring a sense of satisfaction and mastery. Children on the spectrum leave a trail of special interests in the sand, and in our witnessing the sand tray we acknowledge this specialness and gain access to deeper connection.

Sandtray Worldplay offers a nonverbal medium for the expression of feelings, the sharing of experience, and the telling of stories. Attwood (2006) describes the challenges of verbal language for children with Asperger's syndrome as especially complex. Although some children may have a strong vocabulary, challenges with the social pragmatics of language often lead to confusion over meaning, particularly when nuances in speech carry emotional meaning missed by them. Speech may not provide an effective medium for conveying children's own thoughts, leading to mounting frustration and stress for them in the effort to communicate. In Sandtray Worldplay the therapist is able to observe and thus gain an understanding of children without initially needing to talk about what the images in the world mean.

The image language (De Domenico, 2000) of Sandtray Worldplay has the virtue of being a language congruent with the way many people on the autism spectrum "think in pictures," as exemplified in Temple Grandin's (2006) description of her visually based thought process. Similar to Grandin, who describes her thoughts as pictures, Eileen Miller (2008) terms her daughter Kim as "the girl who spoke with pictures" in her book of the same name. Miller describes Kim's expression of her thoughts through drawing as more complete and effective than words. For children and adolescents on the spectrum, this visual language—which is made possible by the Sandtray Worldplay vocabulary of images—values and supports children's interests.

Yet there are other nonvisual and nonverbal components to the image language of Sandtray Worldplay as well, and these have the capacity to engage the other senses fully. Stephen Shore (2006) reminds us of how we need to consider all the senses as contributing to the development of young people with autism. The process of playing in the sand itself provides one such sensory-based opportunity for accessing feelings. The sensory properties of the sand are inviting to many children, who readily plunge into the depths of the sand tray, digging, shaping, and pouring to create a world that holds meaning for them. This play is both developmental and integrative.

Children on the spectrum may need to learn more about how to play, and certainly it is often true that "the type and quality of their play varies from those children who appear to be following a typical developmental trajectory," as noted by Mastrangelo (2009, p. 35). Sensory play in the sand offers children a solid base on which to build as their exploration of play themes, ability to play symbolically, and ability to communicate deepens. For children on the spectrum, especially those with sensory integration or gross motor challenges, this play offers an opportunity to feel grounded in the sand. The kinesthetic process of shifting sand can also evoke sound and movement, offering alternative ways of connecting with children on a sensory and communicative level as well as helping them to feel calm, engaged, and focused.

This calming potential of the sand is highly significant for children on the spectrum, since anxiety and the mastery of distressing affect and sensory experience can provide such a challenge for them. I have repeatedly heard children recognize and express the feeling of relaxation and focus they gain from playing in the sand. In the words of one adolescent girl, well experienced at exploring the challenges of her life in the sand, "The sand tray is a way for us to express our feelings." De Domenico stated, "When we enter into our creations, we explore ourselves" (personal communication, August 5, 2004). Another adolescent gazed into her sand tray world and focused on a mermaid. She then shared that "she feels kind of how I'm feeling. She's feeling free and relaxed" (Richardson, 2009, p.118). These experiences of the safety and support of the sand tray can extend to making it possible to deal with challenging, and potentially overwhelming, feelings and sensations in a concrete and reassuring way.

Attwood (2007) describes how the child with Asperger's syndrome often "has a clinically significant difficulty with the understanding, expression, and regulation of emotion" (p. 29) together with the risks inherent in persistent symptoms of anxiety and depression. Attwood stresses the need for concrete, accessible "tools" (2006, p. 358) for managing anxiety before it threatens to overwhelm. The sand tray and images provide these tools for many children and adolescents.

While older children can describe the relief and understanding they experience through the creation of their sand tray worlds, younger children show the importance of the sand tray and the value of this dynamic, expressive therapeutic tool in different ways. Even when their sessions may focus on play with puppets or making art, young children repeatedly will connect with the sand tray at the beginning or end of a session, sometimes just running their hands through the sand before moving on to other play and sometimes returning to the sand tray to leave a significant image in the sand as an expression of what they have experienced in that day's play. Children also may want to choose an image to show to the parent who has brought them to therapy that day, even when the parent has not been present at the session and they have not spent most of their time playing in the sand. Such is the power of the image and the connection of the children to the images and the process of play.

For children who are tactilely defensive and do not like the feel of the sand, the empty sand tray may offer an alternative safe space to play. One 7-year-old boy, while consistently viewing my sand tray images with great fascination, did not wish to use them in the sand. Instead, he chose dinosaurs and fossils to play on the floor, never choosing a human figure to include in his play. He also created elaborate and sometimes collaborative artworks, using these other ways of playing and creating to explore his presenting issues of perfectionism and anxiety and to explore the relationship with the therapist. One afternoon, when he had made paper boats for us to play with, he asked to fill an empty sand tray with water. The shimmering expanse of water engaged him in a way that the sand had not, and he placed his boat and some shining rocks in the water. He placed a little boy in the boat, sailing on a calm sea in the sunshine. He was smiling and relaxed and pleased with the rightness of his world.

Structure and Flexibility

Flexibility with the materials of Sandtray Worldplay is particularly important in working with children who are, by virtue of their neurological makeup, inflexible (Richardson, 2009). For children on the spectrum, inflexibility may stem from difficulty making generalizations, taking the perspective of another, or moving away from narrowly defined interests or the constraints of literalness and perfectionism. Sand tray and world play offers therapists a way to carefully attend to this movement since we witness the construction of the world in the sand by the child and then have the opportunity to enter into this world with the child and to see it from his perspective. The world looks, and feels, different to the child on the autism spectrum. Wolfberg (2003) suggested the importance of careful observation of the play of children on the spectrum, with particularly close attention to the symbolic dimension of play as well as to the social communication aspects of the play. The Sandtray Worldplay therapist's careful observation of children is an essential part of deepening their ability to play and communicate. As we observe children who are building a world in the sand, we can come to see both the children within the context of this world as well as the world's meaning to them. When we receive whatever they are ready to share about their world or are invited in to play with them, we have another opportunity to see them wholly more clearly and to support them more effectively. Offering children an opportunity to enter into the richness of an image language through play, in the shifting and always responsive sand, allows for a more flexible capacity to express the self and to respond to the therapist within the shared and safe world. The container of the sand tray itself and the careful observation of and joint attention to the world with the therapist provide the support necessary to explore playing, storytelling, problem solving, and integration.

Careful attention to children's process of building the world, the stories shared, and the connections made to their life must be maintained by the therapist. Children need support to stay in contact with the therapist and to avoid the stuckness of repetitive play. Both the child and the therapist, when invited into the play, have to play authentically for there to be movement in treatment. In playing with children on the spectrum, Schuler and Wolfberg (2001) caution:

> The practitioner's dilemma is one of balance. Although more direc-tive adult-structured approaches may be overly controlling, more child-centered approaches that attempt to acknowledge the child's state of mind and try to follow its lead are often too subtle to draw in the child's attention. One of the challenges in the design of effec-tive intervention thus lies in the creation of child-centered structures that are neither too loose nor too rigid. (p. 257)

De Domenico (2000) addresses this dilemma through the consistent reciprocity between child and therapist, supporting movement in the play and new understanding in the child, and also through an approach that can offer more structure or more clarification as needed by the child. Children's play can be amplified with the support of the therapist, with movement, music, or art making. Children may also move into another sand tray. In this way, children can literally take more space to work out a problem before returning the images they are playing with to their original world.

More structured play in the sand tray offers another way of looking at a challenging situation or reframing an experience. An example of struc-tured play, discussed in the next section, is "the bridge to fourth grade," in which I invited a child to specifically focus on the different aspects of crossing this bridge from one grade to the next. Such structured play has some commonalities with the "replays" of Levine and Chedd (2007), who developed a technique for literally "replaying," through structured play with props and storytelling, a situation that has been challenging to a child. Levine and Chedd explain that, through replaying a situation, the child is able to "develop symbolic skills and master upsetting emotions" (p. 18). Similarly, Bromfield (2010) suggests that therapeutic reenactments can help children who are unable to move forward and feel stuck or unsuccessful.

Supporting this inability to move forward was one approach I used in working with an adolescent girl with Asperger's syndrome who had been experiencing escalating anxiety. While she often used the sand tray to explore ways of feeling, in her own wise words, calmer and more creative, on one occasion I suggested that she actually put her anxiety into the sand tray. Initially resisting this idea, she trusted the process of the sand tray enough to give this a try, and proceeded to work with and around the heavy stone she chose to be "my anxiety." Through her play she realized, "It actually helped! When I put all the things I didn't like, then I knew what I wanted to see. And then when I put those in, it was okay."

Whether the play is structured in this way, when needed to create movement for the child or is more open ended, sharing the world together always offers an opportunity to appreciate the child's unique way of seeing and experiencing while staying with the child's growing edge. Children on the autism spectrum seem to understand some of this intuitively. When I first introduced the sand tray to my office, an environment already full of myriad expressive materials congruent with my training both as a play therapist and an art therapist, a 7-year-old boy walked through the door after a tough day of second grade and rushed straight to the alcove with the sand tray. He took in the images arrayed on shelves, and my first sand tray positioned in the light from the window. He bypassed the much-loved puppets, the instruments, the paints, and building materials to stand in front of the sand tray. He then began to jump up and down, chanting, "thank you, thank you, thank you!" He reached his hands into the sand. A journey had begun for him and for me. I will describe this journey of a child building, and a therapist witnessing, worlds in the sand. Sandtray Worldplay will be discussed in the context of addressing core strengths and challenges for children on the spectrum, with a discussion of the particular challenges that bring individual children and adolescents to therapy. I will also discuss how the stages of this journey unfold for children on the autism spectrum, bringing with them movement in therapy and positive outcomes through the flexible medium and multiple languages of Sandtray Worldplay.

Worlds in the Sand

The sand tray may be where a child first moves into symbolic play or shares a story with the therapist. Sometimes the sand tray is a place where children start to explore, creating a world where their special interests are revealed to another. One 6-year-old, in his first sand tray, joined one of his favorite things, a bridge, together with one of his favorite people, a baseball player, and added a little boy looking at them. He did not need to tell this story verbally, it was already a rich expression of his interests and curiosity. Sometimes the sand tray provides the medium through which a verbal story emerges together with the play, and sometimes the play in the sand is where that story takes on a deeper affective dimension.

The World of Animals

When 7-year-old Toby came to see me, his diagnosis seemed incomplete. His high level of tension and anxiety was clear, and he presented with both communication and social challenges. Following continued developmental evaluation, he was given a diagnosis of Asperger's syndrome. His repertoire of expressive play, both at home and in therapy sessions, was limited, although he was curious about the toys and expressive materials available to him. He had difficulty staying in the playroom and initially needed his mother's presence. His very energetic play with puppets and dinosaurs displayed a great deal of anger and frustration as he battled away, testing out the new therapist and sharing some of his own frustrations and fears. Monsters and frightening powerful creatures battled alongside a large dragon puppet even as frightening dreams disrupted Toby's sleep at night.

As Toby became increasingly fascinated by the sand tray, his play changed. He was able to say good-bye to his mother and come into the playroom with the therapist. He was both calmer and more expressive, with a much greater range of affect and a growing ability to share the story of his worlds. These stories revealed a great deal about Toby's own thoughts and feelings. He enjoyed sharing these, and he often shared his worlds with his mother as well.

Dinosaurs and dragons continued to appear in his sand trays, and the "worst guys" got angry and lost control. Wizards stepped in, "to give them bad dreams," and everyone from mummies to minotaurs struggled "to be on the good side." From his initial battling with puppets, he had moved to articulating what was happening in these battles. He could show how animals were "mad: they're not friends" and then go on to find resolution "because they don't really like the battle." This was dramatically different from the repetitive fighting of his earlier play. Toby searched for helpers for his animals and for a place for them to be safe.

His dragons moved into the sand tray and developed a wider repertoire of affect and behavior. Joining them were eagles who "wanted to make a nest, and relax in the nest" as well as to fly and fight. He began to explore the nature of the relationships between the animals and creatures he had chosen. One day he returned to playing with the dragons and decided, "Now the other dragon will have a friend, the same kind he is!" These two dragons were able to work and play together, "building a sand castle, they want to make sure that it's safe." They had a plan for working together and living together since a larger dragon had "taught them how to share."

This play emerged at a time when Toby was struggling with self-control and managing frustration. We were working on ways to support him at home and at school, including sensory supports that helped him to gain comfort and regulate his emotions. Toby moved the dragon from the sand tray into a drawing, to which he added a thought bubble saying, "Thank you," for helping him when he was struggling.

As more affect was present in his play, so too were families of animals and Toby's exploration of how they could communicate and help one another. One day he created a world full of horses. The sand tray portraying this world can be seen in Figure 11.1. He was equally engrossed in building this world and sharing its story with the therapist and then with his mother. In this world, the horses took care of one another. They had enough food and were friends with one another as well as with the smaller animals living in their world. They were even able to help a dragon who had been hurt. Toby was able to connect this world with his own favorite animal, "horses!" and to share horse stories with his mother, feeling relaxed in the office and proud of the world he had created.

He was able to create safe and shared worlds when he was feeling stressed. His animal families were able to work out conflicts that interrupted the peace of their lives together. Toby became increasingly

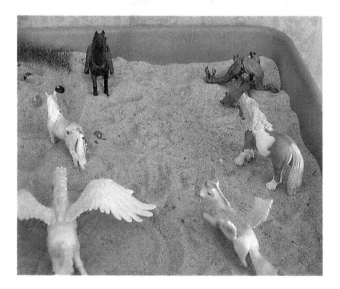

Figure 11.1 The world of horses and help for the dragon.

articulate about what these conflicts were. He was able to explain his understanding of what is hard for his animals. One day, he explained, "They (a chimp family) have a big problem. Other animals won't leave the baby chimp alone." He then told the story of how the family helps their little one: "they're gonna protect him. He can get his mom and dad." Toby had begun to use the whole room for his play, moving animals to fly through the air or travel out onto the floor and back into the tray. He worked on this "problem" together with the chimp family, as he mounted them on horses and moved them to a second sand tray, literally giving them more space to solve their dilemma. Helped by the horses, they were able to return to the first sand tray and live among the other animals with more comfort. They created a safe space for their family, and especially for the little chimp. Figures 11.2 and 11.3 indicate this movement and change, showing the journey of the chimp family and the resolution of the challenge in the original sand tray.

Crossing the Bridge: Structuring Play to Create Movement

Nine-year-old Dylan's delightful, inquisitive demeanor and his absence of meltdowns had led his medical team to question his Asperger's syndrome diagnosis even as they arrived at it. Yet he was experiencing, if internalizing, the stressors and anxieties of children on the spectrum. In spite of his high intelligence, a special interest in history, and behavior that pleased all his teachers, the expectations of school were often daunting for Dylan. He was having headaches and difficulty sleeping coupled with his anxiety. We used relaxation, art making, and eye movement desensitization and reprocessing (EMDR) to address his stress level. While all of these approaches helped Dylan to gain a sense of mastery and control, it was the sand tray that enabled him to focus on the challenges of the coming school year.

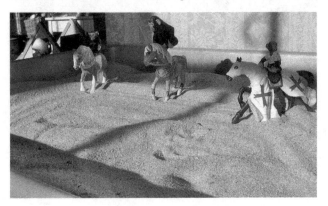

Figure 11.2 The chimp family journeys into a second sand tray.

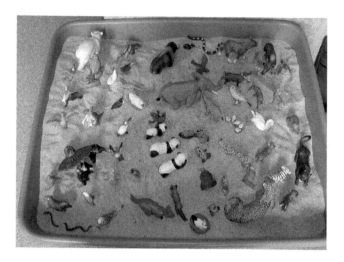

Figure 11.3 The chimps' world at peace.

The shift from third grade to fourth, with an increased emphasis on "reading to learn" and group projects, was frightening to Dylan. Together with his family, we addressed his concerns about the upcoming transition and discussed ways they could find out more about the expectations for the coming year. Anxiety about these expectations was making Dylan feel that he wanted to "go back" to what was known and comfortable, in spite of his academic readiness for new challenges.

Dylan enjoyed the sand tray and was an experienced builder of worlds in the sand. He had often shared or built these worlds with his parents and incorporated his interest in history as well as his experiences into them. One summer day he came into my office with his mother, and they talked about how difficult it was for Dylan to even think about the transition to the next school year. Departing from our usual open-ended play, I took a curved wooden bridge from the shelf of images and dubbed this "the bridge to fourth grade." Dylan found a large book to put on the far side, "a fourth-grade book," and placed a smaller book on the familiar, third-grade, side shown in Figure 11.4.

We talked about the coming year and all the ways he could learn more about what was to come, to help him feel more comfortable. At our next session, we moved the bridge into the sand tray.

"Here's where I am right now," said Dylan, pointing out the "third grade" side of the bridge in the sand. "This is the school," he said, putting my largest building with tightly closed windows on the floor. He pointed out a window on the second floor. "This is the classroom, and I don't even know what classroom I'm going into. Right now it's locked. But when I get over the bridge, I'm going to look for the key." He turned to me and asked,

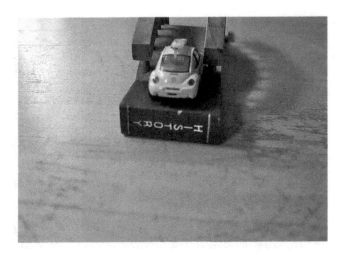

Figure 11.4 The bridge to fourth grade.

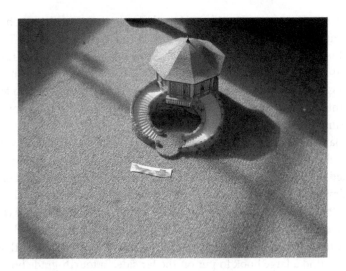

Figure 11.5 The key to the classroom.

"Do we have a key?" He then created a large key of stiff paper, painted with metallic gold paint, as shown in Figure 11.5.

Dylan then placed the key inside a treasure box and covered both with sand. He added people, both children and adults, and a house with a driveway to the sand tray, saying, "I want this to be my house." He placed a car in motion over the bridge as well as trees, water, and birds, as depicted in Figure 11.6. One of the birds, flying and looking for food, was able to "see in the classroom!" In the car, he said, there was a family, driving with their dogs.

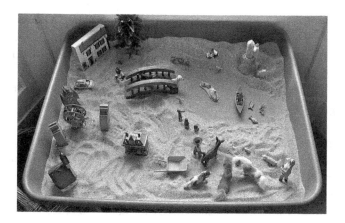

Figure 11.6 Seeing into the classroom and strategies for comfort.

Dylan then talked about the teacher and the children who would be in the new class. He realized that the teacher was on vacation and unable to come and get the key to the school, leaving the kids in her class waiting for her return and wondering what was in store for them in the new school year. Dylan suggested that the children driving in the car could "listen to music and pet their dogs." That would help them to feel better, more comfortable and relaxed, and less worried about the coming school year. Like the children in the sand tray, Dylan has a supportive family and beloved dogs. He realized that he could do the same things as the children in the sand tray, to help him to be more comfortable, and that his parents could help him as well. Before he left the office that day, he asked to keep the key to the school "in a safe place." At the next session he shared the bridge and the key with his father. They talked about supports and coping strategies to help him manage his anxieties about school. He showed his father the school building and said, "I'm waiting to see, can I read fourth-grade books?"

Sharing the Sand Tray With Parents and Reviewing the Worlds

Sharing the worlds built in the sand tray allows parents an opportunity to enter a child's world more fully. As Bromfield (2010) reminds us, "Parents allow us to enter their child's personal world, the one that they and their child have shared" (p. 17). Children can also invite their parents into their sand tray world, whether to build together or to witness the world that has been built by the child. Therapists too can invite parents to share the connections they see to the child's life in the world that has been built or in the worlds built over the course of therapy. Therapists may ask parents how they themselves experience the child's world. Parents recognize that there is something special in the play therapy setting and relationship that allows for movement and change through dynamic expressive play. As Dylan's parents reflected, "We asked ourselves what would happen if we used sand and clay at home, and we realized that this would not be the same as his doing these things in therapy."

The vividness of children's sand tray worlds helps us to focus together on the growth as well as the challenges children are experiencing. When Toby's mother and I reviewed the course of his therapy since beginning in treatment, we discussed his positive transition to a new school program offering him more supports. Toby's perceptive mother experienced him as "happier" and more able to deal with social and learning challenges. We both noted his dramatically increased ability to tell stories, and I shared with his mother how impressed I was by his ability to reflect on what was happening in his worlds, whether this was sharing or discord, and by his ability to attribute emotions to the animals he played with.

His mother noticed how the themes of play sometimes mirrored challenges at home. Toby's exuberant affection for the huge and cuddly family dog sometimes elicited growls, which he had been largely ignoring in his desire to connect and play. But in the sand tray one day, as shown in Figure 11.7, Toby had depicted whales that became angry when they were walked on by smaller animals, saying, "Don't walk on us!"

He had invited his mother in to see this sand tray, and together we were able to broach how the dog too did not want to be "walked on" or squeezed and what had to happen for them both to be happy and safe.

We also saw parallels in his development that were reflected by his play in the sand tray. Toby's mother described him as "making connections" not only in his play but also in his relationships and ability to communicate.

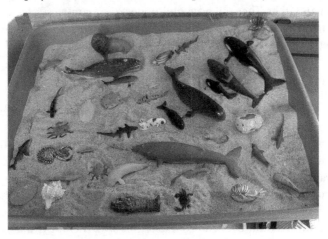

Figure 11.7 The world of the whales mirrors challenges at home.

These new abilities were helping him to build friendships in his new school program. Toby was becoming more observant, more patient, and more willing to share.

For Dylan, his play in the sand tray world helped him to give voice to his fears and anxieties about the coming school year and to share these fears with his parents. Wisely, his parents helped him to find interesting "fourth-grade books" to read during the summer, when there was no stress about book reports or spelling tests. They also explored the fourth-grade expectations with Dylan. They highlighted the new opportunities that he would have, like learning to play an instrument. They continued to practice relaxation with Dylan at home and to explore his suggestions for ways to have fun. He continued to share his play in the sand tray with his parents as well. When the school year began, Dylan was ready to move forward.

When we reviewed how the new school year had begun, Dylan expressed his own feelings of accomplishment and greater maturity. He was an active part of his class, sang in a concert, and had begun to play an instrument, all of which he enjoyed. He told me that he had "done interesting things" in his new class and that he felt that the new opportunities of fourth grade were special and enjoyable now that he was more comfortable at school. As we sat at my art table we looked at a Statue of Liberty he had painstakingly created from clay, basing her on one of his favorite historical sand tray images. We talked about why he liked her so much and why she was so important to him. Dylan decided that the Statue of Liberty gave people an opportunity "to do new things" in a new country, just as he had during this new, fourth-grade school year. "It's fun", he said. "I like it. It gives me the freedom to do new things." The freedom of the sand tray had helped him to find more freedom and flexibility in his life.

For many children on the autism spectrum, as for the children discussed herein, the sand tray is a preferred venue for play, connection, and communication. The sand tray may well be the place where a breakthrough in treatment takes place. For other children, although the images available for play may be fascinating, the sand itself is not appealing. This was the case with the child previously discussed who chose an empty sand tray full of water to create a world and to include for the first time a human figure in his play. The child's sensory profile must be known and understood by the therapist if Sandtray Worldplay is to be successful.

The rich visual language made possible by the images for play is potentially intriguing to children. The images are a wonderful support to the therapist, both in engaging a child's interest and showing the therapist's understanding of and respect for a child's special interests. There is the danger, however, that a child will become absorbed in the images to the exclusion of the therapist and thus will engage in play that closes off the therapist's access to the story of the world in the sand. Supporting the play and the child so that the shared meaning of the world is not lost but rather fosters growth and communication is the responsibility of the therapist. This requires training and experience on the part of the therapist, coupled with a sensitive understanding of the child's comfort level, communication style, and sensory needs. This chapter discussed the balance of freedom and structure possible in Sandtray Worldplay and how vital it is that the therapist maintains an awareness of this full spectrum of possibilities for children who are themselves on the spectrum.

References

Attwood, T. (2006). Asperger's syndrome and problems related to stress. In G. Baron, J. Groden, G. Groden, & G. Lipsitt (Eds.), *Stress and coping in autism* (pp. 350–371). Oxford: Oxford University Press.

Attwood, T. (2007). *The complete guide to Asperger's syndrome*. London: Jessica Kingsley Publishers.

Bromfield, R. (2010). *Doing therapy with children and adolescents with Asperger's syndrome*. New York: John Wiley and Sons Inc.

De Domenico, G. (2000). Comprehensive *guide to the use of sandtray in psychotherapy and transformational settings*. Oakland, CA: Vision Quest Images.

Grandin, G. (2006). *Thinking in pictures: My life with autism*. New York: Vintage.

Greenspan, S., & Shanker, S. (2004). *The first idea: How symbols, language, and intelligence evolved from our primate ancestors to modern humans*. Cambridge, MA: Da Capo Press.

Greenspan, S., & Wieder, S. (2006). *Engaging autism: Using the Floortime approach to help children relate, communicate, and think*. Cambridge, MA: Da Capo Press.

Levine, K., & Chedd, N. (2007). *Replays: Using play to enhance emotional and behavioral development for children with autism spectrum disorders*. London: Jessica Kingsley Publishers.

Malaguzzi, L. (1987). *I cento linguagi dei bambini*. Washington, DC: Reggio Children.

Mastrangelo, S. (2009). Harnessing the power of play: Opportunities for children with autism spectrum disorders. *TEACHING Exceptional Children, 41*, 34–44.

McAfee, J. (2002). *Navigating the social world: A curriculum for individuals with Asperger's syndrome, high functioning autism, and related disorders*. Arlington, TX: Future Horizons Publishing.

Miller, E. (2008). *Autism through art: The girl who spoke with pictures*. London: Jessica Kingsley Publishers.

Myers, M. (2009). Reaching through the silence: Play therapy in the treatment of children with autism. In S. Brooke (Ed.), *The use of the creative therapies with autism spectrum disorders* (pp. 123–138). Springfield, IL: Charles C. Thomas.

Prizant, B., Wetherby, A., & Rydell, P. (2000). Communication intervention issues for young children with autism spectrum disorders. In A. Wetherby & B. Prizant (Eds.), *Autism spectrum disorders a transactional developmental perspective* (pp. 193–224). Baltimore: Paul H. Brookes.

Richardson, J. (2009). Creating a safe space for adolescents on the autism spectrum. In S. Brooke (Ed.), *The use of the creative therapies with autism spectrum disorders* (pp. 103–122). Springfield, IL: Charles C. Thomas.

Schuler, A., & Wolfberg, P. (2001). Promoting peer play and socialization: The art of scaffolding. In A. Wetherby & B. Prizant (Eds.), *Autism spectrum disorders a transactional developmental perspective* (pp. 251–278). Baltimore: Paul. H. Brookes.

Shore, S. (2006). *Beyond the wall: Personal experiences with autism and Asperger's syndrome.* Shawnee Mission, KS: Autism Asperger's Publishing Company.

Wetherby, A., & Prizant, B. (Eds.). (2001). *Autism spectrum disorders: A transactional developmental perspective.* Baltimore: Paul H. Brookes.

Wetherby, A., Prizant, B., & Schuler, A. (2001). Understanding the nature of communication and language impairments. In A. Wetherby & B. Prizant (Eds.), *Autism spectrum disorders a transactional developmental perspective.* Baltimore: Paul. H. Brookes.

Wolfberg, P. (2003). *Play and imagination in children with autism.* New York: Teachers College Press.

PART **III**

Programmatic Play-Based Intervention

III
Programmatic Play-Based Intervention

CHAPTER 12

DIR Floortime

A Developmental/Relational Play Therapy Approach for Treating Children Impacted by Autism

ESTHER HESS

Play is a complex phenomenon that occurs naturally for most children; they move through the various stages of play development and are able to add complexity, imagination, and creativity to their thought processes and action. However, for many children with autism spectrum disorder (ASD), the various stages of play are difficult to achieve. Challenges in motor planning, expressive and receptive communication, imitation and fine and gross motor movements are just some of the many obstacles that children with ASD encounter during play (Mastrangelo, 2009). The Developmental, Individual Difference, Relationship-Based (DIR®) Floortime model is an interdisciplinary framework that enables play clinicians, parents, and educators to construct a comprehensive assessment and intervention program based on the child's and family's unique developmental profile that addresses these core deficits (Greenspan & Wieder, 1999).

Floortime™ is the heart of the DIR® Floortime™ model, and it is the play component of a comprehensive program for infants, children, and their families with a variety of developmental challenges, including autism spectrum disorders. This comprehensive program includes working on all elements of the DIR® Floortime™ model, the functional emotional developmental levels, and the underlying, individual, neurological differences in processing capacities, thus creating those learning relationships that will help the child move ahead in his or her development. These relationships in turn are tailored to the child's individual differences that move him or her up the developmental ladder, mastering each and every functional emotional developmental capacity that he or she is capable of (Greenspan, 2010). The DIR® Floortime™ model involves often not just Floortime but different therapies, such as speech and language therapy, occupational therapy, physical therapy, educational programs, counseling support for parents, and both home and school programs. For the purposes of this chapter, we will focus on the Floortime component, which is the heart of both the home and school component. The chapter will then conclude with a summary of evidence-based research that lends support to this developmental/relational-based play intervention for children impacted by autism and their families.

The DIR Floortime Model

Floortime is a particular technique where the play partner gets down on the floor and works with the child to master each of his or her developmental capacities. To represent this model fairly, you will need to think about Floortime in two ways (ICDL, 2000):

1. A specific technique, where, for 20 or more minutes at a time, a parent gets down on the floor to play with his or her child.
2. A general philosophy that characterizes all interactions with the child. All of the interactions have to incorporate the features of Floortime™ as well as the particular goals of that interaction, including understanding the child's emotional, social, and intellectual differences in motor, sensory, and language functioning; and the existing caregiver, child, and family functioning and interaction patterns.

At the heart of the definition of Floortime are two of what could be called emphases that sometimes work together very easily and other times may appear to be at opposite ends of a continuum:

1. Following the child's lead.
2. Joining a child in his or her world and then pulling him or her into a shared world to assist in mastery of each of his or her functional emotional developmental capacities (Greenspan & Wieder, 1999).

It is critical to be aware of both of these polarities, tendencies, or dimensions of Floortime.

Following the Child's Lead

The most widely known dimension of Floortime is *following the child's lead*—in other words, harnessing the child's natural interests. But what exactly does that mean? By following a child's interests, or his or her lead, we are taking the first steps in making what I call a *great date* with a child—in other words, a validating emotional experience. What are the elements of a great date? For most of us, it includes being in the company of someone who is attentive, available, and fun. And when we are with a person who incorporates all of these emotionally affirming elements, we obviously want the date to go on forever. Conversely, if we are on a bad date with someone who does not make us feel good about ourselves or our experience, most of us would attempt to escape that encounter as soon as possible. Following a child's lead and taking the germ of an idea and making that the basis of the experience that you are about to share with the child actually encourages the child to allow you into his or her emotional life. Through the child's interests and natural desires we get a picture of what is enjoyable for the child. Consequently, the child who stays regulated and engaged longer is able to learn within the experience and ultimately move forward developmentally (Hess, 2009).

Case Example

A child appears not to be able to leave her home without holding onto a stick. This seems like something inappropriate that we might want to discourage. But yet something about this object has meaning for this child. So we first have to ask ourselves, what is it about this activity that is so meaningful for the child? It is minimizing to simply attribute what we assume to be aberrant behavior to the fact that a child has a developmental delay like autism. Not only is this short sighted, but it does little to help us understand the underlying causes that are potentially fueling the odd behavior. The key to understanding the child is to follow her lead as an entry point into her world and create an emotional connection that allows us to pull that child into a shared emotional experience. This might mean that the adult facilitator picks up his own stick and attempts to mimic the gestures of the original item. Then it is up to the adult to expand the initial gesture into something socially appropriate and mutual, say, taking the two sticks and gently pretending to fence with them, or helping the child with developmental delays enter the world of symbolism by pretending that the stick is actually the body of an airplane, the play facilitator guiding this activity by making the appropriate sounds and gestures of a gliding plane.

Here the two philosophies behind DIR® Floortime are at work. We are accepting the child and the beloved object, knowing that there is something intrinsically valuable in the relationship that the child has with the object (I will speak later in the chapter regarding how individual, underlying, neurological processing differences are often guiding a child's choice of play and/or flight) and we are also encouraging a child to leave her preferred world of isolation in favor of an experience where her original idea of holding onto a stick has magically emerged into a shared play experience.

Joining the Child's World

Following the child's lead is only half of the equation; half of this dynamic that we call Floortime. There is another half: Joining the child in his or her world and pulling him or her into a shared emotional experience in order to help him or her master each of the Functional Emotional Developmental Capacities. These are the fundamentals of emotional, social, language, and intellectual development. When we talk about Functional Emotional Capacities, we're talking about the fundamentals of relating, communicating, and thinking (Greenspan, 2010).

The larger goal is to join the child in his or her world. We want to then pull the child into our shared world to teach and help him or her learn how to focus and attend, relate with real warmth, be purposeful and take initiative, and have a back-and-forth set of communications with us through non-verbal gestures, and eventually, through words. We want to teach children how to problem-solve and sequence and get them involved in a continuing interaction with their environment and the people in it. We want to teach them to use ideas creatively and then we want to teach them to use ideas logically and then progress up the developmental ladder until they are not only using ideas logically but actually showing high degrees of reflective thinking, empathy, and understanding of the world so that they can evaluate their own thoughts and feelings. Not every child is capable of achieving the highest level of reflective thinking, but almost all children are capable of moving up the developmental ladder, mastering their own Functional Emotional Developmental Capacities in regards to optimum social, emotional, intellectual, linguistic, and academic growth (Greenspan, 2001). Some concerns expressed by play clinicians are whether or not DIR® Floortime is applicable to children who have moderate to severe forms of developmental delays. The direct answer is yes, even with children who are severely impacted with developmental delays. With the right kind of support, you can move that child forward and upward.

Case Example

Jane is 5 years old, chronologically, although her current developmental age is that of a child about 6 months old. She has no functional language and does not appear to have the interest or capacity to play with toys. In addition to the diagnosis of severe autism, the child also has a co-morbid diagnosis of moderate to severe mental retardation. She enters the playroom mostly aimless and not able to stay engaged with anything or any person for any length of time. Characteristic of the disorder, the child flaps her arms in a self-stimulatory gesture in a continuous horizontal pattern.

The difficulty that play clinicians often face with severely impacted children is the confusion of how to follow a child's lead when the child appears not to be able to offer any lead to follow. This is the art of Floortime. You cannot do Floortime, the play therapy portion of this intervention, unless you understand the child's DIR® (the developmental capacity, the underlying, neurological, processing differences and how to use the child's relationship in the world to woo that child into a shared experience). By knowing a child's DIR®, the interventionist knows how and where to enter the child's world in such a way as to create a validating experience—in other words, the great date. To move a child forward developmentally to become a more complex thinker, despite overt cognitive delays, we need to make sure they possess the basic capacity to be regulated and stay engaged.

Since Jane is only offering her hand movements as "the lead," this is where the clinician must enter. Playfully, the therapist puts her own hands within the child's self-stimulatory hand and arm movements. Notice that the clinician is not entering the play encounter thinking that she is with a 5-year-old child; rather, the therapist joins Jane at the little girl's developmental capacity. In other words, in the clinician's mind, she is now playing with a child who is 6 months old. She must drop her intervention and level of expectation to that level while she uses her relationship to support the child's underlying processing challenges. Consequently, the therapist slows the child's flapping gesture down, creating a regular opening and closing rhythm to what was, a moment before, a chaotic gesture. As the interventionist slows and regulates to the beat of the activity, the clinician also uses her voice and her facial gestures to create a high affective encounter. The clinician begins to sing a classic child's song: "Open shut them, open shut them, give a little clap." Suddenly, Jane, who up until this time appeared not to be able to focus or attend, looks with curiosity into the face of her play partner. She appears intrigued and curious. The clinician has just taught this child the first fundamental game of play, pat-a-cake. The developmental age of this child, and subsequently, her ability to be a more complex thinker, has improved within one play session from 6 months of age to 9 months of age.

Progressing From Following a Child's Lead to Mastery

How do we use "following the child's lead" to actually mobilize and help the child master these critical developmental milestones? To help children master the first stage of shared attention, when they are, for example, wandering away from our interaction with them, we may play a game that places the play partner in front of the child, essentially blocking the child's exit from the interaction. The blocking gesture necessitates the child's creation of some kind of engagement with the play partner, even if it is a gesture of annoyance. This will form the foundation of the first act of shared attention that they are providing. The play partner is encouraged to continue to up the ante by creating more playful obstructions (like asking for a ticket or a token from the child to assure passage). These types of maneuvers create multiple opportunities for shared attention as well as sustained engagement because the child is otherwise involved with the therapist. Interestingly, this is also the beginning of purposeful action because the child is trying to move the obstruction (in this case the therapist) out of the way. As the child continues to attempt to maneuver the obstacle out of the way, the therapist "plays dumb," forcing the child to solve his or her way out of the current obstacle. These strategies are called *playfully obstructive strategies* and they are for the most aimless or avoidant of children.

Case Example

A 5-year-old boy named Ian, impacted with a moderate degree of autism, enters the playroom and appears to absent-mindedly pick up a piece of chalk before dropping the drawing material randomly on the floor. Previously, his mother had expressed concern that her son is not showing any age-appropriate interest in drawing, coloring, or cutting, and she fears that the child is progressively falling further and further behind his classmates. The clinician, keeping in mind the parent's concern, decides to take the play activity out of the playroom and into an outdoor play area. She follows Ian's lead by attempting to incorporate the child's fleeting interest in the chalk and then attempting to expand that germ of an idea into a sustained play encounter by doing some chalk drawings on the sidewalk. Once outside, she places Ian in her lap, both to prevent flight and also to help the child become more regulated and engaged by providing proprioceptive input (deep pressure) around which he can organize and reduce the anxiety that is potentially fueling his resistance to the play activity. She hands the child a piece of chalk, while mimicking hand-over-hand gestures in its use. Ian completely rejects the activity and withdraws his hand from any attempt to handle the chalk.

What is going on in the mind of the clinician? This question arises when considering how far to push this child in terms of his capacity to tolerate further playful obstruction. One of the basic principles of Floortime is "never take *no* for an answer." In other words, try not to back away from the resistance presented when you try to initially move a child forward developmentally. The first step in this case is to clarify the child's actual capacities to see if he has the physical ability to hold a piece of chalk in his hand. Using occupational therapy strategies, the therapist explores whether or not the child has an adequate pincher grasp (the ability to pinch together the thumb and the forefinger) by seeing if the child is capable of handing the clinician's therapy dog a dog biscuit. The thinking behind this is that the child's resistance to drawing can be overcome by his greater love for the clinician's dog. Ian is readily able to feed the dog with the appropriate grasp. This encourages the clinician to further expand the interaction by having the child draw the letters of the dog's name in chalk and then by having him use his pincher grasp to again dot the letters of the dog's name with muffin (left over from a previous social skills baking activity) while instructing the dog to "eat up her name" on command. This time around, the request to draw with the chalk is met with absolutely no resistance as Ian delights in the use of this "living puppet" to playfully overcome his resistance to the task and ultimately move him forward developmentally.

The goal of playfully obstructive strategy is to follow the child's lead on one hand but then create opportunities and challenges that help the child master each of his functional emotional developmental goals on the other. That is the dialectic, the two opposite polarities of Floortime: Joining the child in his rhythms while creating systematic challenges that pose opportunities to master new developmental milestones. It is in those systematic challenges that many of the specific techniques and strategies of Floortime come into play.

We, as play clinicians, are always trying to broaden the child's capacities in terms of his or her current level of development. In other words, the basic axiom of Floortime is that if children show the capacity to be a little bit purposeful, the next step is to encourage them to be very purposeful. If they can open and close a series of back-and-forth encounters (circles of communication) then we want to playfully enlarge this capacity until the child is able to sustain a series of 50 or 60 of these reciprocal interactions (Greenspan, 2010).

In order to engage in these Floortime interactions where we are following a child's lead while continually challenging him or her to master each functional emotional developmental milestones we must be aware of his or her individual, underlying, neurological processing differences. A particular child's unique developmental challenge, be it sensory, social, or motoric, creates an awareness in the clinician and a starting point for intervention. If, for example, a child is underreactive to touch and sound, this necessitates the play partner to be very energetic as he pulls the child into the shared world. Conversely, if another child is oversensitive to touch and sound (e.g., covering her ears to avoid sudden noises, easily becoming agitated), the play partner may have to be extra soothing while still being compelling. Many children have a *mixed profile*, a combination of reactivity under different circumstances where he or she can be both under- and over-reactive to environmental stimuli. In this situation, the rhythm of the play clinician needs to match both the internal and external "beat" of the child by being both soothing and compelling (e.g., using a soft yet energetic whisper while approaching these children) (Greenspan, 2001).

The clinician must also be aware of children's auditory processing capacities and language abilities, because the more pleasurable their play encounter is, the more likely they will be to invest in future emotional experiences. Auditory processing has less to do about hearing and more to do with the way that the brain processes auditory messages. I often ask clinicians to imagine being on a bad cell phone line, where the message is not necessarily being dropped, but rather incessantly interrupted (Hess, 2009). Likewise, the children with a form of auditory confusion may symptomatically resemble children who are tuned out to the world because the auditory message is too confusing to follow. Too often, the play partner does not take into account that area of processing distortion and speaks too rapidly or at a level that is far too complex for their developmental level. This is where keeping in mind DIR® is critical. Rather than demand that children meet the play partner with regards to auditory regulation, it is up to the play partner to realistically assess where they are developmentally, take into consideration the individual, underlying, neurological differences (in this case auditory processing concerns), and then use the relationship to help support the children's differences. For example, the practitioner may woo the child with simple energetic phrases such as "Open door?" rather than either a monotone request or command.

With visual spatial processing, some children may have good visual memory but may not be good visual problem solvers. Therefore, the clinician may need to use a great many visual cues while building visual memory skills to help children join into a shared world experience. Additionally, many children have both motor problems and sequencing concerns. To address these issues, we need to start with simple actions and progress to more complex action patterns. By tuning in to children's underlying, neurological, processing differences, we can then challenge them to master more complex levels of development (Greenspan & Weider, 1999).

Case Example

A 4-year-old boy named Joseph, who is impacted by high-functioning autism, is in a total inclusion class where the teacher-to-student ratio is 1:16 and in which there is no teacher's aide. Our first sign of alert that there may be underlying, neurological, processing differences is that despite the fact that the month is November and his mother has started out the day by dressing him in long pants and long sleeves, Joseph has stripped down to tennis shorts and a T-shirt and stuffed his original outfit into his cubby. This is the uniform that he wears each day in class. While not necessarily indicating some kind of pathology per se, we have a "red flag" regarding Joseph's ability to tolerate different textures against his body and we need to be thoughtful as to how his potential for tactile defensiveness could impact his ability to learn. Joseph is now in class and looks somewhat interested in joining his peers on the floor during morning circle time. Although he has been in school for over 2 months, he appears lost and does not know exactly where he is supposed to sit. There are no definitive markings that show his "spot" on the carpet. Consequently, Joseph spends much of his initial time in the class trying to figure out exactly where he belongs. The teacher then begins the lesson. While he is reminding the students about last evening's homework assignment, in which the children were supposed to bring something from home that started with the letters H, M, or B, the overhead PA system goes off, announcing the lunch specials for the day. The conflicting auditory messages of the PA system and the teacher's instruction appear to create total confusion in Joseph. However, he does have certain coping skills. He is looking around, earnestly trying to copy the actions and gestures of his peers. He even raises his hands as he sees his classmates do to ask the teacher if he can go to his cubby. Joseph's hand-raising gesture and question comes about a beat and a half after his classmates ask their questions. This is called a processing delay, and although not a critical issue at this point in his academic career, it is a potential harbinger of future learning challenges. When finally given permission to join his classmates, Joseph proceeds to the area of his cubby. He appears quite lost. Not only is he confused about what the teacher wants from him, but he also appears to have no idea where his unmarked cubby has gone to. He returns to the carpet appearing disoriented.

One of the many ways that clinicians can use DIR® Floortime™ is by first identifying a child's strengths. Joseph is clearly a visual learner. He is trying very hard to copy his peers and overall he is quite compliant. Why do we want to focus on a child's strengths before moving ahead to treatment? If you remember the idea of a great date, a validating emotional experience that you have with children that reinforces their desire to stay engaged with the therapist, learn from the therapist, and ultimately move forward developmentally, then focusing on their present ability, whatever that may be, is the entrance into both treatment and that reinforcing relationship.

Once children feel validated, they are more likely to allow the therapist to challenge them without fleeing the experience (Hess, 2009).

In the case of Joseph, many strategies can be incorporated to support his underlying neurological differences. As a visual learner, he could benefit from several visual cues that the teacher could have placed strategically around the classroom, including a textured and color-coordinated spot on the carpet to support his challenges regarding motor planning capacities, particularly when he is stressed and overwhelmed. Likewise, his cubby could have his picture at the entrance to help him locate his place for his assignments. The teacher could also be more cognizant of Joseph's auditory processing challenges. Instead of exclusively giving his instruction orally, the teacher could also supplement the lesson with various visual maps and schedules around the classroom that give additional direction and assure that at least one type of message (either oral or visual) is understood by the child. There is also a suggestion that although he does not really understand how to use his peers for support, Joseph does indeed appear curious about his classmates and seems to want to try to imitate their gestures and movements. "Soft souls" are the children who we find in every classroom who understand children with developmental concerns. They are neither intimidated by autistic self stimulatory gestures nor put off by some of the more esoteric movements of children with special needs. In contrast to kind adults who might be more inclined to feel sorry or excuse the behavior of an atypically developing child, a typical peer generally demands that the child on the spectrum fully participate in social activities. Teachers need to identify to the parents of children impacted by autism these "soft souls" so that typical peer play dates can be arranged as part of the therapeutic process (Hess, 2009).

A Caveat About the Caregiver

We also need to pay attention to ourselves as caregivers, as families, as family members, and as therapists. What are our natural strengths and weaknesses? What do we do easily? Are we high-energy individuals, great with underreactive children who need lots of energizing and wooing, but who have a hard time soothing? Or are we great soothers—we are good with hypersensitive children who need calm and a lot of soothing, but have a hard time energizing up for the child who is underreactive? In regards to our own personal foibles, do we take the child's avoidance of our overtures as a personal rejection and therefore shut down? Or do we take the child's avoidance as a challenge and try too hard and become too intrusive as we demand that the child involve himself in the relationship with us? By paying attention to our own individual personalities, our family patterns, our therapeutic skills and strategies, we are ultimately going to make better clinical decisions that fine-tune our abilities and help us create the learning interactions that help our children succeed (Greenspan, 2010).

Clinicians are constantly asking how to create and sustain an interaction. The key point is to harness the child's initiative and both receptive and expressive processes and to avoid feeling pressured to come up with a particular product at the end of each encounter. The goal is to observe what they are doing and then find the right rhythm, the right moment, that allows you to join them in doing what they are already involved in. The next step is to take a gesture where children are merely tolerating your presence and turn the encounter into imitative gestures that can be taken to the next level by challenging the child to move forward developmentally.

Once the interaction is reciprocal and there is a nice back-and-forth rhythm, including attention, engagement, and purposeful communication, then we need to work to ensure that the communication continues to expand. The hardest thing for children with developmental concerns like autism is to engage in back-and-forth communication that moves forward in a continuous flow of intentional verbal and non-verbal gestures. To achieve this goal, the play clinician is encouraged to create numerous obstacles so that children must interact with the clinician on a continuous basis to get what they want.

Case Example

Sally is a 3-year-old child brought to the clinic by her aunt and uncle, who are her legal guardians. She continually wants to go out the door. Rather than simply acquiesce to the request, the clinician makes that objective much more complex by creating a 10-step process, rather than just a 1-step objective. As Sally approaches with her need to go outside, the aunt resists, saying, "Go get Daddy if you want me to open the door, it's too heavy." Sally must now find her uncle, who additionally offers his own playful obstruction to the process to prolong the social interaction. The uncle says something like, "Can you show me where to turn the knob?" The child shows her uncle the knob, and he then adds, "Help me pull on the door," and begins to make sounds of exertion. Sally begins to mimic the sounds of exertion as she supports the process of getting herself outside. The adult play partner has just added the beginning of language, making the whole process all the more complex. Clinicians should vary their own movements and gestures as a response to the clinician's process. (Greenspan, 2010)

In conclusion, DIR® Floortime™ requires clinicians, and the parent or caregiver whom they are training to appreciate the polarity between following the child's lead and entering their world. Only then can children be "pulled" into a shared world, by finding their pleasure and joys while continually challenging them to master each of the functional developmental capacities. That means paying attention to the child's underlying neurological differences in the way that they process sound, sights, and movements, and modulate sensations. It also means paying attention to the family patterns and to your own reactions as the play clinician. This encourages both self-awareness and improved techniques as one enters a child's world and tailors interactions to the child's specific nervous system. That is the basis of this play intervention. That is why DIR® Floortime™ is more than just a technique that scripts 6–10 times a day for 20 minutes at a time of reciprocal play interaction; rather, it is a lifestyle and philosophy for school, home, and every time you have the opportunity to interact with a child.

Evidence Base for the DIR® Floortime™ Approach

Evidence-based practice integrates the best available scientifically rigorous research, clinical expertise, and the therapist's characteristics to ensure the quality of clinical judgments and delivery of the most cost-effective care (Weisz & Gray, 2007). A starting point to measure effectiveness of intervention is to determine the factors to be measured. With developmental programs like DIR® Floortime™, in contrast to behavioral approaches that tend to measure specific targeted behaviors or target underlying capacities or "core deficits" as the focus of intervention, progress is evident in a complex array of changes in interactive behavioral patterns.

Developmental capacities seek to measure changes in an individual's capacity for shared attention, the ability to form and have warm, intimate, trusting relationships and the ability to initiate using intentioned actions and social engagement that leads to spontaneous communication. Additionally, developmental capacities look at problem-solving strategies by assessing the ability to have coregulation and consequently be able to adapt to the feelings of others. Developmental capacities also determine an individual's ability to be creative as well as the capacity to have logical and analytic thought while developing a sense of self or core values (Cullinane, 2009).

Developmental models emphasize individual processing differences and the need to tailor intervention to the unique biological profile of children as well as the characteristics of the relationship between parent and child. Because both of the factors being measured are complex and because of the wide range of individual neurological processes in the population, research on the effectiveness of a developmental framework has progressed by examining the subcomponents of the overall approach. The subcomponents can be summarized by looking at the three major aspects of the DIR® Floortime™ approach:

D for developmental framework
I for the underlying, neurological, processing differences of a child
R for relationship and subsequent affective interactions

D: The Developmental Framework

A developmental approach considers behavior and learning in the greater context of a developmental or changing process. In 1997, evidence first showed the promise of the DIR® Floortime™ approach when 200 charts of children who were initially diagnosed with autistic spectrum disorder were reviewed. The goal of the review was to reveal patterns in presenting symptoms, underlying processing difficulties, early development, and response to intervention in order to generate hypotheses for future studies. The chart review suggested that a number of children with autistic spectrum diagnoses were, with appropriate intervention, capable of empathy, affective reciprocity, creative thinking, and healthy peer relationships (Greenspan & Wieder, 1997). The results of the 200-case series led Greenspan and Wieder to publish in 2000 the full description of the DIR® Floortime™ model (ICDL, 2000). In 2005, Greenspan and Wieder published a 10- to 15-year follow-up study of 16 children diagnosed with ASD that were part of the first 200-case series. The authors described that 10 to 15 years after receiving DIR® Floortime™ as a treatment method, these children had become significantly more empathetic, creative, and reflective adolescents with healthy peer relationships and solid academic skills (Greenspan & Wieder, 2005).

The DIR® Floortime™ model has provided a developmental framework that has been studied and found to be accurate in understanding behavior. A common pediatric assessment tool, the Bayley Scale of Infant Development, has adopted the DIR® milestones, specifically configured as the Greenspan Social–Emotional Growth Chart (SEGC) as the measure by which social and emotional development is measured (Greenspan, 2004). In 2007, Solomon et al. published an evaluation of the Play Project Home Consultation (PPHC), an in-home–based version of the DIR® Floortime™ model that trains parents of children with autism spectrum disorder in the DIR® Floortime™ model. The results showed significant increases in the child subscale scored on another pediatric assessment tool, the Functional Emotional Assessment Scale (FEAS; Greenspan and DeGangi, 2001), after an 8- to 12-month program using DIR® Floortime™ (Solomon et al., 2007).

I: Individual Underlying Neurological Processing Differences

In 1979, Jean Ayres, an occupational therapist from Torrance, California, pioneered discoveries about the way in which a child's sensory processing capacities could impact the way in which children learned and integrated themselves into their worlds (Ayres, 1979). This revolutionary idea provided a new way to understand the importance of movement and regulatory behaviors in children and began to offer explanations for some of the more worrisome behaviors impacting children with developmental concerns like autism. Over the last 40 years, a large body of research has further illuminated the impact of biologically based differences in regards to both sensorimotor processing and the impact on emotional regulation. In 2001, the National Research Council of the National Academy of Sciences published a report, entitled "Educating Children with Autism," which called for the tailoring of treatment approaches to fit the unique biological profile of the individual child (Committee on Educational Intervention for Children with Autism, 2001). Lillas and Turnball (2009), in their published text, describe how all behavior is influenced by the sensory systems in the brain. They indicate that an infant's sensory capacities are genetically prepared to respond to human interaction and are shifting in direct relationship to the parent's touch, facial, vocal, and movement expressions. Child–parent interactions and sensory activities create nerve cell networks and neural pathways in the development of the child's brain. The exchange of that takes place during child–parent play interactions and are seen as an ongoing loop of sensorimotor transformations (Lillas & Turnball, 2009).

R: Relationship and Affect

Developmental models have evolved from many years of discovery in the field of infant mental health. Beginning in the 1950s, there was a new understanding of the importance of parent–child interaction (Bowlby, 1951). Building on these years of research in developmental psychology that underscores the importance of early relationships and family functioning, Dr. Stanley Greenspan and his partner, Dr. Serena Wieder, began their work together studying the interaction of mothers and their babies in the context of infants who were at high risk for attachment problems (National Center for Clinical Infant Programs, 1987). Subsequently, there have been numerous research studies confirming the importance of parent–child interaction and the value of intervention programs that focus on supporting the parent–child relationship, particularly in the areas of joint attention and emotional attunement (Mahoney & Pearles, 2004). In 2006, Gernsbacher published a paper that showed how intervention itself between a parent and child could change the way in which parents interact, in turn increasing reciprocity, and that these changes correlated to positive changes in social engagement and language. In 2008, Connie Kasari and colleagues at the University of California–Los Angeles (Kasari, Paparella, Freeman, & Jahromi) used a randomized controlled trial to look at joint attention and symbolic play with 58 children with autism. Results indicated that expressive language gains were greater for treatment groups where a developmental model was utilized as compared with a control group that was based on exclusive behavioral principles. Most recently, psychobiologist Colwyn Trevarthen (Malloch & Trevarthen, 2009) introduced the concept of infants' relational intentionality with their primary caregiver that prompts musical exchanges. He has coined a phrase *communicative musicality* to describe babies' natural musical aptitude that gets them emotionally in sync with their mothers. He further describes the social and emotional problems of children who have mothers with severe emotional problems that inhibit the natural rhythmic relationship between themselves and their children.

Conclusion: Integration and Application of DIR

Autism is now recognized as a disorder of integration among various distinct brain functions. Research investigation is currently focused on understanding deficits in neuronal communication as a basis of the wide array of behavioral manifestations of the disorder (Cullinane, 2009). Developmental intervention has advanced to incorporate the use of affect to enhance integration of sensory-regulatory, communication, and motor systems. With that in mind, neuro-imaging research is beginning to provide a deeper understanding as to how emotional experiences are actually impacting developing brain growth. Siegel (2001) showed how attuned relationships in infancy change brain structure in ways that later impact social and emotional development, and recently, a research study by Casenhiser, Stieben, and Shanker (2010) through the Milton and Ethel Harris Research Initiative at the York University in Canada investigated the behavioral and neuro-physiological outcomes of intensive DIR® Floortime™ intervention, using both event-related potential (ERP) and electroencephalography (EEG) measurements. Discussion is also continuing on ways to apply the basic principles of DIR® Floortime™ towards an adult developmentally delayed population (Samson, 2010).

While research efforts continue to reveal a better understanding of the etiology, pathophysiology, and efficacy of treatment approaches for autism, clinical experience also continues to accumulate. DIR® Floortime™ is one of two approaches formally recognized by the American Academy of Pediatrics in its Toolkit for Autism as treatment options for children impacted by autism (Myers & Johnson, 2007). There are now more than 10 active school programs in six states rooted in the DIR Floortime approach for the treatment of children and adolescents with autism: California, New York, New Jersey, Georgia, Florida, and Utah (ICDL, 2010). As recently as September 2010, a judge in Los Angeles, California, approved a settlement allowing families of children with autism in Eastern Los Angeles County to receive state funds for DIR® Floortime™ intervention (Zarembo, 2010).

Efforts continue to deepen our understanding of the complexities of autism. The alarming increase in the diagnosis of autism worldwide (Kogan et. al., 2009), as well as the lack of specific information about etiology of the disorder demands that play therapists increase their knowledge and understanding of how a child's development is impacted by the individual, underlying, neurological processing differences and the interaction of the relationships that the child has in the world (Greenspan & Wieder, 2005). In September 2009, *Zero to Three* focused an issue on the importance of play, specifically on the role of spontaneous, child-led, social play experiences that support social, emotional, and cognitive growth (Hirschland, 2009). Although research continues, it is imperative that developmental approaches like DIR® Floortime™ remain a viable option for play intervention for children with developmental delays and their families.

References

Ayres, J. A. (1979). *Sensory integration and the child*. Los Angeles: Western Psychological Services.

Bowlby J. (1951). *Maternal care and mental health*. World Health Organization (WHO) Monograph Series, no. 51. Geneva: World Health Organization.

Casenhiser, D., Stieben, J., & Shanker, S. (2010). *Learning through interaction*. Retrieved from http://research.news.yorku.ca/2010/08/11/ontarios-lieutenant-governor-visits-yorks-Milton-Ethel-Harris-research-initiative

Committee on Educational Intervention for Children with Autism. (2001). *Educating children with autism*. C. Lord & J. P. McGee (Eds.). Division of Behavioral and Social Sciences and Education, National Research Council. Washington, DC: National Academy Press.

Cullinane, D. (2009). Evidence base for the DIR®/Floortime approach. Retrieved from http://www.drhessautism.com/img/news/EvidenceBasefortheDIR®Model Cullinane0901 09.pdf

Gernsbacher, M. A. (2006). Toward a behavior of reciprocity. *Journal of Developmental Processes*, 1, 139–152. Retrieved from http://psy.wisc.edu/lang/pdf/gernsbacher reciprocity.pef

Greenspan, S. I. (2001). The affect diatheses hypothesis: the role of emotions in the core deficit. In autism and the development of intelligence and social skills. *Journal of Developmental and Learning Disorders*, 5, 1.

Greenspan, S. I. (2010). Floor Time™: What it really is, and what it isn't. Retrieved from http://www.icdl.com/dirFloortime/newsletter/FloortimeWhatitReallyis andisnt.shtml

Greenspan S. I., & DeGangi, G. (2001). Research on the FEAS: Test development, reliability, and validity studies. In S. Greenspan, G. DeGangi, & S. Wieder (Eds.), *The Functional Emotional Assessment Scale (FEAS) for infancy and early childhood: Clinical and research applications* (pp. 167–247). Bethesda, MD: Interdisciplinary Council on Developmental and Learning Disorders.

Greenspan, S. I., & Wieder, S. (1997). Developmental patterns of outcome in infants and children with disorders in relating and communicating: A chart review of 200 cases of children with autistic spectrum diagnoses. *Journal of Developmental and Learning Disorders*, 1(87), 141.

Greenspan, S. I., & Wieder, S. (1999). A functional developmental approach to autism spectrum disorders. *Journal of the Association for Persons With Severe Handicaps, 24*(3), 147–161.

Greenspan, S. I., & Wieder, S. (2005). Can children with autism master the core deficits and become empathic, creative and reflective? A ten to fifteen year follow-up of a subgroup of children with autism spectrum disorders (ASD) who received a comprehensive Developmental, Individual-Difference, Relationship-Based (DIR®) approach. *Journal of Developmental and Learning Disorders, 9*, 39–61.

Hess, E. (2009). *DIR®/Floor Time™: A developmental/relational approach towards the treatment of autism and sensory processing disorder.* Paper presented at the American Psychological Association Annual Conference, Toronto, Canada.

Hirschland, D. (2009). Addressing social, emotional, and behavioral challenges through play, *Zero to Three, 30*(1), 12–17.

Interdisciplinary Council on Developmental and Learning Disorders. (ICDL). (2000). *ICDL clinical practice guidelines: Redefining the standards of care for infants, children and families with special needs.* Bethesda, MD: The Interdisciplinary Council on Developmental and Learning Disorders.

Interdisciplinary Council on Developmental and Learning Disorders. (ICDL). (2010). Interdisciplinary Council on Developmental and Learning Disorders annual conference, poster sessions.

Kasari, C., Paparella, T., Freeman, S., & Jahromi, L.B. (2008). Language outcome in autism: randomized comparison of joint attention and play interventions. *Journal of Consulting and Clinical Psychology, 76*(1), 125–137.

Lillas, C., & Turnball, J. (2009). *Infant/Child mental health, early intervention and relationship-based therapists: A neuro-relationship framework for interdisciplinary practice.* New York: Norton & Company, Inc.

Mahoney, G., & Perales, F. (2004). Relationship-focused in early intervention with children with pervasive developmental disorders and other disabilities: A comparative study. *Journal of Developmental and Behavioral Pediatrics, 26*, 77–85.

Malloch, S., & Trevathen, C. (2009). *Communicative musicality: Exploring the basis of human companionship.* London: Oxford University Press.

Mastrangelo, S. (2009). Harnessing the power of play: Opportunities for children with autism spectrum disorders. *Teaching Exceptional Children, 42*(1), 34–44.

Myers, S. M., & Johnson, C. P. (2007). Council on Children's Disabilities. *Pediatrics, 120*, 1162–1182.

National Center for Clinical Infant Programs. (1987). *Infants in multi-risk families. Case studies in preventative intervention.* In S. I. Greenspan, S. Wieder, R. A. Nover, A. Lieberman, R. S. Lourie, & M. E. Robinson (Eds.), *Clinical Infant Reports, Number 3.* International Universities Press.

Samson, A. (2010). Applying DIR®/Floor Time™ principles to a developmental disabled adult population. Paper presented at California Association for Disabilities, Los Angeles.

Siegel, D. (2001). Toward an interpersonal neurobiology of the developing mind: attachment relationships, "mindsight," and neural integration. *Infant Mental Health Journal, 22*, 67–94.

Solomon, R. S., Necheles, J., Ferch, C., & Bruckman, D. (2007). Pilot study of a parent training program for young children with autism: The P.L.A.Y. Project Home Consultation Program, *Autism*, *11*(3), 205–224.

Weisz, J., & Gray, J. S. (2007). Evidence-based psychotherapy for children and adolescents: Data from the present and a model for the future, *ACAMH Occasional Papers*, *27*, 7–22.

Zarembo, A. (2010). Judge finalizes autism therapy. *Los Angeles Times*, September 14.

CHAPTER **13**

The PLAY Project

*A Train-the-Trainer Model of Early Intervention
for Children With Autism Spectrum Disorders*

RICHARD SOLOMON

Introduction

The development of an evidence-based, cost-effective, and easily dissemi-nated form of intensive intervention for children with autistic spectrum disorders (ASD) is a major priority for both the health and education sys-tems in this country. The most recent prevalence estimate for ASD from the Centers for Disease Control and Prevention is 1 in 110 children (CDC, 2007). According to the National Research Council (NRC) (cited in Lord, Bristol-Power, & Cafierol, 2001), these children need intensive interven-tion—25 hours per week of engaging, comprehensive intervention with a high 1:1 or 1:2 adult-to-child ratio—which most states do not provide because (1) there is a national shortage of trained personnel, (2) such inter-ventions when provided by professionals are very expensive ($25–60K annually) and (3) a cost-effective model has not yet been developed and tested for national distribution. The unmet national need is enormous.

The P.L.A.Y. (Play and Language for Autistic Youngsters) Project (http://www.playproject.org; hereafter referred to as PLAY) systematically trains professionals to coach parents to use PLAY principles, strategies, methods, and techniques with very young children (14 months to 6 years of age) with autism spectrum disorders. Its ultimate aim is to help parents be their child's best play partner. The project has research evidence (see the "Evidence Specific for Play" section, below) to support its developmental and interactional methods (Solomon, Necheles, Ferch, & Bruckman, 2007), has recently (2009) received a National Institutes of Health (NIH) grant to do a randomized controlled effectiveness study of the model, and has been successfully disseminated in hundreds of sites in dozens of states in the United States and internationally. PLAY's train-the-trainer model has the potential to address this growing unmet national need for intensive early intervention for young children with autism spectrum disorders and their families.

This chapter first describes the PLAY model and then presents the theoretical and empirical foundation for this intensive developmental intervention (IDI) approach. A case study is then offered, along with conclusions and a set of guidelines for using the approach with children with ASD.

Overview of the PLAY Project Model

Over the last 10 years, under the medical direction of developmental/behavioral pediatrician Richard Solomon, MD, PLAY has established itself as "a community based/regional autism training and early intervention center dedicated to empowering parents and professionals to implement intensive, developmental interventions (IDI) for young children with autism spectrum disorder in the most cost-effective and efficient way" (from the project's vision statement). PLAY trains child development professionals to coach parents, typically at home, to help their child with ASD make developmental gains through play-based interactions.

The PLAY Project uses Greenspan's Developmental, Individual Difference, Relationship-Based (DIR) framework (Greenspan, 1992; Greenspan & Wieder, 1997a), which describes six increasingly complex functional developmental levels (FDLs) through which children gain the ability to fully relate to others:

1. Self-regulation and shared attention (FDL 1) (Birth–3 months)
2. Engagement (FDL 2) (4–8 months)
3. Two-way communication (FDL 3) (9–14 months)
4. Complex two-way communication (FDL 4) (15–24 months)
5. Shared meanings and symbolic play (FDL 5) (2–3 years)
6. Emotional thinking (FDL 6) (3–5 years)

An appreciation of these levels is important in understanding the PLAY Project model; they are briefly described next.

In infancy, babies learn to regulate themselves to stay calm and attentive for longer and longer periods of time (FDL 1). By 4 to 9 months of age, this shared attention extends to full engagement (FDL 2) in games such as peek-a-boo and patty-cake. A key element of Greenspan's theory is the importance of interactional *circles*, or the back-and-forth contingent reciprocal exchange of communication. At each FDL, the number and complexity of circles increases. Soon, then, infants as young as 9–15 months begin two-way communication as partners in the relationship (e.g., chase, catch) and can sustain playful, back-and-forth interactions (FDL 3) that become increasingly complex. By 15–24 months toddlers develop complex two-way problem-solving communication with a combination of gestures and words; simple pretend play (e.g., feeding dolls, phone to ear) is emerging; and back-and-forth interactions take on the quality of simple conversations (FDL 4). By age 2, communication becomes progressively more and more symbolic with shared meanings allowing young children to understand routines and one- and two-step commands (FDL 5). From ages 3 to 5, children become amazingly sophisticated emotional thinkers. They can answer why and when questions and recall the past in detail. They talk in complex sentences and bridge ideas such that rich imaginative play becomes one hallmark of their functional communication (FDL 6).

This developmental framework also incorporates key elements common to most play-based models (see "Methodological Framework and Empirical Evidence" in this chapter for a full discussion). These include promoting parental sensitivity (i.e., reading the child's gestural cues) and responsiveness to the child's cues, lead, and intentions (i.e., following the child's lead) to increase the number of contingent reciprocal social exchanges (i.e., circles of communication). We also use Vgotsky's (1978) construct of the *zone of proximal development* to help parents play in ways that are not too high or too low developmentally but at the *just right* level where they follow the child's lead and challenge the child at the same time. Finally, the coaching model has been structured with the PLAY Project Skill Sequence, which includes dozens of activities and techniques to provide parents with guidance on what to do when following the child's lead is difficult.

In short, PLAY has incorporated developmental and interactional theory and evidence into a train-the-trainer model that makes the theory practical for professionals and parents. Figure 13.1 shows the key components of the PLAY Project model.

Identification and Referral (Michigan)

PLAY Central, home of the PLAY Project, is located in Ann Arbor, Michigan, at the Ann Arbor Center for Developmental and Behavioral Pediatrics. The founder, Richard Solomon, a board-certified developmental and behavioral pediatrician, serves as a regional resource to help families obtain a diagnosis of and referrals for their children with autism.

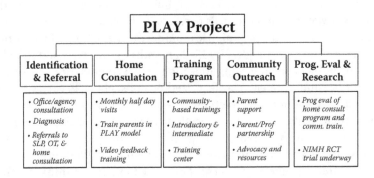

Figure 13.1 The PLAY project.

Experience gained through the "laboratory" in Michigan has helped the PLAY Project training directors learn about the networking process in communities and the importance of community in helping families no matter where they live.

As medical director, Solomon oversees the Ann Arbor PLAY Home Consultation program and longitudinally follows hundreds of children on the spectrum. He works in close collaboration with community-based referral sources that provide medical services, special education, speech and language therapy, occupational therapy, and psychiatric interventions. The goal is to help families obtain services that are consistent with the National Research Council. (In Michigan, as in the large majority of states, there are no publicly funded services that routinely and consistently provide 25 hours per week of intensive intervention for the children). Altogether, 15 independent PLAY Projects in Michigan, in total, serve nearly 15% of all young (14 months to 5 years old) children with autism spectrum disorders in the state. Solomon also works closely with the Michigan Chapter of the American Academy of Pediatrics and educates pediatricians about the importance of early identification, referral, and intervention. This local, regional, and statewide experience has served to disseminate the model in other states and regions where difficulties with diagnosis, referral, and intervention are also widespread.

The PLAY Project Home Consultation (PPHC) Program

The centerpiece of The PLAY model is the Home Consultation program, which is designed to train parents to be their child's best play partner.

PLAY Consultants (PC), who have degrees in child development fields (occupational therapy, speech/language pathologists, early childhood educators, social workers, recreational therapists, child psychologists), receive structured, intensive, year-long training in the model (see "Training"). A full-time PC can care for 25 new families, though most consultants are part time and will serve 5–15 families. Families typically receive 10 half-day (3 hours) home visits per year (though office-based adaptations of PLAY have also been successful). During home visits caregivers' interactions are videotaped. Between home visits, families get written feedback and suggestions for ways to improve their playful engagement. A training manual guides PC fidelity to the model. Families are expected to provide 2 hours per day using a combination of 15- to 20-minute PLAY sessions and a focus on PLAY-ful interaction during daily routines. PCs may travel up to an hour radius from the service center to serve families. Thus, large regions of a state can be served by a small group of PC providers (see "Guidelines" for cost of and settings for PLAY services). PLAY is an alternative to having professionals provide all of the intensive intervention in which case costs can range from $25,000 to $60,000 per year. This makes the PLAY parent training model a cost-effective alternative.

PLAY is outcomes oriented. During the *first visit*, home consultants collect baseline information that not only informs clinical judgment but also can be used to evaluate outcomes (see Appendix 1 for a list of evaluation instruments). In subsequent visits, home consultants train and coach parents to play with their child by teaching them to use The PLAY Project Skill Sequence (Figure 13.2) as their main training tool.

PLAY Skill Sequence: Summary

1. List Principles & Strategies Based on Comfort Zone (CZ) Sensory Profile (SP) & Fuctional Development Level (FDL)

2. Assess Child's unique: CZ Activities, SP & FDL

3. Define Daily & Weekly Curriculum/Activities

4. Follow Child's Cues, Lead & Intent to Increase Circles

5. Create Menu of Specific Techniques

6. Video Tape/ Critically Review Interactions and Progress

7. Refine Curriculum, Methods & Techniques

Figure 13.2 A summary of the PLAY Skill Sequence.

The Skill Sequence introduces the parents to PLAY's key principles:

1. The importance of "affect (the feeling life) in the context of relationship" (i.e., the importance of having "fun with people")
2. Providing the right dose (i.e., 2 hours per day of engaging intervention)
3. Profiling the child accurately to make sure that parents are
4. Playing at the right developmental level (not too high or too low).

We familiarize parents with the key concepts of comfort zone, sensory-motor profile, and functional developmental levels:

- Children's comfort zone is defined as what they will do when you let them do whatever they want to do. Comfort zone activities are repetitive, stereotyped, dominating interests.
- Sensory-motor profile is children's unique set of responses to the world based on their perceptions. Some children are overreactive to the world, sensitive to noises and sights; others are underreactive and may be hard to engage or arouse. Some children, for example, become overfocused on visually stimulating objects and will watch spinning toys over and over again. Many have poor auditory processing abilities and will not turn to their names. Most children with autism love deep pressure. So it makes sense that, if we want to engage children, we will limit the modes that bother or absorb children and focus on the sensory modes that engage them.
- Greenspan's functional developmental levels were described previously. How these levels are used to help children climb the developmental ladder will be detailed in the following case study.

The Skill Sequence guides the home consultant in accurately assessing the child's unique developmental profile, developing a curriculum of activities for the parents and teaching them the methods that promote contingent reciprocal interactions (i.e., following their lead and intention to increase circles). It also provides families with dozens of specific techniques that help them implement the approach. Most importantly, video feedback offers parents the perfect blend of theory and concrete specifics. They can see themselves in interaction, which can be analyzed to improve their approach. As children (hopefully) make progress, the curriculum must be refined. So the sequence starts all over again in this iterative developmental process.

Two other educational tools—*The PLAY Project DVD* and *Parent Training Manual*—are built around the Skill Sequence. The DVD is a replica of the 1-day PLAY Project Workshop I and explains the Skill Sequence by showing over 30 video clips of parents playing with their children. A second DVD, to be released this year, will describe ways to help young children with high-functioning ASD gain higher-level social skills.

Each half-day/3-hour home visit uses modeling, coaching, video feedback, and written feedback to help implement and then refine the Skill Sequence. Modeling involves PLAY Consultants (PC) demonstrating strategies, methods, and techniques of the Skill Sequence; coaching involves observing the parents as they play with their child and giving them positive feedback about their performance; video feedback involves analyzing a 15-minute segment of film taken at the home visit. The video is reviewed back at the office and subsequently used to give detailed written feedback.

Community Training Programs

Key to the PLAY Project's mission is educating communities about the science of autism spectrum disorders, the importance of the National Research Council recommendations for intensive early intervention, and the PLAY model. Community-based trainings include grand rounds presentations for medical professionals and community lectures and workshops. The basic and advanced workshops introduce professionals and parents to the PLAY Project methods for lower- and higher-functioning children with autism spectrum disorders, respectively. Over the last 10 years over 100 communities in dozens of states have been served, with thousands of parents and professionals attending community-based trainings. Evaluations of lectures and workshops have been generally positive.

Agency Training Programs

Agency training programs are much more intensive and extensive than the community trainings. Over the last 10 years, 162 agencies (private rehab services, schools/preschools/early intervention programs, hospitals and community mental health agencies) in 34 states and eight countries have been trained to provide the PLAY consultation program in their communities (see http://www.playproject.org for a listing).

Agency trainings occur in two phases. First agency personnel attend an intensive 4-day training (usually in Ann Arbor, Michigan) where future home consultants are taught to use the PLAY model and Skill Sequence, and how to set up a PLAY consultation program within their agencies. In the second supervision phase, PCs return to their agencies, start making PLAY consultation visits, and then send videos of their visits and their write-ups to PLAY supervisors who give them audio feedback. The use of Internet downloaded video and audio feedback allows for efficient, effective, long-distance supervision. Agency personnel can, with good planning, start serving families within a month of being trained (Figure 13.3, Agency Trainings).

The PLAY supervisors, who have at least 2 years of experience in the model, use a detailed fidelity-training manual to assess all aspects of the PC performance. Supervision is provided for 20 videos and write-ups,

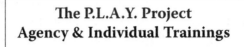

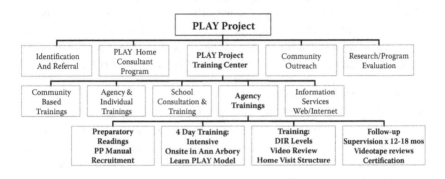

Figure 13.3 The PLAY Project trainings.

which takes about 12–18 months to accomplish. Assuming successful completion of supervision, agency staff will be certified. The complete cost of training to certification ranges from $4500 to $5500 depending on the number of personnel trained per agency.

Community Outreach

PLAY helps agencies start up their community-based programs by bringing PLAY workshops to the community, connecting them to physician/referral sources, and offering technical assistance (e.g., letters, brochures, fact sheets, flyers, YouTube clips, media packages, TV and radio interviews). PLAY has established a close working relationship with Easter Seals National and is disseminating home consultation programs through their national affiliates all over the United States.

Program Evaluation

As mentioned, the PLAY Project is outcomes oriented. Baseline and repeated measures are built into the clinical model so a child's progress can be evaluated objectively (see Appendix 1 and the Case Study). An evaluation of the PLAY Home Consulting program has been peer reviewed and published by the journal *Autism* (Solomon, 2007), and in 2009 the project received a large $1.85 million National Institute of Mental Health (NIMH) grant to implement a 3-year, multisite, randomized, controlled trial of the PLAY versus standard community services in collaboration with Easter Seals National and Michigan State University (see "Theoretical and Empirical Rationale"). PLAY's clinical and training programs are based on a growing body of empirical research, which is described in the next section.

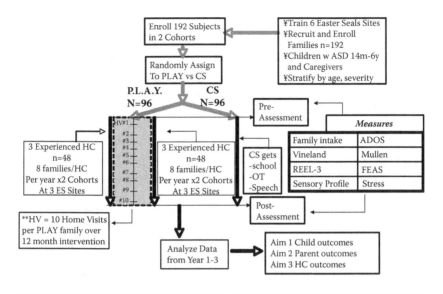

Figure 13.4 The PLAY Project NIH research design.

Theoretical and Empirical Rationale

Among the intensive interventions for young children (14 months to 6 years of age) with autism, two broad types—behavioral and developmental—are typical (Prizant & Wetherby, 1998). Though the approaches differ deeply in their fundamental theoretical underpinnings (Ingersoll, 2010), they share the key elements recommended by the National Research Council (e.g., 25 hours per week, high adult-to-child ratio).

In behavioral approaches—also known as applied behavioral analysis (ABA), early intensive behavioral intervention (EIBI), applied verbal behavioral (AVB) intervention, and pivotal response therapy—the children are typically taught 20–40 hours per week using an operant learning (Skinnerian) paradigm to increase language, social, and cognitive skills (Eikeseth et al., 2007; Howard, Sparkman, Cohen, Green, & Stanislaw, 2005; Lovaas, 1987; Lovaas, Koegel, Simmons, & Long, 1973; McEachin, Smith, & Lovaas, 1993; Sallows & Graupner, 2005; Simpson, 2005; Smith, 1999). These largely drill-based methods have been carefully evaluated and repeatedly shown, in research settings, to be efficacious in helping children learn discrete skills leading to improved cognitive abilities and language skills. Their impact on social skills is less certain (Shea, 2004), and the consistency of efficacy has been questioned in a recent meta-analysis (Krebs-Seida, Ospina, Karkhaneh, Hartling, Smith, & Clark, 2009).

In the intensive *developmental* interventions (IDI), on the other hand, drills and techniques are secondary to following the child's lead and promoting joint attention and contingent interactions to promote high affect ("fun") interactions. This focus on interaction and functional development make it more difficult to operationalize and quantify outcomes than the more commonly used behavioral approaches (Rogers, 2000). As a result, until recently the scientific evidence for IDI for very young children (14 months to 6 year olds) has been limited (Greenspan & Wieder, 1997b; Myers, Johnson, & the Council on Children with Disabilities, 2007; Rogers & Delalla, 1991; Tannock, Girolametto & Siegal, 1992; Wallace & Rogers, 2010). Over the last several years, however, a number of studies have been published that support IDI (Drew et al., 2002; Green et al., 2010; Kasari, Gulsrud, Wong, Kwon, & Jocke, 2010; Mahoney & Perales, 2004; McConachie, Randle, Hammal, & Le Couteur, 2005; Siller & Sigman, 2002; Solomon et al., 2007), and a number of new studies are under way that promise to provide empirical evidence for specific models like Mahoney's Responsive Teaching model (http://www.crainscleveland.com/article/20090925/FREE/909259974/1007), Prizant's SCERTS model (http://www.scerts.com/research-corner), and the PLAY Project. Some of these recent models combine teaching, behavioral, and developmental methods (Dawson et al., 2009; Ingersoll, 2010). Most of the IDI studies train parents to mediate child functioning. Parent training has the advantage of decreasing costs and promoting the use of intervention in natural environments, thus increasing the likelihood of generalization (Diggle, McConachie, & Randle, 2003). The empirical evidence—from early case studies to more rigorous research—for IDI in general and then the PLAY Project in particular will be briefly presented.

Evidence for IDI

The prototypical IDI model is represented by Greenspan and Wieder's DIR approach (Greenspan, 1992; Greenspan & Wieder, 1997a; Greenspan & Wieder, 1997b; Wieder & Greenspan, 2005). Greenspan's case series (Greenspan & Wieder, 1997b) involved a cohort of 200 children. This sample had a highly motivated, middle-upper income parent population. While this groundbreaking early study can be considered only observational, as there were no controls and no detailed description of the specific intervention protocols used, nonetheless, after 2 years of intervention, 58% of treated children—a very high rate of success—showed substantial improvements clinically, and many of the children no longer met the criteria for autistic disorder on key measures (e.g., CARS).

Four other studies, using various design methods and various IDI approaches, are of interest here. In a fascinating, longitudinal study, Siller and Sigman found that caregivers who synchronized their behaviors to their children's attention and activities helped children with autism develop superior joint attention and language when compared to parents who were less contingent or synchronized (Siller & Sigman, 2002). Mahoney and Perales (2004) used a controlled design and a parent-training model very similar in hours and methods to PLAY. His group found highly significant improvements in the intervention group ($N = 20$ children with pervasive developmental disorder [PDD]) on social reciprocity and language measures compared with the control group ($N = 30$ children with other types of developmental delays). In another controlled trial, McConachie et al. (2005) studied the Canadian *Hanen* model. Parents of 51 children aged 24 to 48 months received either immediate intervention or delayed access to the course. A significant advantage was found for the intervention group in parents' observed use of facilitative strategies and in children's vocabulary size. The training course was well received by parents and has a measurable effect on both parents' and children's communication skills (McConachie et al.).

Recent randomized controlled designs include the work of Green et al. (2010), Kasari, Gulsrud, Wong, Kwon, and Jocke (2008), and Kasari, Paparella, Freeman, and Jahromi (2010). Green and his coworkers in England implemented a large-scale ($n = 152$) randomized, multisite, controlled trial with young children (ages 2–4 years old) with ASD. This structured, home-based, 1-year intervention program was parent mediated and communication focused. Parents were asked to play with their child a half-hour per day. Even though the program did *not* meet the NRC definition of intensity, parents on a blinded observation measure showed statistically and clinically significant improvement in their sensitivity and responsivity to child cues. The children significantly improved attention, engagement, and initiation behaviors. Whereas the direct measure of language using the Pre-school Language Scale (PLS-4) was not different from the control group, language acquisition as measured by the MacArthur Child Development Inventories showed statistically significant improvement.

Kasari et al. (2008, 2010) assessed an intervention to promote joint engagement between caregivers and toddlers with autism. The intervention consisted of 24 caregiver-mediated sessions with follow-up 1 year later. Compared with caregivers and toddlers randomized to the wait-list control group, the immediate treatment (IT) group made significant improvements in targeted areas of joint engagement. The IT group demonstrated significant improvements with medium to large effect sizes in their responsiveness to joint attention and their diversity of functional play acts after the intervention with maintenance of these skills 1 year postintervention. These are among the first randomized controlled data to suggest that short-term parent-mediated interventions can have important effects on core impairments in toddlers with autism.

Evidence Specific for PLAY

In our study titled "Pilot Study of a Parent Training Program for Young Children with Autism: The P.L.A.Y. Project Home Consultation Program" (Solomon et al., 2007), 68 2- to 6-year-old children with ASD were evaluated using a pre- and postdesign at the start and at the end of the first year of intervention. Results from the Functional Emotional Assessment Scale (FEAS; Greenspan, DiGangi, & Wieder, 2001), a valid and reliable age-normed clinical rating scale, served as the primary outcome. The FEAS is a videotape observation scale that measures (1) changes in caregiver nurturing and contingent reciprocal interaction and (2) children's functional development (i.e., Greenspan's 6 Functional Developmental Levels [FDL]). FEAS raters were blinded and trained to reliability.

Child FEAS scores showed a highly statistically significant increase over the 12 months of the project (p £ .0001). When FEAS scored were translated clinically, 45.5% of children made good to very good clinical gains. There was no statistical relationship found between initial ASD severity and FEAS scores. Clinical ratings found that 66% of children made very good (1.5 FDLs or better) or good progress (1.0 FDL). In terms of "the dose" of intensity, there was a trend ($p = .09$) suggesting that the more hours a parent put in playing the better the child did on the FEAS scores.

Without a control group, it is not possible to say that changes in post-FEAS scores are directly attributable to the home-based training. The current controlled study funded by the NIMH plans to address this important issue.

Summary of the NIMH RCT PLAY Project Study

Following publication of our pilot study, the PLAY Project was granted a Phase 1 small business innovations research (SBIR) National Institutes of Health (NIH) grant to assess the feasibility of a multisite, randomized, controlled trial study. Our collaborators were Easter Seals National, who provides the sites, and Michigan State University, who provides independent evaluation. The Phase 1 trial showed feasibility, and the PLAY received a $1.8 million grant to implement a Phase 2 effectiveness trial in 2009. We are now in the second year of the 3-year study. In the first year we successfully recruited 60 children ages 3–5 years, matched by age, gender, and severity, and then randomized into community standard services (special education preschool with school-based language and occupational therapy services) or community standard *plus* PLAY Project Home Consultation.

The children are followed for 1 year. A rigorous, pre- and postevaluation design addresses whether (1) parents learn and implement the model, (2) PLAY children improve their functional, cognitive, and adaptive development when compared with control children, and (3) HCs show fidelity to the model. Altogether 120 children will be studied, making this one of the largest effectiveness trials of its kind. If the PLAY Project model proves to be effective, it will offer a replicable method of early intensive developmental intervention for young children with ASD. The train-the-trainer model provides an efficient, low-cost system for quick dissemination to serve a growing, unmet, national need.

Case Study

When Logan (not his real name), who was almost 3 years old, first came to my office it was sadly easy to see that he had the triad of autistic characteristics: delays in language, problems with social interaction, and dominating, repetitive interests. A beautiful, chubby little boy with black curly hair that framed a pixie face, he had 15–20 single words (a substantial delay), which reflected his interests: *book, up, out,* (1-2-3) *go, juice, train, Barney.* He seemed to understand routines but couldn't follow a simple command to "get that train." He spent much of his time looking through books, lining up trains, cars, and trucks and "would watch videos all day long if you let him."

I made the diagnosis of *mild* autistic disorder because Logan had expressive language before age 3, no dysmorphic physical features, evidence of intelligence (his interests were symbolic, such as books, trains, Barney), some engageability, and a solid, supportive family. Importantly, he had a good sense of humor. His older brother, Drew, loved to engage him. His father, Tom, was an engineer who made a good living, and his mother, Ann, was a stay-at-home mom who could put in the time for PLAY. In fact, he had all the good prognostic signs except one—response to intensive intervention. Currently his only service had been the public special education preschool, which did not provide much intensity.

I referred him to the PLAY Project Home Consulting program nearest to the family home and also recommended additional speech and language and occupational therapy. Jennifer, our trained PLAY consultant (with a master's in education), began her once-a-month, half-day home visits. She modeled, coached, and gave video feedback as previously described. Logan's initial profile is shown in Figure 13.5, Visit 1.

He was, according to Greenspan's developmental profile (see previously outlined FDLs), a child who was only fairly well regulated; for example, he threw a lot of "fits" when things didn't go his way, and he spent about half of his time in his "comfort zone" absorbed in lining up cars and ignoring his family (FDL 1, attention and self-regulation). Thus, his Level 1 on the bar graph was rated, in a rough clinical estimate, as only 50% of what would be typical for a child his age (Figure 13.5, Visit 1). He was not hard to engage (FDL 2, engagement) (75% of typical). He did not often initiate interactions on his own, however. When children reach a solid 100% FDL 3 (two-way communication) they will not leave you alone. This was our

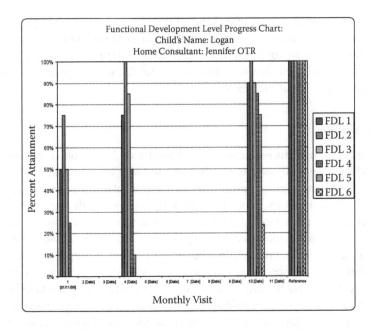

Figure 13.5 Logan's functional developmental level progress chart.

goal for Logan, but he was far from it (thus, 50% at Level 3). We gave him a little credit for FDL 4 (25%) because he showed intelligence by doing some problem solving (push a chair over to the cupboard to get food); he could open and close several "circles" (contingent reciprocal exchanges) of interaction when rough-housing with his dad; and he had a little pretend play (he would make car sounds)—all of which are characteristic for FDL 4.

After the first play session, Jennifer developed a curriculum of activities for Logan (Step 3 in the Skill Sequence)—rough-and-tumble play, chase, simple pretend activities (e.g., animal sounds, feeding a baby)—all designed to get him having fun with people. His parents limited "train time," TV, computer, and videos. They put in about 2 hours per day total, with a few 15- to 20-minute play sessions and "interacting all day long," trying to engage him.

In the second and third (Figure 13.5, Visits 2 and 3) sessions, Jennifer taught the family to get more and more circles of interaction (Step 4 in the Skill Sequence). *Opening a circle* means initiating an interaction (the first volley). *Closing a circle* means responding contingently. We coach parents to "woo" their children into interaction by recognizing subtle cues to "read" their intentions moment to moment so as to follow their lead (see Step 4 in the Skill Sequence). This method is at the core of early play. The

PLAY Project has over 50 techniques (Skill Sequence Step 5), which help parents answer the question: what do I do next?

By his fourth visit, his parents did what Logan loved, and now he loved being with them and would not leave them alone. He was more regulated and available (FDL 1 = 75%), always engageable (FDL 2 = 100%), and frequently initiating (FDL 3 = 85%). As connectedness increased, words became more meaningful, and Logan's words started pouring out. He had over a 100-word vocabulary, and, more importantly, he could follow spontaneous one- and two-step commands: "Logan, go get the trains in your bedroom and bring them to me." He was using gestures along with words to communicate more complex intentions, which is the hallmark of FDL 4, and he was playing simple pretend. He understood longer sentences ("Let's get ready. We're going to visit Grandma and Grandpa"; FDL 5 = 10%). This was major progress. See his profile at Visit 4 on Figure 13.5.

Over the next four visits, Jennifer worked on FDL 4 and 5 activities: pretend play with puppets, cars (even trains could now be played with interactively), and little dolls in a dollhouse. Logan loved sword fighting with cardboard tubes from wrapping paper. He was enjoying hide-and-seek. And, more importantly, he was *with* us, engaged and fluid in his interactions.

Relatives noticed the "new" Logan. He no longer sought out isolation (unless it was really noisy and chaotic). He could join his cousins in simple chase games and *wanted* to be around other children.

At about the 9-month mark, despite Logan's wonderful progress, Jennifer noticed that Logan's mother, Ann, was looking weary and overwhelmed. The PLAY Project trains home consultants to be very sensitive to the emotional challenges of families raising a child with autism. Jennifer recognized and supported Logan's mother's feelings. She referred the family for counseling visits. Ann and Tom allowed extended family to help by babysitting. Ann started going out once a week with "the girls." Dad had a weekly "fun day" with Drew, Logan's brother, to alleviate a growing jealousy, and the family, at least for the time being, got back on track emotionally.

With renewed energy, the family was able to support Logan as he marched up the developmental ladder. We were making more and more demands for longer and more meaningful interactions. A very important technique is "Speaking for the Child." When he would gesture, we would articulate his gesture verbally. For instance, when he would cry about having to stop doing something, we would teach him to recognize his own feelings and negotiate:

Consultant: Logan, you don't want to stop playing.
Logan: (Would stop crying and shake his head no.)
Consultant: You want to watch a little more TV.
Logan: (A smile would shine through his tears.)

Consultant: OK. A little more TV?

Logan: More TV? (his little voice rising in request.)

Consultant: OK. A little more. Just 5 more minutes.

He was now able to understand abstract experiences (FDL 5 and emerging 6).

By home visit 10, Logan was continuing his climb up the functional developmental levels while maintaining integrity at the lower FDLs. His play grew truly imaginative as his fixation on lining up trains evolved into dramas about trains crashing and then needing help from the "train doctor." Other trains worried about him and so modeled empathy. This is the beginning of FDL 6 (see Figure 13.5, Visit 10). He was beginning to take another's perspective, all of which would serve him well in his interaction with peers as Logan headed toward kindergarten.

When we reviewed Logan's last videos with a group at my office, many of the therapists there questioned Logan's diagnosis. Indeed, to an outsider, play at FDL 6 would look like typical play with any child. This is a far cry from where Logan had started. Stuck as he was initially, Logan, with the help of his family, was able to follow the long and winding road out of his isolation through the allure of play.

Guidelines for Using the Approach

Age and Severity

As the overview and the case study suggest, the PLAY Project's parent coaching and home consultation program are suitable for very young children—14 months to 6 years of age—with ASD regardless of the severity of their condition. Given its developmental focus, PLAY is uniquely designed for very young children less than 3 years of age though strong evidence for intervention with children less than 3 years of age is sparse (Rogers, 2010). In terms of severity, young children with ASD have unpredictable courses regardless of initial presentation. Children who appear to have a severe form of autism may make rapid progress, whereas others who appear to be mildly affected may stagnate. Greenspan's developmental framework allows for a sophisticated analysis of the child's profile, allowing PLAY consultants to "fill in the holes" of functional development and promote the developmental progress of most children. There are of course children who will not be helped with this model, as it is clinically effective in two-thirds of children with ASD. Children least likely to benefit are those with low affect where it is difficult to "follow their lead," poor receptive language, and those whose initial response to intensive intervention is poor. Generally, children with this profile do poorly regardless of therapeutic approach.

Costs and Implementation

Because the PLAY Project model is adaptable, efficient, cost-effective, and easily disseminated, it has been implemented in multiple settings in both private and public sectors. The cost of the PLAY Home Consultation program for families is between $3000 and $4000 annually depending on the number of visits and local economic standards. The efficient train-the-trainer design—with a 4-day initial training and then year-long, long-distance supervision approach—allows for rapid dissemination. The total cost of training a PLAY Consultant to certification is approximately $5000. Agencies that adopt PLAY are licensed at a cost of $750 per year starting in the second year.

In terms of the types of agencies that use PLAY, currently two states (Utah and Ohio) have implemented the PLAY Project in Birth to Three (Early Intervention Part C IDEA law) programs statewide. Easter Seals, a private nonprofit organization, has trained over 20 agencies and now serves hundreds of children with ASD nationally. For-profit rehabilitation centers have successfully adopted PLAY, billing the program through speech and language pathology and occupational therapy codes. The business model is profitable. In Michigan, Community Mental Health Centers (i.e., public sector agencies) use PLAY for low-income families who have a child with ASD. They have adapted the parent consultation approach to the office setting using an hourly office visit (and billing codes) once weekly instead of the half-day once-monthly home training model that is more typical. In Ohio and Washington State, PLAY has been incorporated into hospital services.

Limitations of the Model: Families

The PLAY Project model has clear limitations in terms of the families it can serve. Since the model depends on parents putting in enough time, stressed, overwhelmed, multiproblem families will not do well with this model; however, low-income families as a rule have done very well with PLAY. We now have extensive experience with families where cultural background influences attitudes toward playing with the child. We have found that when the PLAY consultant raises the issue for discussion and the model is modified to fit the family and/or the family's language limitations, most families regardless of culture can implement the model. There is of course a subset of families, focused more on academics and language, that is not interested in play-based models. And finally, in states where intensive services are not covered, even the low cost of PLAY is prohibitive. In some states where services are covered publicly the PLAY model has been expanded to train PLAY tutors, who provide 6–15 hours of play per week that supplements parents' time. This obviously increases the cost of

PLAY, but such a program gives parents a break from the full responsibility of providing intensive intervention.

Limitations of the Model: Trainees and Agencies

The PLAY Consultation model depends on translating the approach to families. This is a complicated task. Through experience, we have found that master's-level child development specialists (e.g., MEd., SLP, OT, MSW) are best at translating the model in a family setting. Furthermore, the agencies that hire these child developmental specialists must be committed to serving this group of children, must have a reliable diagnostic and referral source that will refer young children with ASD to the agency, and must be supportive administratively.

Conclusion and Future Directions

> Play is so important to optimal child development that it has been recognized by the United Nations High Commission for Human Rights as a right of every child. Ginsburg (2007).

For children with autism this birthright is denied twice over. First, the vast majority of states don't offer intensive behavioral or developmental services, and insurance companies don't pay for them. Second, children with autism thwart our efforts to play with them because they prefer self-isolation. The PLAY Project, described in this chapter, offers a cost-effective, evidence-based option for states, communities, and parents. Through its community-based trainings, train-the-trainer agency programs, and home consultation model PLAY can be disseminated broadly and efficiently.

As a physician it is my duty to educate parents about *all* appropriate intervention options, but it is my bias that parents should be their child's first and best play partners, especially if their child has autism. So, I introduce them to the PLAY Project. I tell them that autism is a genetic condition—not the fault of their parenting—that responds to intensive play-based intervention most of the time. I explain that the brain of the child with autism is like a loose net that cannot capture the complexity of the world in its web, and it is our job to tighten that net through rich, playful, engaging interventions. As a pediatric professional, it is a relief to be able to refer families to an evidence-based program in their community that can help. And it is the great satisfaction of my work to hear parents say that, for the first time, they feel connected to their child and their child feels connected to them through play.

Appendix 1. The PLAY Project Evaluation Measures

• Childhood Autism Rating Scale (CARS), diagnostic confirmation of autism (Schopler, Reichler, & Renner, 2010).
• Greenspan Social–Emotional Growth Chart, a parent report of their child's functional development (Greenspan, 2004).
• Functional Emotional Assessment Scale (FEAS), a videotaped observation measure of the parents' nurturing interactions and sensitivity to child cues as well as the child's functional developmental level (Greenspan, DeGangi, & Wieder, 2001).
• Functional Developmental Level (FDL), progress chart (see the case study).
• Receptive Expressive Emergent Language (REEL-3), a parent report language measure (Bzoch, League, & Brown, 2003).
• Sensory Profile, a parent report of sensorimotor issues (Dunn, 1999).
• Satisfaction Surveys, at 3 months and 1 year.

References

Bzoch, K. R., League, R., & Brown, V. L. (2003). *Receptive–expressive emergent language test*, third edition. PRO-ED, Inc.
Centers for Disease Control and Prevention. (CDC). (2007). Prevalence of autism spectrum disorders. *MMWR, 56*, 1–40.
Dawson, G., Rogers, S., Munson, J., Smith, M., et al. (2009). Randomized controlled trial of an intervention for toddlers with autism: The early start Denver Model. *Pediatrics*, Online, November 30.
Diggle, R., McConachie, H., & Randle, V. (2003). Parent-mediated early intervention for young children with autism spectrum disorder. In: *The Cochrane Library*, Issue 2. Oxford: Update Software.
Drew, A., Baird, G., Baron-Cohen, S., Cox, A., Slonims, V., Wheelwright, S., et al. (2002). Original contribution: A pilot randomized control trial of a parent training intervention for pre-school children with autism. Preliminary findings and methodological challenges. *European Child & Adolescent Psychiatry, 11*(6), 266–272.
Dunn, W. (1999). *Sensory profile*. NCS Pearson.
Eikeseth, S., Smith, S., Jahr, E., & Eldevik, S. (2007). Outcome for children with autism who began intensive behavioral treatment between ages 4 and 7, *Behavior Modification, 31*(3), 264–278.
Ginsburg, K. R. (2007). The importance of play in promoting healthy child development and maintaining strong parent-child bonds. *Pediatrics, 119*(1), 182–191.
Green, J., Charman, T., McConachie, H., Aldred, C., Slonims, V., et al. (2010). Parent-mediated communication-focused treatment in children with autism (PACT): A randomized controlled trial. *Lancet*, Online May 21.

Greenspan, S. I. (1992). *Infancy and early childhood: The practice of clinical assessment and intervention with emotional and developmental challenges*. Madison, CT: International Universities Press.

Greenspan, S. I. (2004). *Greenspan social–emotional growth chart*. NCS Pearson.

Greenspan, S. I., DeGangi, G., & Wieder, S. (2001). The functional emotional assessment scale (FEAS). The Interdisciplinary Council on Development and Learning Disorders (ICDL).

Greenspan, S. I., & Weider, S. (1997a). An integrated developmental approach to interventions for young children with severe difficulties in relating and communicating. *Zero to Three National Center for Infants, Toddlers, and Families, 15*(5).

Greenspan, S. I., & Wieder, S. (1997b). Developmental patterns and outcomes in infants and children with disorders in relating and communication: A chart review of 200 cases of children with autistic spectrum disorders. *Journal of Developmental and Learning Disorders, 1*(1), 87–141.

Greenspan, S. I., DeGangi, G., & Wieder, S. (2001). *Functional Emotional Assessment Scale: Clinical and research applications*. Bethesda, MD: Interdisciplinary Council on Developmental and Learning Disorders.

Howard, J. S., Sparkman, C., Cohen H., Green G., & Stanislaw H. (2005). A comparison of intensive behavior analytic and eclectic treatments for young children with autism. *Research in Developmental Disabilities, 26*, 359–383.

Ingersoll, B. (2010). A comparison of naturalistic behavior and development, docial pragmatic approaches for children with autism spectrum disorders. *Journal of Positive Behavioral Interventions, 12*(1), 33–43.

Kasari, C., Gulsrud, A., Wong, C., Kwon, S., & Jocke, J. (2010). Randomized controlled caregiver mediated joint engagement intervention for toddlers with autism. *JADD*, February 10, Online, Springer.

Kasari, C., Paparella, T., Freeman, S., & Jahromi, L. B. (2008). Language outcome in autism: Randomized comparison of joint attention and play interventions. *Journal of Consulting and Clinical Psychology, 76*(1), 125–137.

Krebs-Seida, J., Ospina, M., Karkhaneh, M., Hartling, L., Smith, V., & Clark, B. (2009). Systemic reviews of psychosocial interventions for autism: An umbrella review. *Developmental Medicine & Child Neurology, 51*, 95–104.

Lord, C., Bristol-Power, M., & Cafierol, J. (2001). *Educating children with autism*. Washington, DC: National Academy Press.

Lovaas, O. I., Koegel, R., Simmons, J. Q., & Long, J. S. (1973). Some generalization and follow-up measures on autistic children in behavior therapy. *Journal of Applied Behavior Analysis, 6*, 131–166.

Lovaas, O. I. (1987). Behavioral treatment and normal educational and intellectual functioning of young autistic children. *Journal of Consulting and Clinical Psychology, 55*, 3–9.

Mahoney, G., & Perales, F. (2004). Relationship-focused early intervention with children with pervasive developmental disorders and other disabilities: a comparative study. *Journal of Developmental & Behavioral Pediatrics, 26*, 77–85.

McConachie H., Randle, V., Hammal, D., & Le Couteur, A. (2005). A controlled trial of a training course for parents of children with suspected autism spectrum disorder. *Journal of Pediatrics, 147*, 335–340.

McEachin, J. J., Smith, T., & Lovaas, O. I. (1993). Long-term outcome for children with autism who received early intensive behavioral treatment. *American Journal of Mental Retardation 97*, 359–372.

Myers, S. M., Johnson, C. P., & the Council on Children with Disabilities. (2007). Management of children with autism spectrum disorders. *Pediatrics, 120*(5), 1162–1182.

Prizant, B., & Wetherby, A. (1998). Understanding the continuum of discrete-trial traditional behavioral to social-pragmatic developmental approaches in communication enhancement for young children with autism/PDD. *Seminars in Speech and Language, 19*, 329–351.

Rogers, S., & Delalla, D. (1991). A comparative study of the effects of a developmentally based instructional model on young children with autism and young children with other disorders of behavior and development. *Topics in Early Childhood Special Education, 11*, 29–47.

Rogers, S. J. (2000). Interventions that facilitate socialization in children with autism. *Journal of Autism and Developmental Disorders, 30*(5), 399–409.

Sallows, G. O., & Graupner, T. (2005). Intensive behavioral treatment for children with autism: Four-year outcome and predictors. *American Journal on Mental Retardation, 110*(6), 415–438.

Schopler, E., Reichler, R. J., & Rochen Renner, B. (2010). *Childhood autism rating scale, second edition*. Western Psychological Services.

Shea, V. (2004). A perspective on the research literature related to early intensive behavioral intervention for young children with autism. *Autism 8*(4), 349–367.

Siller, M., & Sigman, M. (2002). The behaviors of parents of children with autism predict the subsequent development or their children's communication. *Journal of Autism and Developmental Disorders, 32*(2), 77–89.

Simpson, R. (2005). Evidence-based practices and students with autism spectrum disorders. *Focus on Autism and Other Developmental Disabilities, 20*(3), 140–149.

Smith, T. (1999). Outcome of early intervention for children with autism. *Clinical Psychology: Science and Practice, 6*, 33–49.

Solomon, R., Necheles, J., Ferch, C., & Bruckman, D., (2007). Pilot study of a parent training program for young children with autism: The PLAY Project Home Consultation program. *Autism, 11*(3), 205–224.

Tannock, R., Girolametto, L., & Siegal, L. (1992). Language intervention with children who have developmental delays: Effects of an interactive approach. *American Journal on Mental Retardation, 97*, 145–160.

Vygotsky, L. S. (1978). *Mind in society*. Cambridge, MA: Harvard University Press.

Wallace, K., & Rogers, S. (2010). Intervening in infancy: Implications for autism spectrum disorders. *Journal of Child Psychology and Psychiatry, 51*(12), 1300–1320.

Wieder, S., & Greenspan, S. (2005). Can children with autism master the core deficits and become empathetic, creative, and reflective? A ten to fifteen year follow-up of a subgroup of children with autism spectrum disorders (ASD) who received a comprehensive developmental, individual-difference, relationship-based (DIR) approach. *Journal of Developmental and Learning Disorder, 9*, 1–29.

CHAPTER 14

The ACT Project

Enhancing Social Competence Through Drama Therapy and Performance

LISA POWERS TRICOMI AND LORETTA GALLO-LOPEZ

The group of eight children, two facilitators, and eight student interns assembles and begins to get ready for their drama therapy session. They move the chairs into a tight circle and take their seats. The energy is anxious and bubbling over. There is a combination of rocking, hand flapping, and chattering, at a louder-than-normal level—a typical scene for a group of children diagnosed with autism spectrum disorders (ASD). Andy enters and aimlessly roams the perimeters of the room. He is a sturdy tow-headed boy, who appears much younger than his 10 years, with thumb in mouth and carefree movement. Seemingly unaware of the proper protocol to begin group, seemingly uninterested in the others, he takes his seat only when repeatedly redirected to do so. Andy is considered to be on the severe end of the spectrum. He is nonverbal and requires a 1:1 facilitator during group. The warm-up begins. The ball is passed person to person with eye contact as the targeted skill. Eventually names are added to the exercise. Andy accepts the ball, he passes the ball, but the aim of the exercise seems lost on him. He is participating to the best of his ability. The warm-up takes on a more interactive and multimodal approach, as the group gets on their feet, passing a feeling, and possibly passing a phrase that would communicate a feeling. Andy becomes increasingly disinterested and wanders off, with his assigned 1:1 intern following close behind, attempting to connect with him and keep him engaged. He touches the piano, lies on the gym mats, and very briefly glances at himself in the mirror. He is in constant motion, as he plays cat and mouse with his 1:1. He walks in and out of the circle, at times stopping in front of someone, then moving on. He is not disruptive, and the others continue the exercise without a hitch. He is fully accepted and allowed to participate at his own level. As therapists, we of course want him to be more connected, to use words, to be interested in the activities, and ultimately to be interested in the others.

The general warm-ups are complete, and it is time to move on to the action part of the drama therapy session. This is the place of pretend play, taking on roles, developing characters, working with story. The props and costume pieces are brought to the middle of the room, and out come the wands, the capes, the glasses, and the hats. The others swarm and sort through the items to find the right object to assist with their transformation. Andy wanders through, stopping briefly to look at the objects. He picks up a black top hat. He places it on his head. He walks over to the mirror, observes himself wearing the hat. Then—he begins to dance. The transformation is complete.

This chapter explores the use of drama therapy techniques and nondirective role play in play-building with children and adolescents diagnosed with ASD. It outlines the drama therapy approach used by the ACT Project, a weekly group drama therapy program for children and adolescents diagnosed with ASD that focuses on communication and social skills development. First, we outline the principals and practices fundamental to drama therapy and present rationale as to why drama therapy, specifically group drama therapy, is a powerful and effective treatment modality for children and teens diagnosed with ASD. Next, we provide examples of the practical application of drama therapy techniques to children diagnosed with ASD and discuss its specific benefit. We will then offer a detailed description of the ACT Method of drama therapy and its application within the ACT Project groups. Finally, through case presentation, we present the journey of a preteen named Sammy as we follow his participation in an ACT project group over a 2-year period.

Drama Therapy

Drama therapy is the practical and intentional use of drama and theater practices, such as plays, rituals, and stories, for therapeutic purposes. It is action oriented and experiential and provides a context for participants to express emotion, tell their stories, explore dramatic roles, set goals, and solve problems. Drama therapy can be a platform for behavior change, skill-building, emotional and physical release, and integration (Long, Haen, Zaiser, & Beauregard, n.d.).

Typically, the drama therapist first assesses a client's developmental and clinical needs and then determines an approach that might best meet those specific needs. Drama therapy is a versatile therapeutic modality and can be used in groups, with individuals and with families. It may take many forms depending on the established therapeutic goals as well as individual and group needs and the skill and ability levels of the participants. Techniques and processes used in drama therapy are varied and many and may include theater games, improvisation, puppet and mask work, storytelling, and enactment. Drama therapists may use elements such as performance, text, or ritual to support and enrich the therapeutic and creative process. "The theoretical foundation of drama therapy lies in drama, theatre, psychology, psychotherapy, anthropology, play, and interactive and creative processes" (National Association for Drama Therapy, n.d.)

All drama therapy sessions begin with a warm-up. The warm-up is preparation for the session and is multifunctional. It provides emotional distancing for the participant, from either a more distanced to a less distanced state, and it can also serve as a means to elicit a sense of calm from a previously anxious or excitable state. The warm-up engages the creative imagination, brain connection, as it uses the body, feelings, senses, thoughts, and intuition (Bailey, 1994). It prepares the participant for the action part of the drama therapy session.

Following the warm-up, a drama therapy session moves into the action phase. This is a deeper level of enactment that the warm-up facilitates. The participants are warmed up to their roles and feelings and begin connecting with others. The action is the actual dramatization that occurs within the session. This is where the development of space, characters, plot, conflict, and resolution takes place. The children are encouraged to create ideas from "their own imagination" rather than stories or movies that are well known or mainstream. This requires spontaneous and creative interaction as well as abstract thinking. This form of play is where the script and play shaping begin to take form.

Drama therapy sessions always end with a closure experience. Closure in this instance is not necessarily about resolving the issue of the client or participant but rather about providing a centering or grounding, a transition from action back into the everyday world of the client (Landy, 1994).

Several theoretical terms and principals are unique to the use of drama therapy. The idea of *aesthetic distance* is a main tenet. Aesthetic distance is the balance between emotion and cognition, between thinking and feeling, between experiencing and reflecting. It is inherent when one takes on a role or engages in the "me/not me" experience of becoming a character other than self. It allows individuals to think and feel at the same time. If individuals are thinking too much, or rationalizing, they are considered to be overdistanced. By the same token, the flooding of emotion indicates that individuals may be underdistanced (Landy, 1994).

One way drama therapists offer aesthetic distance is by creating a safe space for participants to explore their experiences. In this safe space, the fear circuits of the brain within the amygdala are calmed so that emotions and cognitions can interact (Bailey, Bergman, & Dickinson, 2010). This is accomplished by using drama therapy techniques that balance thinking and feeling through multimodal experiences: moving, talking, seeing, hearing, and thinking simultaneously. Whenever we are engaged with drama and theater, we are functioning on several levels simultaneously. We have an emotional response to a scene because we have accepted the premise of the story presented. "The power of the theatre is our engagement with it, with both of our brain hemispheres; the left hemisphere to appeal to our logic and intellect and the right hemisphere to engage our intuition, creativity, artistry, and dramatic imagination" (Jennings, 1994, p. 2).

Drama Therapy and Autism Spectrum Disorder

The flexibility of drama therapy and its capacity to adjust to the special interests and ability levels of clients make it an ideal treatment modality for use with children and teens diagnosed with ASD. Tony Attwood (2008) identifies drama as an effective approach to teaching social skills to teens with Asperger's syndrome. He details the work of Viktorine Zak who, at the Vienna Children's Hospital in the 1940s, developed the first treatment programs for children with Asperger's syndrome. Zak, a nurse who was the sister of Hans Asperger, the pediatrician who first identified children with this disorder, used drama activities to teach social skills to the children in her program.

In the book *Pretending To Be Normal*, Liane Holliday Willey (1999) indicates that as a child with undiagnosed Asperger's disorder she learned to use acting and imitation to develop social skills. Attwood (1998, 2008) recommends the use of role play and drama activities to help individuals with Asperger's disorder learn reciprocal conversation skills and vocal tone and inflection as well as how to read facial expressions and body language, all fundamental skills necessary for the basic understanding of social cues and the development of social communication (Attwood, 1998, 2008).

Beyer (1998) points out that children with autism benefit from a play environment that is specifically geared to their needs. Such an environment should include opportunities for nondirective play and play that is spontaneous and varied. Play that requires interaction between two or more people and that focuses on connectedness is often difficult for children with autism due to their deficits in reciprocal communication and social interaction (Wolfberg, 2009). While interactive play is intuitively understood by neuro-typical children, children on the autism spectrum may require specific direction, reinforcement, and support to engage fully in socially interactive play (Beyer, 1998). Drama therapy affords children with autism spectrum disorders the opportunity to engage in play specifically geared toward supporting connectedness with others in an environment that can easily be tailored to meet their needs.

Greenspan and Wieder (2006), in their book *Engaging Autism*, clearly espouse the benefits of drama for children with autism spectrum disorders. They assert that role playing enhances flexibility and creativity and provides opportunities to learn to improvise in difficult or uncomfortable situations. They also maintain that drama is a particularly effective intervention for individuals with autism spectrum disorder as it uses a wide range of developmental abilities.

Simon Baron-Cohen is one of the preeminent leaders in the field of autism studies. Through his research, he has developed important theories in autism studies, most notably that individuals with autism exhibit a significant deficit in Theory of Mind (ToM). Baron-Cohen also supports the notion that the absence of joint attention skills in children at 18 months may be a prime indicator of autism. The term Theory of Mind refers to "the ability to put oneself into someone else's shoes, to imagine their thoughts and feelings, so as to be able to make sense of and predict their behaviour. It is sometimes also called mind-reading or mentalizing" (Baron-Cohen, 2008, p. 57). Joint attention skills encompass the ability to follow someone else's gaze, to show interest in what another person is interested in, and to begin to engage with another in shared, simple interaction (Baron-Cohen, 2008; Greenspan & Wieder, 2006; Wolfberg, 2009). Baron-Cohen also describes the *Triad of Autism* as comprising three areas of atypical development: social, communication, and repetitive behaviors. Baron-Cohen supports the notion that the social and communication domains are inextricably linked. Drama therapy is unique in its ability to integrate and support the development of these various elements of social learning and social communication within a natural setting (Chasen, 2011).

Symptoms related to repetitive behavior and narrow interests are found in both individuals with autism and Asperger's syndrome. These include hand flapping, rocking, spinning of the body, obsessive interests (e.g., repetitively touching specific things, collecting items, collecting information on a narrow topic), lining things up, and repetitive, nonpurposeful play (e.g., spinning the wheels of a car, becoming mesmerized by spinning objects such as washing machines, fan blades) (Attwood, 2008; Baron-Cohen, 2008). Drama therapy enables children and teens with ASD to use those special interests and repetitive behaviors as a starting point— a way to begin within their comfort zone—while consistently challenging them to broaden those interests through new and engaging experiences, continually guiding them beyond their highly controlled worlds. Autism and Asperger's disorder also share common communication abnormalities such as echolalic speech (echoing phrases), neologisms, literal understanding of speech, varying degrees of language delays, and using speech inappropriately for the social context. Also included are highly repetitive movement and behaviors, difficulty with change and transitions, the need for sameness, rigidity, splinter skills, and atypical, often remarkable memory (Attwood, 1998, 2008; Greenspan & Wieder, 2006). Individuals with autism spectrum disorders also experience difficulties with interpersonal interaction, such as being unable to anticipate how someone will feel or what they might think, how to react to another person's behavior, reading other people's emotional expressions (face or voice), and accepting there may be other perspectives, not just a single correct perspective. Drama therapy is an interactive intervention that relies on verbal and physical interplay. It provides children and teens with ASD the opportunity to move from solitary to joined experiences and in so doing supports the development of pragmatic language, reciprocal conversation skills, social understanding, and meaningful social connections (Corbett et al., 2011).

Although it is well recognized that characteristics of individuals with ASD vary widely across the spectrum, the deficit areas where there seems to be the most congruity are those of social communication, social interaction, and social imagination. The application of drama therapy directly addresses each of these areas. Drama enables one to explore and express human feeling through voice, language, and body. It fosters true and spontaneous, communication, interaction, and imaginative thought and activity. As noted already ToM refers to the ability to "put oneself into someone else's shoes" (Baron-Cohen, 2008, p. 57). As "putting oneself in someone else's shoes" is at the core of drama and theater work, it makes sense that drama would be a highly effective way to address deficits in this area.

Kase-Polisini (1988), an educator in creative dramatics, contends that engaging in creative drama helps children to develop skills in creative thinking, communication, and physical and emotional development. "When you create a play you are also learning about basic theatre elements, as you also develop such basic skills as verbal and nonverbal communication, socialization, creative problem solving, and the acquisition and retention of new information. It is important to remember that learning through drama is accomplished through role taking or the imaginative projection of oneself in to the 'shoes" of others, and hypothetical situations" (p. 107).

Drama therapy is a multimodal therapy, as it engages us on several levels at the same time. It requires engaging both hemispheres of the brain: the left to appeal to logic and intellect; the right, to engage creativity, dramatic imagination and intuition (Jennings, 1994). One unique advantage of drama therapy for children with autism spectrum disorders is that it provides a body–brain connection. The fear circuits of the brain are over-ridden when one is engaged in enactment, as both the limbic system and the prefrontal core is involved. The recent focus on the neuroplasticity of the brain suggests that it is possible to create new neuropaths through repetition of the drama techniques, targeted to increase understanding of abstract language and nonverbal communication (Chasen, 2011), described in this chapter. This is especially true into the teen years as pruning of the synapses continues.

Drama therapy techniques are ideal for enhancing identification and appropriate expression of emotions for children and teens diagnosed with ASD. By using role play and character development exercises, clients are able to discharge anxiety and increase empathy. Group drama therapy is an excellent vehicle for engaging in and sharing experiences related to emotions around specific common themes (Chasen, 2011).

Drama therapy provides sensory integration through the use of costuming, music, movement, and visual arts with set and prop building. The use of script development, storytelling, and drama games increases the clients' ability for planning, synthesizing, and organizing. The use of the executive functions is highlighted when clients write their own dialogue and explain intricate plot lines. Through this work the child becomes confident, competent, and capable.

The use of abstract thought, critical to the development of ToM and the ability to "put oneself in another's shoes," is developed in drama therapy through the use of humor, joke-telling, character development, role-taking, and plot development. These techniques help to improve the clients' ability to understand and express language.

Visual spatial and motor coordination are also targeted using drama therapy exercises such as mirroring, space walking, and other theater warm-ups. In mirroring, participants pair up and alternate taking on the role of leader and follower. The leader creates movements using hands, facial expression, or full body, and the follower mirrors those movements. This exercise fosters eye contact, attention skills, social interaction, and connection. In space-walking, participants move through the therapy space based on specific instructions such as walking as if it is windy, snowing, you are on hot sand, floating in space, or walking a dog. At some points participants are instructed to interact in different ways with others who are also "moving through space." This is an especially popular activity as it is always energizing and great fun. Memory and attention are used and enhanced through the same exercises of mirroring, storytelling, and performance of scripted work. Processing speed is improved through activities such as the *freeze game,* and improvisation. The freeze game involves asking participants to move freely and then to quickly freeze. At times participants are asked to identify what they are frozen as, such as a football player catching a pass, a person walking a dog, a dancer, or a dinosaur. Improvisation builds on some of the themes, thoughts, and ideas that may have been the focus of previous games and activities by allowing the actors to spontaneously develop the characters and plots. The Improvisation, Brainstorming Enactment, and Scriptwriting portion of the sessions, as described next, also target reasoning and problem-solving ability.

The ACT Project

The All Community Theatre (ACT) Project is a drama therapy and performance program for children and teens with autism spectrum disorders. The ACT Project was founded by registered drama therapist Loretta Gallo-Lopez. Gallo-Lopez and fellow registered drama therapist Lisa Powers Tricomi, along with approximately 12 theater students from a university theater department, work with four groups totaling approximately 30 children and adolescents diagnosed with ASD. Each group develops, scripts, and performs two plays per year. The weekly one and one-half hour sessions involve specific drama therapy exercises to develop social skills and relationship-building, improve communication and relatedness, and enhance spontaneity and creativity.

The program applies the ACT Method©, which was developed by Gallo-Lopez and Powers Tricomi based on their many years of clinical experience with children and teens with ASD. The ACT Method uses a wide range of drama and theater exercises and activities including dramatic play, improvisation, role play, theater games, puppet and mask work, the use of costumes and props, scripted readings, playwriting, movement, music, visual arts, and performance to achieve group and individual therapeutic goals. The program meets weekly throughout the school year. It culminates in a performance conceived and created by the participants, allowing them to feel a sense of validation and acceptance and to experience the sense of pride that comes from encouraging and appreciative applause.

The student interns play an integral role in the ACT Project groups. They are for the most part undergraduate theater majors who participate as part of a service learning or internship experience in connection with their Introduction to Drama Therapy course. Many are so moved and motivated by the experience that they continue on even after their course is completed. The interns participate fully in the activities and in some ways take on the roles of peer models helping to establish a supportive and playful atmosphere. They cheerfully take on roles in group improvisations and are thrilled when cast by the group members in supporting roles in the plays. Their presence allows the ACT Project to provide a minimum of a 2:1 child-to-adult ratio, ensuring an environment that provides both freedom and safety.

Participants in the ACT Project engage in a method of group therapy that follows what Jennings identifies as the Creative–Expressive model of drama therapy (Jennings, 1994). This model, which focuses on the healthy aspects of each participant, is preferred to the Task and Skills model, which uses dramatic play as more of a rehearsal for living. In the Task and Skills model the play activities are geared toward accomplishing specific tasks rather than enhancing creativity and expression (Jennings, 1994). A primary goal of the Creative–Expressive model is to help the individuals and the group to discover their own creative potential through drama. Dramatic exploration is both verbal and nonverbal and uses embodiment, projected and symbolic, as well as role play. In this manner clients are allowed to move freely through the activities and at their own pace and comfort level. There is no specific focus on resolving issues from the past; rather, the focus is to highlight the skills of the individual within the group to increase self-esteem and establish a stronger sense of self. Confident, competent, and capable are the qualities that are encouraged using drama therapy via the ACT Project.

There are many theater companies and theater artists who use theater and drama for nontheatrical purposes and produce excellent and creative work. The significant difference, however, between a mainstream drama group and the application of drama therapy is that in drama therapy we establish and work toward specific therapeutic goals. Because the ACT Project was developed and is facilitated by trained and credentialed drama therapists, the work maintains the element of a therapeutic as opposed to a recreational encounter. This is an important distinction, and it is intended that the interventions presented here be facilitated by trained drama therapists. An examination of drama therapy as used in the ACT Project and its purposeful and practical application of drama therapy techniques are provided herein and are followed by an outline of a typical 90-minute drama therapy session used by the ACT Project implementing the ACT Method (Gallo-Lopez & Powers-Tricomi, 2010).

As noted earlier, a crucial element of the drama therapy warm-up for children diagnosed with autism spectrum disorders includes establishing the safe space. Using the ACT Method, the safe space is created physically by placing the chairs in a tight circle and making sure the room is clear and clean. Then the space is made safe through continuity and consistency of place, time, and routine such as familiar and repetitive warm-up drama exercises. These are intended to alternately energize or relax the group members, develop group cohesion, and use multimodal experience (moving, talking, thinking, and feeling). The exercises are also organized to calm participants through repetition and safety and to target symptoms and build skills specific to the ASD diagnosis. ACT Method warm-ups focus on the following: understanding nonverbal communication, use of eye-to-eye gaze, vocal tone, facial expression and body language, movement and physical coordination, social/group interaction, self-awareness and awareness of others, and relationship building.

Typical drama exercises such as passing a feeling or a sound, the Name Game, (Bailey, 1994), and other games using a ball to provide focus and establish a routine are part of the weekly warm-up ritual. The objective of this repetition is to help provide a feeling of safety and structure for the child with ASD. To enhance the group's ability to tolerate transitioning between activities, the same warm-ups are practiced for several weeks in a row. As the group develops more cohesion and confidence, there is greater challenge added, such as an extra ball or changing sound to words. This is a good way to monitor improved flexibility and frustration tolerance.

Using the ACT Method, the action phase is designed to incorporate the next three segments: Brainstorming, Scriptwriting, and Enactment. Brainstorming is targeted toward the executive functions of the brain, with the goal of developing and enhancing skills including group interaction, collaboration and compromise, spontaneous reciprocal conversation, emotional flexibility, social interaction and social competence, creative thinking and problem solving, and frustration tolerance and relationship building.

During the Brainstorming session, the clients are asked to begin to think of the "who what, when, and where" of a story. This typically begins with a discussion about places group members have been or would like to go. The discussion may then move on to characters group members would like to play, time periods they would like to explore, or myriad other topics.

As the sessions progress, the children or teens are separated into smaller groups or (depending on the ability of the child/teen) work individually teamed with an adult. The process of Scriptwriting begins. The group members are encouraged to develop ideas from their own imaginations, rather than from television shows or movies, to foster creative thinking. This is sometimes very difficult for children with ASD, who are often obsessively focused on a particular movie or television show to the point where they can recite scenes verbatim. But with practice and support this becomes a creativity enhancing and confidence-building experience. The scripts and dialogue are wholly developed by the group members, with adults in the role of scribes, asking questions only for clarification. This process instills feelings of competence and builds confidence and a sense of capability.

The group members rejoin, and the Enactment phase of the session begins. This is when stories are "put on their feet" and improvisations are introduced as a way to further develop the stories and scripts. Both Scriptwriting and Enactment exercises include techniques that develop the executive functions of the brain through reasoning and plot development and are targeted to develop and enhance skills such as group interaction, collaboration and compromise, understanding abstract, humorous and figurative language, perspective taking, creative thinking and problem solving, empathy, assertiveness, emotional flexibility, relationship building, pride, and self-esteem.

It is the job of the facilitators to assist the group members in finding creative ways to merge the different stories together into a unified whole. This of course is an exercise in flexibility, negotiation, and compromise—typically so difficult for children and teens with ASD. But because of the depth of group cohesion and acceptance and the level of motivation of the group members to generate and perform a cohesive play, this experience supports the development of these skills in a way that very few other activities can. And in many ways, this is some of the most important and behavior altering work accomplished via the program.

ACT Method sessions always end with de-roling, or stepping back into their "real-life" identities, and a cool-down. This facilitates reflection of the work that was done and instills a sense of accomplishment and provides closure. It reinforces competency and restores balance to the individual group members allowing them to safely and comfortably return to the world outside the group. This may be accomplished in a variety of ways, depending on the group members' ability to engage in discussion or other needs stemming from the talking, moving and thinking that occur during an active session. The goals of the de-roling, cool-down, and closure phase include improving frustration tolerance, emotion regulation, and modulation as well as enhancing social competence and perspective taking.

An essential element of the ACT Project is the use of performance. Although performance in front of a live audience is not typically part of most drama therapy programs, we believe that for individuals with ASD the performance itself serves multiple purposes. Although the ACTors are obviously presenting a final product in the form of a play, the play is merely the conduit or bridge, as it is the connection between the actors and between the actors and the audience that is the ultimate goal. For children and adolescents with autism spectrum disorders, the experience of performing, of feeling valued and heard, of bowing to appreciative applause can be quite unique and truly transformational. The story of Diana provides a clear illustration of the power of performance and highlights the various elements of the ACT Project noted previously.

Diana

Diana is a 19-year-old with low-functioning autism and severe receptive and expressive language delay. Much of her speech is echolalic in nature or involves verbalizations that are inappropriate to the social context. She has difficulty with change and transition and will often flap her hands and rock back and forth whether sitting or standing. She loves to spin around and to sing, especially songs from Disney movies, and is drawn to her image in any mirror that happens to be within her sight. When she first began attending the ACT Project 2 years ago, Diana had difficulty participating in the group activities, was easily confused and frustrated, would cry and make grunting sounds to communicate displeasure, and spent much of the group time responding to internal stimuli. Her favorite activities involved music and dancing, and we used this preoccupation to foster her engagement with group members and in group activities. In improvisations, Diana would always take on the role of a movie princess such as Snow White, Cinderella, or Sleeping Beauty. Diana loved to try on princess costumes from our costume trunk and chose her character for our first play based on her favorite princess dress. She named her character Princess Diana and incorporated qualities, movements, and actions from various movie princesses into Princess Diana's persona. As we developed and rehearsed the play, Diana became more and more motivated to participate in group activities, to connect with other group members, and to use words to communicate. She smiled constantly and, according to her mother, anxiously awaited her Wednesday evening ACT group. But it was the actual performance that seemed to have the greatest impact on Diana. Princess Diana had a magnificent fainting scene and sang a song that concluded the play. Both scenes always produced rousing applause during rehearsals, as Diana smiled a wide, proud smile. As the day of the performance approached we decided to rehearse the group bow. Diana eagerly took her place in line, grabbed the hands of the group members on either side of her, and performed a spectacular bow—arms up, smile to the audience, deep curtsy. Diana became our bow leader from then on, waiting for her cue and then confidently leading the group in a bow at the end of the performance.

Diana thrived on the experience of performing and constantly asked when we would be in the theater again. In improvisational play, Diana continued to expand her repertoire of princess roles. She engaged more fully in group drama games and reciprocal conversation and responded more appropriately to social and communication cues. She responded less to internal stimuli, appeared more present in the sessions, and interacted more playfully with the other group members and interns. In our second play Diana sang several duets with one of the boys in the group. This was a first for Diana, for although she loved to sing she could not tolerate someone singing along with her or singing as part of a group. She loved this experience so much that we began to raise our expectations of Diana and to gently push her further and further beyond her comfort zone. We used her love of the hand-holding bow to challenge her to engage physically with her singing partner by holding hands and walking arm in arm as they sang. We added simple choreography, including a few twirls of course, and worked with Diana on expressing emotion via her voice and facial expression. She loved practicing this in the mirror both in group and at home. And of course after each song Diana and her partner bowed together to rousing applause.

As illustrated in the case of Diana, as we focus on each individual's strengths and interests, participants use characteristics that may typically be viewed as deficits in a more positive manner. An obsession for scripting dialogue from television shows or movies, for example, can be a skill that supports the memorizing of dialogue. Some participants have actually memorized the entire script in a week, including every actor's lines and all the stage directions. Obsessive interest in Disney characters can lead a voiceless and essentially nonverbal client to sing a familiar song during performance. A passion for cartoons can be redirected and used in making story boards for the play. A love of dance can lead to a piece of choreography that a participant teaches to all the other group members and interns, thus providing her a moment to direct the action and connect in a new way. According to Attwood (1998, 2008), the special interests or passions of individuals with Asperger's syndrome serve a variety of functions. For many individuals, these special interests or passions provide comfort and relaxation, help to overcome anxiety through a sense of certainty and predictability, and create a sense of identity. These interests may also help to occupy time and provide a focus for conversation and a means of displaying intellectual ability. Attwood also suggests that there may be benefit in working with and engaging the special interest rather than working to try to change it. It is the philosophy of the ACT Project to always begin where the individual is and to use those special interests to motivate, to stimulate creativity, and to validate the importance of the special interest and its value to the individual. This concept of attributing value to the interests or passions of the group participants is indeed a unique and significant element of the program as it is typically the experience of most individuals with ASD that those special interests are frowned upon, ignored, or viewed as something to be diminished or eliminated by others. Through engagement in the ACT Project, we follow individuals' lead and begin where they are. We work toward expanding and broadening the interests and focus and, in so doing, the view of self and the world. In the case of Emma, the acceptance and inclusion of her special interest by the facilitators and the group was the catalyst for a truly transformational, interactive experience.

Emma

Emma is a 16-year-old teen group member diagnosed with high-functioning autism. For the past 3 years, Emma has had a passionate interest in all things related to the cartoon Sponge Bob Square Pants. She carries plush dolls and figurines of characters from the Sponge Bob cartoon, has dozens of drawing pads filled with her renderings of the characters, and writes original stories about Sponge Bob and the other characters. Emma began attending the ACT Project 2 years ago. She arrived for her first group session with a large plush Sponge Bob doll that her mother was attempting to get her to surrender prior to entering the studio. Emma refused, sat down on the floor, and began to cry. She loudly informed her mother that she didn't want to come to this group, that she hated acting, and that she wanted to go home. One of the group facilitators walked over to Emma and her mom and invited both Emma and Sponge Bob to join the group waiting in the circle in the studio. Emma's mother informed the facilitator that Emma was not allowed to bring Sponge Bob to school or to any other activity in which she participated. The facilitator explained that the ACT Project was a very special kind of group and that everyone—including Sponge Bob—was welcome. Emma slowly stopped crying, and she and Sponge Bob cautiously joined the circle of participants eagerly waiting for the group to begin. The first warm-up activity involved a beach ball and a name game. When group members took turns throwing the big colorful beach ball across the circle calling out the name of the recipient, both Emma and Sponge Bob were included in the activity. When the group got on their feet and practiced passing a sound and movement around the circle, Sponge Bob helped Emma to reach beyond her comfort zone and use her voice and body more freely. She loudly proclaimed, "I'm not making eye contact so don't even go there!" But Sponge Bob made eye contact whenever it was his turn to pass a sound or movement to the person next to him. The attitude of acceptance engendered by the adults in the room allowed the group members to welcome Sponge Bob without judgment or teasing. Sponge Bob attended weekly. At first he spent each session in Emma's arms, but over time he often became an observer as Emma propped him in a chair and eventually even allowed others in the group to hold him. He has participated in warm-up activities, drama games, and script- and songwriting and has been assigned roles in group improvisations. Sponge Bob has participated in most of the ACT Project plays, often speaking dialogue that Emma had written but could not bring herself to recite. Sponge Bob's presence enabled Emma to comfortably assimilate into the group, to take risks by trying new and different activities, and to connect with others in ways she would never have been able to without Sponge Bob's support. She will even make eye contact from time to time both in group activities and on stage. In our most recent production Emma for the first time allowed herself to be the center of attention, dancing a solo she had choreographed while the other actors and interns followed as her backup dancers. Sponge Bob participated in the number but in the arms of another group member. And at the end of the performance Emma took her bow center stage while Sponge Bob looked on from the wings.

The Significance of the Group Experience

The specific use of group as opposed to individual therapy was an important and deliberate choice when establishing the ACT Project. Group therapy for children diagnosed with ASD directly challenges many of the exact symptoms that are considered deficits. As in all groups, social interaction is a primary focus; however, in ACT Project groups participants move beyond simple skills of interaction to more complex skills including negotiation and compromise as they decide how to merge each person's story into one coherent whole and discuss who will play what role, where the play will be set and, how to move the story along. This process not only increases the participants' social abilities of engagement, interaction and relatedness but also helps them develop skills in compromise, reciprocity, frustration tolerance, acceptance (of self and others), and perspective taking—in other words, Theory of Mind. What follows is a more detailed case presentation describing the journey of Sammy, who has participated in the ACT Project for 2 years. It outlines many of the activities and interventions that helped move Sammy along his journey toward social competence.

Sammy

Sammy began attending the ACT Project 2 years ago when he had just turned 10 years old. He was diagnosed with high-functioning autism and presented with typical physical indicators of autism such as rocking, hand flapping, lack of eye contact, and avoiding peer interaction. Sammy was not particularly interested in acting, but he liked to draw stories and repeat lines from his favorite television shows and movies; his mother wanted him to participate in a program where he might improve his lagging social skills. Sammy had no friends and in school would typically eat his lunch alone as there was no one he knew well enough to sit next to. He was an only child and spent most of his time at home alone in his room, watching television, playing video games, or drawing.

Sammy spent his first group session with The ACT Project rocking in his seat and flapping his hands uncontrollably. He refused to participate in group activities and responded to questions or requests with a single word, in a monotone voice, void of any emotion. He made no eye contact, did not smile or laugh, and appeared to be distracted by his own thoughts. He spent much of the first few months just trying to get comfortable with his own body. His gait was awkward and unsteady. When we played ball games in a circle, Sammy rarely caught the large colorful beach ball when it was thrown to him and did not go after the ball when he missed it as the other children in his group did. Whenever Sammy threw the ball he had difficulty getting the ball to reach someone across the circle.

Sammy ignored attempts at interaction from other group members though he continued to respond to adults with one-word answers in a monotone voice. He could not (or perhaps would not) remember the names of other group members, facilitators, or interns—even though we played a name game at the start of each group session. When we engaged in drama games such as passing a sound or movement, Sammy rarely looked at the person on either side of him and would often forget the sound or movement being passed, needing to have it repeated for him. When he repeated a sound, it was typically done in a monotone fashion, devoid of emotion, even if he was being passed a loud or angry sound. When the group was asked to bring in jokes—either from friends or family members, books, or on line sources—for our Jokes Extravaganza (an activity done several times a year to give group members an opportunity to perform jokes for their peers and to work on enhancing their understanding of humor and figurative speech), Sammy complained that he didn't know any jokes and didn't know anyone who could tell him a joke. During the Jokes Extravaganza he agreed to perform a knock-knock with one of the interns and appeared surprised and even smiled when their performance drew laughter and applause.

During group activities, we use a pretend microphone that is passed around and used for character interviews and other activities. The group members know it doesn't really work but are willing to pretend that it does because the facilitators and interns participate fully in the pretense. The first time Sammy used the microphone he tapped the top and said, "Hey, is this thing on?" Everyone laughed, and Sammy smiled. From then on anytime someone used the microphone Sammy's words, "Hey is this thing on?" were playfully repeated, and each time Sammy smiled, establishing a small but significant connection.

Improvisation

As the group moved on to improvisation work, Sammy appeared equally uncomfortable. During an improvisational scene in which group members pretended to be people at a hotel, either guests or employees, Sammy chose to be a complaining guest. He expressed a few angry words about the condition of the hotel and his displeasure with his accommodations but engaged primarily in monologue, speaking out loud but not to anyone in particular.

When one of the adults in the room would attempt to engage him in play or conversation, Sammy would either walk away or ignore the interaction. He did, however, remain in character and within the scene throughout the improvisational experience and moved through the space a bit more comfortably than he had previously. As we continued each week with similar improvisational play experiences Sammy began to slowly expand his role repertoire, taking on characters with a wider variety of characteristics.

When we began to brainstorm ideas for our first show, Sammy was reluctant to become involved in any scenes that would require him to interact with his peers. He asked if he could play a character who was not on stage or who could say his lines from behind the curtain. He eventually chose to play the role of an angry store owner whose main goal was to chase away his customers or kick them out of his store for not buying anything. Sammy had difficulty maintaining focus or following the script during the initial rehearsals and had to be consistently reminded when it was time for his line. "Oh I forgot" was his typical response. He spoke his lines softly and with little emotion but eventually began to listen to the other actors and to remember his lines and his stage cues. He reluctantly chose a hat and other objects to be part of his costume, and as the rehearsals progressed the hat and props assisted Sammy in beginning to take on some ownership of his character. He worried about how many people would be in the audience but performed his part without complaining, and though he could barely be heard he seemed to enjoy the experience and the applause.

When preparing for our second play, Sammy asked to work one on one with an intern and indicated that he wanted to play the role of the announcer in the play. He wrote lines for himself and the intern announcing each upcoming scene in the play and then decided to create several commercials that would be used between scenes. He was able to tap into his own thoughts, ideas, and imagination and to create a script that included things of interest to him. Although Sammy did not engage in much character development, we welcomed the departure from the angry old man character, as Sammy began to explore some other emotions such as excitement and surprise. Eventually Sammy and the intern created several commercials that required Sammy to interact and engage in dialogue with the intern. He chose to use the pretend microphone for one of the scenes and began to project his voice further and further. During our dress rehearsal in the theater Sammy surprised himself when he realized that even from the back row he could be heard.

When Sammy returned from summer vacation to begin his second year with the ACT Project, we worried that any progress he had made in the previous year might have dwindled away. Surprisingly, Sammy was excited to be back and from the start seemed more at ease and at home in the space than he had all of the last year. The familiarity of our routine and the initial activities appeared to be comforting and motivating. He asked to play some of the games we had played the previous year and actually greeted the other actors as they arrived for the group session. We continued to see progress throughout the first few months: less rocking and flapping, greater vocal range and expression of emotions, and an ever increasing level of playfulness. When we did our Jokes Extravaganza, Sammy brought in two jokes to share and happily waited for laughter and applause from his audience. When we played the transforming object game, Sammy was able to use a ladle as a wand, a cup as a hat, and a stick as a fishing pole. When it was time to begin working on our next script Sammy was filled with ideas. He created a character with magical powers who wanted to take over the world. He enlisted a group of interns as his henchmen and had them sitting around him taking notes as he brought life to his story. He created dialogue, names for each of the characters, and a cohesive story line. At the start of the next week's session group members were asked to pass a sound or word around the circle that their character might say in the play. When it was Sammy's turn he used his whole body and exploded in a deep, loud, evil laugh. He smiled proudly as in turn each person in the circle mimicked his evil laugh. Later in the session as we worked to bring the various divergent stories together Sammy negotiated and compromised with the other group members, and together they found a path to merge their stories into one. Sammy performed his character with a level of emotion and connection that we had never seen him reach before and, indeed, we doubted he was capable of. During one scene he patted one of his henchmen on the head and proudly proclaimed, "Good job." And throughout the performance Sammy incorporated his body into the action and used his voice fully and dramatically. The audience was awed.

After that performance, Sammy continued to become more social and more involved in group. For the first time, in our most recent production Sammy played two roles—including a role in someone else's story. Playing two roles in one performance is often difficult for children with ASD as it requires them to make a transition from one character to another. However, Sammy moved seamlessly between the two characters, even creating different accents and body movements for each. He used his body to express emotion, pain, sadness, strength, and power and for the first time even incorporated humor into his character and his scene. The evolution of Sammy's performances over the past 2 years has closely mirrored the development of his social awareness, understanding, and competence.

Sammy still rocks in his chair and flaps his arms from time to time, but he also engages in conversation, responds to questions, participates in all group activities, and expresses emotions and has developed a newfound level of comfort in his body. Beyond the safety and familiarity of the ACT Project environment, Sammy's developing social skills continue to generalize and expand. His teacher's describe him as "more connected" to the world and the people around him. His mother reports that he seems happier, more motivated, more talkative, and more positively engaged with others. He no longer sits alone at lunch, as he has found a friend to eat with and to talk to about movies, video games, and the pictures and stories he creates from his imagination. Each week our hearts are warmed as he amazes us with his continuing metamorphosis into a more social and emotionally connected individual. He still avoids making eye contact if he can get away with it and rarely understands the humor in a joke, but he smiles and laughs often and he knows everyone's name.

Conclusion

Many children and adolescents with ASD live what appear to be very solitary and isolated lives—devoid of friendships or connections to others. The ACT Project seeks to offer the ACTors who participate an opportunity to experience the beauty of connection, the joy of developing relationships, and the unique understanding of self and others that accompanies social growth. Through the experience of creating original work, sharing with and being heard by others, and engaging with others to develop their ideas into a functioning whole, ACT Project participants practice flexibility, compromise, communication, and a host of other skills that move them ever closer to becoming socially competent individuals. The element of performance allows participants to share their thoughts, dreams, and accomplishments with others, further breaking through those walls that have previously kept them isolated and alone.

As we work with these young people and watch their growth and progress, we must rely on what we see and on our anecdotal evidence of the effectiveness of the ACT Project approach to therapy with individuals with ASD. Although there is currently no evidence-based research to support what we believe to be a uniquely engaging and transformative intervention, the ACT Project and ACT Method on which it is based are derived from empirically supported research in the field of drama therapy. Our hope in the near future is to be able to provide research results that will corroborate the outcomes that we continue to observe and that our families regularly report. In the meantime we are informed by the experiences of the children and teens such as those we have shared in this chapter and by special moments like those that follow.

Postscript

Following a dress rehearsal for an upcoming performance, Diana continued twirling and singing in the waiting area. A facilitator asked her how she liked performing in the dress rehearsal. Diana smiled broadly and in her typically soft voice responded, "I am magnificent."

For many ACT Project ACTors, performing in front of an audience is particularly challenging, making any accomplishment on the stage that much more satisfying. David is 15, struggles with reading and writing, is frustrated by school, and gets in trouble often for avoiding school work, not staying focused, and wandering alone around the school campus. He had a major role in our spring play and had more lines than usual. Since he had written the lines himself, however, David was able to improvise successfully in rehearsals when he needed to. The night of the performance he paced and practiced his lines. David went on to perform beautifully in the play and had remembered all of his lines, expressing them with great emotion and zeal. His mother could not stop smiling as she watched the amazing transformation of this typically solitary and quiet young man. As the audience filed out of the theater David paced back and forth across the stage, grinning and repeating some of his lines from the play. He then walked over to the two facilitators and handed one a note on a scrap of paper. David warmly hugged each of them and proudly reported that he already had ideas for next year's play. As David left the theater the facilitators opened the note that read, "Thank you for making us performers. It makes me happy how much I feel that you believe in me."

References

Attwood, T. (1998). *Asperger's syndrome: A guide for parents and professionals.* London: Jessica Kingsley.

Attwood, T. (2008). *The complete guide to Asperger's syndrome.* London: Jessica Kinglsey.

Bailey, S. D. (1994). *Wings to fly: Bringing theatre arts to students with special needs.* Rockville, MD: Woodbine House.

Bailey, S., Bergman, J., & Dickinson, P. (2010, November). *Researching brain-based concepts in drama therapy without a brain scanner.* Paper presented at the meeting of the National Association for Drama Therapy, Chicago, IL.

Baron-Cohen, S. (2008). *Autism and Asperger syndrome: The facts.* Oxford: Oxford University Press.

Beyer, J. A. (1998). *Autism & play.* London: Jessica Kingsley Publishers.

Chasen, L. R. (2011). *Social skills, emotional growth and drama therapy.* London: Jessica Kingsley Publishers.

Corbett, B. A., Gunther, J. R., Comins, D., Price, J., Ryan, N., Simon, D., et al. (2011). Brief report: Theatre as therapy for children with autism spectrum disorder. *Journal of Autism and Developmental Disorders, 41,* 505–511.

Frequently asked questions about drama therapy. (n.d.) Retrieved May 5, 2011 from http://www.nadt.org/faqa.htm

Gallo-Lopez, L., & Powers Tricomi, L. (2010). *The ACT method.* Unpublished manuscript.

Greenspan, S., & Wieder, S. (2006). *Engaging autism.* Cambridge, MA: De Capo Press.

Holliday Willey, L. (1999). *Pretending to be normal: Living with Asperger's syndrome.* London: Jessica Kingsley Publishers.

Jennings, S. C. (1994). *The handbook of dramatherapy.* London: Routledge.

Kase-Polisini, J. (1988). *The creative drama book: Three approaches.* New Orleans: Anchorage Press.

Landy, R. (1994). *Drama therapy: Concepts, theories and practices.* Springfield, IL: Charles C. Thomas.

Long, K., Haen, C., Zaiser, J., & Beauregard, M. (n.d.) *Drama therapy with children and adolescents.* Retrieved May 5, 2011 from http://NADT.org/upload/file/childrenfactsheetfinal.pdf

National Association for Drama Therapy. (n.d.). *Frequently asked questions about drama therapy.* Retrieved May 5, 2011 from http://www.nadt.org/faqa.htm

Wolfberg, P. J. (2009). *Play and imagination in children with autism* (2nd ed.). New York: Teachers College Press.

PART **IV**

Expressive/Creative Interventions

CHAPTER 15

Art Therapy
Connecting and Communicating

CATHY GOUCHER

Amid the clatter of colored pencils being returned to containers and voices repeatedly asking for point sheets to be addressed, art therapy group leaders closed the day's session with a final review of the activities. From within this din emerged the mechanical voice of a usually silent group member, seemingly incongruous with the passionate statement that followed: "Art therapy can change your life. It's about people doing things—getting better." Despite lingering opinions to the contrary, exploring multisensory materials and making visible thoughts, feelings, or beloved special interests on paper, canvas, or in three dimensions is generally embraced by those with autism. The act of engaging in one's environment through creative means or through use of traditional art media requires an individual to be, even for a moment, in the social world, open to interaction with another, even if only to further access needed objects in the environment. This process, witnessed and guided by an art therapist, offers rich opportunities for social-emotional growth.

I look at art therapy with clients with autism through a wellness lens. Client-artists are introduced to materials, process their own expressions and, as developmentally appropriate, diagnosis as a means of helping them discover their latent selves. As an art therapist, I encourage this engagement for the purposes of making and expanding social connections. Case examples to be presented reflect my practice of enthusiastically following client-artists' creative lead. Within an inviting and predictable studio space, I coax expansion of passions and preferred ways of creating through the introduction of novel methods. I capitalize on opportunities to enhance an individual's ability to better differentiate color and form. We partner to develop symbols and better communicate ideas. I also provide therapeutic supports as necessary, such as artificially slowing artists' process (e.g., by drawing with pencil first, tracing with permanent marker, and then adding color to an image) for improved narrative quality. As flexibility, tolerance of a shared creative experience, and communication of ideas grows over time, membership in a community of peers with similar strengths and needs, such as in a group, is made possible.

Art Therapy: An Overview

The mental health profession of art therapy uses the creative process of art making to improve and enhance the physical, mental, and emotional well-being of individuals of all ages. The creative process involved in artistic self-expression helps people to resolve problems, develop interpersonal skills, manage behavior, reduce stress, increase self-esteem, foster self-awareness, and achieve insight (American Art Therapy Association, 2009). Art therapy is typically used with clients for whom words or traditional modes of communication are difficult for a variety of psychological, social, and developmental reasons. There is a growing body of research examining relationships among learning, the arts, and the brain that might offer data-driven insight into why and how art therapy is effective (Gazzaniga, 2008).

In the effective treatment of individuals, an art therapist thoughtfully synthesizes their knowledge of art media and training in psychology and counseling theories, both realms serving to identify methods that might best meet their needs, and works to promote growth from that point onward. Artistic talent is not a prerequisite for individuals seeking or being referred for art therapy services, although they should at least be somewhat interested in artistic or creative self-expression. Art therapists are master's or doctorate-level professionals who hold a degree in art therapy. Art therapists might also hold master's degrees in related fields but would have completed additional training to achieve a continuing education certificate of study in art therapy from an accredited art therapy program. Art therapists are also trained in the application of a variety of art modalities for use in assessment and treatment including drawing, painting, and sculpture (American Art Therapy Association, 2009).

In the United States, art therapists who meet rigorous requirements are credentialed by the Art Therapy Credentials Board (ATCB). The Art Therapist Registration credential (ATR) is granted upon completion of graduate education and post-graduate supervised experience. Board Certification (ATR-BC) is granted to registered art therapists who pass a written, nationally standardized examination and is maintained through stringent continuing education requirements (American Art Therapy Association, 2009).

Art therapy was established as a professional discipline in the 1960s, and its early pioneers were particularly influenced by the child art movement of the 1930s and 1940s, which stressed the importance of facilitating children in spontaneously creating art (Cizek, Viola, & Richardson, cited in Arguile, 1992). This process was considered a vehicle by which children might tell their stories using symbolic language. According to this line of thinking, as children grow and develop they experience a shift from sensory exploration of their world to communicating and interpreting their world through representation and the making of images: "For children, art is a way of learning, and not something to be learned" (Lowenfeld & Brittain, 1987, p. 47). Images reflect and interpret experiences, evoke memories, and communicate ideas to others. Art becomes pleasurable, integrative, and expressive of sensory and life experiences and offers opportunities for mastery and developing a greater sense of competency. One of the early contributors to the field of art therapy, Florence Cane, stated that every individual is "born with the power to create" (1989/1951, p. 9). In an internal world without words or, at best, a significantly limited vocabulary as with a typically developing young child or an individual with autism, images are "the primary containers of experience" and, as such, have the power to convey experience to others and serve as a bridge to language (Wood, 1984). Making a picture is a communicative act, one that the maker hopes is understood when it is viewed (Evans & Dubowski, 2001).

Along similar lines, John Dewey, a contemporary thinker to the pioneers of art therapy, regarded art making with particular relevance in considering the function of art in the treatment of individuals with autism. He believed that "individuality itself is originally a potentiality and is realized only in interaction with surrounding conditions…through resistances encountered, the nature of the self is discovered. The self is both formed and brought to consciousness through interaction with environment. The individuality of the artist is no exception" (1980/1934, pp. 281–282). Further, Dewey posited that the physical process of working with art materials develops imagination through the "progressive organization of 'inner' and 'outer' materials in organic connection with each other" (1980/1934, p. 75).

Similarly, Winnicott (1971) defined play as a transitional space between internal and external reality where a child's sense of self is generated. The essential human activities of play and creative art endeavors define and help to refine the self, even when the presenting self appears diffuse. A child or individual's path to self-expression, charted through developmentally-appropriate creative activities, is by nature idiosyn-cratic and cannot be distilled down into replicable curriculum for wide application.

Art Therapy and Autism

In considering rationale for the use of art therapy with children and young adults with autism, many successful case examples have been offered over the last few decades (Bentivengna, Schwartz, & Deschner, 1983; Betts, 2001; Emery, 2004; Evans, 1998; Gabriels, 2003; Glaaser, Goucher, Miller, & Scheibler, 2007; Kellman, 1999; Martin, 2009; Noble, 2001; Scanlon, 1993; Schleien, Mustonen, & Rynders, 1995; Seifert, 1988). In a review of the literature on art therapy and autism, Gilroy (2006) concluded that its use in long-term group and individual treatment for children can be considered an effective means to promoting cognitive and emotional development, enabling relationships, and lessening prob-lem behaviors.

Despite the fact that art therapy offers potential for enhancing emo-tional, social, and cognitive skills, there is a paucity of empirical and controlled research on the efficacy of art therapy with these individuals through either individual or group intervention. The following constitute the few notable studies that have been published. Structured participation in art and music therapy "lessons" with concurrent behavioral assessment led Parker-Hairston (1990) to discover that children with autism increased in their confidence, allowing verbal and nonverbal social interactions to occur; however, gains were not found to be statistically significant specific to the targeted behaviors of work, unintelligible verbalizations, acceptance of physical contact, play, and observation of teacher. As a result, Parker-Hairston encouraged additional research examining effectiveness, offering that music and art therapy seemed to increase potential for socialization by decreasing the threat of failure.

Using a social skills group format incorporating art therapy and cogni-tive behavioral techniques for children between the ages of 11 and 18, Epp (2008) found significant improvement on social skills measures related to self-assertion, internalization, hyperactivity, and problem behaviors. Due to the blended therapeutic technique format, she cautioned against consid-ering art therapy the sole reason for the gains. It is also important to note that this research was conducted by a social work professional and not a trained art therapist.

In a randomized control trial, Got and Cheng (2008) found preliminary evidence in support of "art facilitation" serving to improve communica-tion and social relationships in individuals with developmental disabili-ties. Although the aforementioned findings are in general promising, there is still a critical need for expanded qualitative and quantitative research on the efficacy of art therapy treatment with individuals with autism.

Despite the lack of empirical studies, connections can be drawn between art therapy and recent research in neuroscience. The current widely accepted characterization of autism as a neurodevelopmental disorder provides a factual framework on which creative intervention might be layered. One might extrapolate from a selective synthesis of what has been discovered about the brains and minds of individuals with autism how art therapy treatment might capitalize on the brain's relative strengths while addressing functional deficits. This is consistent with prominent art therapy leaders' assertion of neuroscience's centrality to better understanding how and why art therapy works (Malchiodi, 2003).

Drawing on Cognitive Strengths

With autism, the way the brain responds to environmental input results in an array of difficulties with social functioning and learning. Areas of the brain typically connected by neural pathways for the function of processing complex information, such as language and social cognition, are not effectively communicating with one another (Minshew, 2010). This functional underconnectivity results not only in difficulties with social functioning but also in an information-processing problem. In a related model, the Parieto-Frontal Integration Theory of Intelligence (P-FIT; Haier & Jung, 2008), intelligence and creativity are realized through a "highly distributed brain system," including the parietal and frontal lobes. Information is gathered through sensory means (the temporal and occipital lobes, among others, found in the posterior of the brain), fed to the parietal cortex, and passed on to the frontal brain regions responsible for applying meaning and taking appropriate, flexible action. This mechanism suggests that breakdowns of the highly distributed brain system result in significant difficulties with language, social function, and cognition.

Using functional magnetic resonance imagery (fMRI) technology examining brain activation during participants' processing of low and high imagery sentences, Kana and colleagues (Kana, Keller, Sherkassky, Minshew, & Just, 2006) found that those with autism predominantly used parietal and occipital brain regions, located in the posterior of the brain. The data of participants with autism, when compared with that of controls, confirmed that language and spatial centers, the frontal-parietal network, in those with autism were not as well synchronized as in the control group. Put more simply, individuals with autism frequently seem to be using mental imagery as a primary means of information processing rather than only when necessary. The overreliance on these areas of the brain provides evidence of the underintegration of language in autism as well as increased reliance on visuals to support comprehension of verbal information. Further, there has been found to be a decreased size of a portion of the corpus callosum, critical to the connectivity of frontal and posterior brain areas, in the autistic brain (Kana, Keller, Cherkassky, Minshew, & Just, 2008). This may be an additional reason for the adaptation toward posterior regions, or those associated with imagery, for information processing.

Gleaned from their research, Williams, Goldstein, and Minshew (2006) offer a profile of cognitive strengths and weaknesses for individuals with autism. Abilities include sensory perception, elementary motor, and visuo-spatial processing. Relative cognitive weaknesses include concept formation and tasks involving complex sensory and complex motor function.

The intact strengths of sensory perception and visuo-spatial processing would seem of particular relevance to art therapy. The use of visuals in treatment of individuals with autism has been found to facilitate processing across brain regions, resulting in changed brain structures and improved communication with higher-order brain circuitry (Williams et al., 2006). In light of this finding, it follows that engagement with art processes, visual and sensory by nature, might facilitate the acquisition and meaningful integration of information.

"Thinking in pictures," as Temple Grandin (1995), well-known writer and scientist with autism, so aptly referred to her processing system, may be an adaptation to the autistic brain's underconnectivity in which the brain makes increased use of the parietal and occipital areas, relying less on compromised pathways to the frontal regions for processing. Perhaps compromised neural pathways might be mitigated and communication between higher- and lower-order brain circuitry might be sparked by concrete, visually based, sensory, predominantly nonverbal art therapy interventions. The visible object or piece of art from this process might be named or used as a point of connection with another, wherein the therapy of the art intervention challenges involvement of the frontal lobes in processing the experience and working to assign meaning. Without involvement of the frontal cortex, abilities to appropriately socially interact, to demonstrate judgment and planning, and to adequately assess the mental states of others will remain impaired (Stuss, Gallup, & Alexander, 2001). Research designs that can examine areas of activation in the brain during the application of art therapy techniques and processing of the art product are critical to assert this. Of additional value would be the longitudinal investigation of demonstrated enhanced mental flexibility, verbal communication, and decreased problem behaviors over baseline as a result of prescribed art therapy interventions.

Even with the lack of a complete research picture, art making has the capacity to have a profound impact on the functioning of individuals with autism. Art involves the activation of places of cognitive strength in the brain, resulting in tangible art forms that might be responded to by the client-artist, art therapist, and, where deemed appropriate, a larger community such as a classroom, school, or neighborhood. The externalization of the internal, sensory experience offers a wealth of opportunity for promoting parieto-frontal lobe connectivity. The artist with autism is challenged to find a word or phrase to accompany the art, and the art is emotionally and cognitively responded to in the company of the artist. The sensitive, thoughtfully framed external response to the art, either by the art therapist or another trusted member of the maker's community, effectively models for the artist what should be an internal, frontal-lobe driven process: seeking meaning in the visual communication and connecting emotion to the work. Perhaps such repeated modeling and mediated opportunities for showing art and receiving feedback in response supports honing of the artist's own brain pathways. Such priming might lead to increased ability to integrate and creatively express experiences, allowing an individual with autism the opportunity to begin to build a more fully realized self.

Lack of integration among areas of the brain may leave individuals vulnerable to emotional and social problems (Noble, 2001). Belkofer and Konopka (2008), examining neurological activity before and after art making, discovered increased activity in the temporal lobe or "what pathway"—where images and meaning are linked—contributing to one's experiences of joy, greater clarity of purpose, and sense of belonging to a community (Belkofer & Konopka, 2008) (see Figure 15.1). Interventions aimed at enhancing connectivity or integrated activities of the brain may improve individuals' internal and interpersonal lives (Siegel, 1999). Challenged with autism or not, humans need "to have another individual simultaneously experience a state of mind similar to our own," (Siegel, p. 22) much like art and the creative process affords. Life might then become more deeply meaningful.

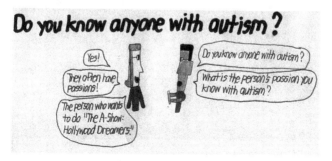

Figure 15.1 Art can help individuals with autism visualize social interactions and communicate as yet an unspoken desire to be understood and part of a community.

It has long been generally asserted that individuals with autism are not creative (Craig & Baron-Cohen, 1999). Creativity is defined as the production of something both novel and useful within a given social context (Flaherty, 2005). It combines the elements of emotion, planning, and sensory perception layered with linguistic, graphic, or motor skills (Jung et al., 2010). Art therapy seeks to help individuals with autism toward underlying potential for creativity. The visuo-spatial and sense perception brain strengths of individuals with autism suggest this potential. Using the Torrance Creativity Tests, Craig and Baron-Cohen (1999) found evidence in support of creativity, discovering that individuals with autism were able to generate possible novel changes to objects, although fewer and with less imaginative fluency than compared with neuro-typical peers.

Creative potential is realized in the application of the creative product, regardless of sophistication, within the community in which individuals function. In art therapy, social connections are developed through the sharing of unique sensory and previously internal experiences concretized in the art product that is deepened over time and nurtures a sense of social competence. Seeking to facilitate creativity in the artist with autism, the art therapist provides developmentally appropriate art materials and interventions to engage the cognitive strengths of the client-artist. The art therapist then invites individuals with autism to attempt or practice engaging their frontal lobe capacity toward assigning language or meaning to the work or art process, identifying and integrating emotions toward fuller community participation.

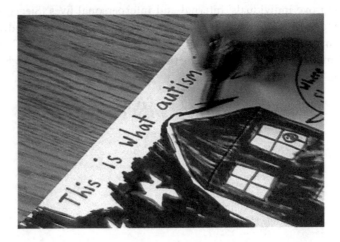

Figure 15.2 "This is what autism is," the drawing declares, depicting a small boy in a red house looking out of his window saying, "Where is Mother! She was supose [sic] to be home hours ago!" and thinking, "It's hard to wait."

"Artmaking is a valued activity that permits individuals on the margins of society to contribute meaningful work to the very culture that excludes them" (Lentz, 2008, p. 14). Art acts as a potentiator as well as a mediator and facilitator of social reciprocity. Art production or sensory experiences with art materials, while often experienced as enjoyable, are not sufficient to promote the social, emotional, and cognitive growth in the autistic brain sought through art therapy. Art therapy interventions go further by specifically providing repeated, often long-term, verbal, and nonverbal opportunities for exploration of topics and concerns of importance to individuals with autism. This exploration attached to the art experience is critical for growth to occur and for a more defined self to emerge.

Art therapy is set apart from other related fields and methods of treatments as art therapists use the process to stimulate individuals' drive to communicate and engage in the novel experience of shared reality (Osborne, 2003) unlike sensory integration, which targets the process alone. Another field frequently confused with art therapy, art education, does not identify the facilitation of social-emotional growth as central to its curriculum, even though it is important to individuals' creative developmental growth and understanding of aesthetics and art production. Moreover, the current treatment landscape for autism largely consists of adult-led pedagogy (TEAACH, PECS[1]), based in cognitive-behavioral theory, which positions the adult in a role of teacher, leader, creator, and solicitor of order and routine. It is presumed that treatment will progress along a steady, linear path of built on responses that initially are externally elicited but become internalized and generalized over time. Art therapy, when viewed as a treatment within this context, appears distinctly out of place. It is a person-centered methodology based on joining with the individual, by providing feedback and challenges in an effort to connect sensory experiences with meaning. Art therapy offers creatively mitigated opportunities for social reciprocity and competence building while celebrating idiosyncrasy and the capacity for individuals to learn and grow at their own pace. The art therapy session is a place in which the therapist and individuals with autism collectively experience possibility. Joining with the artists in a shared sensory process concretely demonstrates this commitment. Respecting and seeking to better understand individuals' special interest areas as expressed through art sends this same message of potentiality. Long-term modeling and providing practice opportunities for socially interacting with peers engaged in the same art therapy group and process allows for individuals to advance at their own pace and build competencies.

The art therapist whose approach to treatment is respectful, developmentally attuned, and person centered can become a powerful intervention. "Art therapy provides a 'communicative scaffold' onto which further development including an increase in the use of verbal language can hang"

(Evans & Dubowski, 2001, p. 101). Authentic selves are brought forward by a thoughtfully mediated creative process rather than imparted by rote means focused seemingly on promoting predictable, socially appropriate responses.

The visible language spoken in art therapy offers individuals with autism regular opportunities for meaningful play, social interaction, and expression of the self. It can be an effective means of treatment due to its ability to interface with areas of relative cognitive strength. Its treatment power is fully realized through the developmentally attuned art therapist, witness to the sensory experience, and facilitator of socioemotional meaning. Through this intervention, internal experiences might be communicated, acted upon, integrated, and competencies built.

Case Examples

In the nonpublic special education facility in which I work, art therapy is an integral part of the related services provided. The school, located in a major city on the East Coast, serves students ages 11–21 with multiple disabilities. Art therapy is valued for its unique methodology, providing, in many cases, a preferred means to tolerating clinical work demands. Growth is reflected in students' steady progress toward counseling goals established by a multidisciplinary clinical team. These goals are annually written or revised by clinical case managers and, where appropriate, in consultation with the art therapist. During each school year, treatment progress is also assessed through prescribed use of the Person Picking An Apple from a Tree drawing assessment (Gantt & Tabone, 1997) that aids in the tracking of developmental growth and periodically the Face Stimulus Assessment (Betts, 2003) used to evaluate self-representation and ability to sustain series' expectations with progressively decreased stimulus. Video is also used in the groups that I run for the purposes of self-reflection and self-assessment of behaviors as well as an art modality of its own in the expert company of a social work colleague who is also a videographer.

While select students receive individual art therapy treatment, most receive art therapy administered in groups. Considerations for referral to art therapy include a curiosity for sensory materials, tolerance of at least a minimal level of interaction with the art therapist around materials, and reactivity to the creative experience or the experience of peers. Treatment might target deepening awareness of self and others that might, dependent on cognitive functioning, ultimately lead to psychoeducation; enhancement of symbolic thought; improved sensory and emotional regulation; developmental growth, such as capacity for sequencing experiences; mental flexibility; and awareness of pleasure derived from a shared, mutually enjoyed experience.

Some individuals with autism are not ready for group art therapy at the beginning of treatment, if at all, even if social skills building and mediated opportunities to practice emotional regulation are clinically indicated. This is most clearly the case with individuals for whom impulse control and affect regulation are not well managed. Behaviors stemming from such issues can prove highly disruptive to a group, leading to frustration and impeded social learning for all. This was true of the following two individual case examples. (Names have been changed to protect identities.) Treatment focused first on building trust in the predictable space of the art therapy studio, allowing for expression of the chaotic, emotionally charged internal world without censorship or immediate push to change. Over time, the creative process was slowed, materials providing for greater control and narrative quality were introduced, and measured modeling of how the art might be emotionally responded to and named was offered. The student's own experience and the social world were bridged.

Adam

My work with Adam, diagnosed with Asperger's syndrome at time of treatment, focused on self-persecutory themes for several years, at times debilitating anxiety, and, on good days, his deep love of family, famous actors, and movies. (This pseudonym was chosen in honor of his passion for old Hollywood—Adam West.) He visually and verbally referred to himself as a "fugitive," socially and emotionally under attack and always on the run. The repetitive themes seemed an effort to deal with overwhelming anxiety following a series of recently failed school placements. The anxiety-laden repeated topics also alerted the treatment team to his critical need for predictability in his environment.

Given the therapeutic space to create reams of drawings of evil characters, punishments, the crucifixion of Jesus Christ, and past school situations in which he had felt threatened, Adam was gradually able to make affective room for positive imagery. This gradual shift was his own. It was not brought forth through any specific art therapy intervention other than the maintenance of a predictable, safe studio space that offered permission for authentic expression and dialogue. Allowed to connect his experiences and feelings with personal historical context through the creation of his own "Bible" of drawings and writings, Adam's fear-based images became less frequent. He began to write and draw about "anything being possible" and began to reflect on his daily socioemotional "bravery" in a journal format that he regularly shared in art therapy. Toward the end of the second year of treatment, Adam verbalized that he felt lonely and expressed an interest in making friends as well as anxiety in the recognition that he wasn't sure how to do so. In further processing these feelings through art themed on the classic movie, *Babes in Toyland* (Ford & Maffeo, 1986), specifically when he imagined the evil character Barnaby shrunken and caged, Adam chose to take on the social challenge of participating in an art therapy dyad. He repeatedly began to state as if reassuring himself as to having made a good decision: "You can't just shrink away your problems."

The art therapy dyad, in addition to continued individual treatment, offered playful opportunities to build on social skills first introduced and practiced in individual sessions. Under the guidance of a particularly skilled art therapy intern, Adam was able to share his special interests with a same-aged peer with autism. The two practiced skills of compromise in developing mutually satisfying shared art activities, such as murals of commonly loved characters. The stage was set for Adam's successful transition to an art therapy group.

The art therapy group into which Adam transitioned was psychoeducational in nature and one in which all members were diagnosed with autism. Within this context, he was able to review his own growth and share his found competencies with others through collaborative video production. The resulting videos, created over 2 years, focused on operationalizing the diagnosis of autism into the challenges and strengths identified by group members. The videos included art, spontaneous creative movement, self-reflective narratives, student-designed and conducted interviews of select staff about the diagnosis, and popular songs with lyrics of personal relevance. The editing was done with the active involvement of group members. The completed videos served as art forms in their own right. They were viewed within the school community and beautifully showcased the abilities of the group members. Through art therapy, in concert with expert individual counseling and case management, family support, and proven safety of the school environment, Adam was able to progress from a place of internal experience, filled with anxiety and self-persecutory imagery, to one of increasingly confident social engagement.

Exemplifying the significance that self-discovery through art can play throughout the life span, Adam elected to continue building on his competencies by making art part of his vocation. He currently works part time as an artist in a supported art studio, creating pieces about his passions, which are for sale to the public. Though this is a new endeavor for him, he has shown the ability to discern creative content that might serve to connect him with others versus art that is of a personal nature and might better be used as a tool for emotional regulation. He has also come to delight in the positive effect his now playful art has on others.

Chris

For another client-artist, Chris, individual art therapy progressed slowly over the span of several years. Diagnosed with autism, Chris frequently engaged in self-talk that featured the scripting of favorite scenes from animated movies, mostly Disney. He also paced and would rapidly write with his finger in the air. He was difficult to engage when he was responding to his internal world, laughing aloud and smiling as presumably the images, songs, and stories streamed by in his mind. He did not initially have counseling hours scheduled, seemingly as a result of his difficulty with traditional means of social interaction. Because of his parents' advocacy, the highly individualized and student-centered philosophy of the school, and his demonstrated interest in engaging with art materials, he was referred to art therapy despite this situation.

Initially Chris sought out a variety of materials including paint, masks, and collage items, seeming to embrace their creative possibilities. He eventually settled on paint and spent months filling various sized papers with "rainbows." The pace at which he would work, layering random, rapidly applied colored brush strokes, would routinely leave the "rainbows" a muddled brown. In an effort to help Chris more fully realize his verbalized intention of creating "rainbows," I offered him permanent markers with which to fill the picture plane, as I knew the colors would remain distinct even when overlapped. Chris seemed to delight in this new process that seemed to bring a bit more order to his self-expression. When asked, he began to offer simple titles in response to his color-filled pages, naming what appeared to be abstractions: "an ocean," "the jungle," "a forest." The images seemed to reflect dense, fluid realms of experience. I responded with increasingly sophisticated interventions aimed at facilitating differentiation and greater symbolic representation, further seeking to engage higher cortical processes. He was challenged to fashion objects that might be found in such environments, returning to the use of a variety of materials. Among them, he created snakes, flowers, people, and elephants. Chris was able not only to practice flexibility in accepting different methods of work but also to demonstrate developmental growth through symbol formation and expanded narrative. He began to spontaneously engage me in play with the objects and invited family and select staff to view his efforts. He became so excited about his growing success in conveying thoughts and feelings that he would blow kisses at me as he left sessions.

After 1 year of demonstrated benefit from the modality, counseling hours, goals, and objectives were added to Chris's Individualized Education Program (IEP). While his progress was by no means fluid over the years that followed, after 4 years Chris had become fully engaged with me in designing calendars of weekly session activities, offering paragraph-length narratives in response to my questions and inserted speech bubbles, and inviting guests to see and respond to his work. Clearly still challenged by the symptoms of his autism as evident in his continued self-stimulatory behaviors and difficulty with routine engagement, art therapy had become a consistent venue for expression of self and a platform for expanding social competence. His

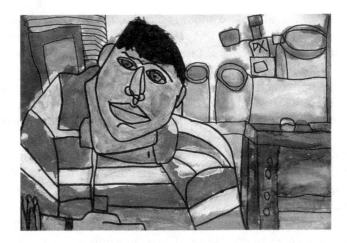

Figure 15.3 The several-year process of moving from undifferentiated color and line to supported development of symbols and better impulse control allowed this student to identify and depict those individuals of greatest support to him as well as to create this image of himself in the art therapy studio.

"scribbles" as he now termed them, formerly known as rainbows, provided a strategy he used in stressful times to self-soothe and reorganize.

Just before his final school year, Chris returned to painting, the medium he had previously struggled to control. He self-selected significant supportive staff and carefully drew and painted each piece. Recognizing the great challenges he had set in motion for himself in this undertaking, I provided Chris with the visual support of a photograph of each person to be painted. As I would trace the lines of the face with black marker, he would draw the highlighted feature with pencil and then "trace his success" on his paper with the same black marker. The process of quickly making permanent his successful pencil lines seemed to help him control his demonstrated impulsive urges to self-sabotage his effort. In choosing to display the finished works in the school and later in a community show, he showcased his overwhelming growth and provided himself concrete opportunities for expressing gratitude for beloved staff before graduating. He completed a final self-portrait his senior year. Once finished, he bounded from the room portrait in hand, declaring to those who happened to be in the hallway at the time, "I'm a painter!" (Figure 15.3).

A Spectrum of Groups

Art therapy groups for young people with autism are best conceptualized along a continuum, with membership determined on the basis of the adolescent's current level of internal distraction and willingness to engage with the social world. In my experience, select students whose greatest need is to develop awareness of self and others and who present as largely internally distracted, if not nonverbal as well, might be served best in a group of peers making art in the company of one another. Social interactions then might be introduced slowly over time and focus on members' interactions within the studio environment. The art therapist's role is to capitalize on opportunities for pointing out a shared thematic interest revealed in the art or similar art processes among peers.

My "parallel process group," initially conceived of in 2003, was developed with these goals in mind. The group began as a result of a cohort of students (ages 13–17) with an innate drive to create art without the need or desire for any creative stimulus or invitation on my part. Much like an art therapist might be in an open studio format, I was then free to help the students use the safe space and the art made within to build social connections. This happened through practiced greetings at the start and end of group, facilitation of shared materials, and routinely hanging their artwork up in the studio for comment. This group continues to be offered each year with differing membership. At times, the group has also had the benefit of co-treatment with a speech-language pathologist, who brings to bear her expertise in mapping language onto the art product put to social use.

Over the years, the quality and level of social interaction between members has varied. Members have been introduced to new supplies for use in creating art about special interests,[2] expanding their repertoire of creative responses beyond their preferred material. This also served to challenge mental flexibility and emotional regulation, as peers' reactions to their artwork and beloved topics was not always positively framed. During other years, the students have also been supported in creating aesthetic environments with their art. For example, one member's repetitive creation of multicolored paper "jellybeans" was used to make a cave-like, sensory space in which the jellybeans and other imagery were hung. Similarly, they have been helped to turn isolated images into simple puppets or elements of a cut paper animation and further guided through the process of developing a basic story and dialogue. Most recently, several group members demonstrated a routine interest in drawing miscellaneous portraits. Playing on this interest, I invited them to draw self-portraits and portraits of each other over several weeks (Figure 15.4).

These successful mixed-media portraits were excitedly received by the group members, who then accepted my offer to help them enter the artworks into a local art competition organized around the theme of self. To the group's delight, their entry was accepted and the framed portraits were hung for the larger metro-area community to appreciate. The members were then helped to further process the experience through the creation of a video sharing their thoughts and feelings in response to seeing themselves

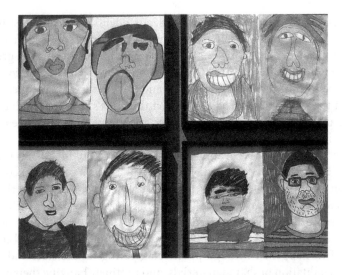

Figure 15.4 Self- and other portraits completed by group members were framed side by side and displayed as a part of a citywide youth media festival celebrating self-awareness.

and their art in a public space. Over the years, I have consistently sought to engage members first with their own art forms and then worked to help them toward a place of social interaction. It is from this place that organically derived collective use of the art product might further move members toward enhanced self-awareness and social competency.

Other autism-exclusive art therapy groups that I facilitate are composed of students who are socially engaged more easily, with intense passion for special interests and associated difficulties with emotional regulation. One of these groups has also folded in psychoeducational goals. "Autism: The Movie" and "Autism: The Book" groups have specifically focused on identifying strengths and abilities as well as psychosocial challenges relevant to autism. The learning process has unfolded through active involvement in the creation of two videos and altered books. Creating altered books involves the transformation of secondhand volumes into art pieces that showcase self-discoveries (Figure 15.5).

Both formats have allowed the group members to incrementally digest diagnostic information about autism and to address their own relevant personal experiences. The students have been given the freedom to reject diagnostic pieces that they feel do not accurately reflect them and to emphasize areas of particular personal strength or weakness. The videos, as detailed a bit earlier in Adam's case, led to student-designed fact-finding interviews about the diagnosis and subsequent delivery of personal narratives exemplifying socioemotional growth. The group members who created the first year's video, inspired by what they had discovered through

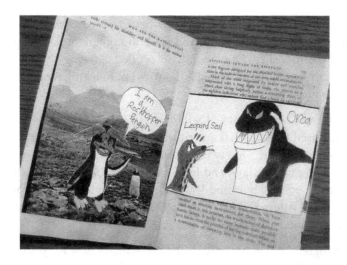

Figure 15.5 In Autism: The Book group, students transform antiquated books about disability and handicap into altered books, visually exploring challenges and personally identified strengths related to autism. Here, a student explores his experience of difference through the metaphor of a Rockhopper penguin and the resultant social anxiety he feels, which he experiences both as the Leopard Seal depicted, as well as at other times the Orca, aggressing before being aggressed upon.

interview and in creative response to learning more about the diagnosis, spontaneously chose to record final thoughts about what they wanted people to "please remember" about autism:

> Just because someone has autism, doesn't mean you are insane or in trouble. People with autism want to get out of misunderstanding [sic] in school. We want to be understood. People with autism need to understand that other people have different tastes which gets on our nerves. People with autism need a break sometimes. Please treat people with autism with dignity and respect.

Student-chosen songs and lyrics were also compactly woven into the video, including short clips from Bruce Hornsby's "The Way It Is" (1986) and The Cars' "You Might Think" (1984), which insightfully offers: "You might think I'm foolish, but baby it's untrue. You might think I'm crazy. All I want is you." Along with other selected song lyrics used in student-made videos, this line has repeatedly given this writer pause to question just how "mindblind" those with autism truly are, provided adequate neuro-connective creative experiences.

In year 2, group members returned to their video as well as the video *Autism and Me* by Rory Hoy (2007) that had lent initial inspiration. Through watching both repeatedly and further creative processing of the experiences offered in each, the students identified the subject of change as one they wished to explore further. Toward the end of the school year spent making art, writing, and selecting poignant songs, members recorded their journeys in a second video titled *Growing Up and Looking Back*. Adam shared the following humorous but touching thoughts during his appearance in the video:

> I am blessed with autism. It will keep me out of jury duty and the army. I used to feel bored and misunderstood before I came to (my school). Now, I write in my journals, e-mail, use my razor to make a quick shave on Sundays, and I am on my own in school. My autism used to go off in school and I would raise my voice. I am in control now. The B sisters and Ms. R lit up my life. I am no longer bored or misunderstood. Thank you.

The progress of therapy tends to be exceedingly slow for young people diagnosed with autism spectrum disorders, and the path of therapy can be frustrating in its oft nonlinear evolution. If the therapist is willing to embrace these challenges and is fortunate enough to be allowed the opportunity to provide long-term treatment, engagement with art can offer concrete and joyful inroads toward activating latent neural pathways. Art can and does facilitate greater connectivity and communication in individuals with autism—a repeated, clinically derived conclusion that desperately calls out for greater empirical study.

Endnotes

[1] TEACCH, or Treatment and Education of Autistic and Communication related handicapped CHildren, was developed by the Department of Psychiatry, School of Medicine, University of North Carolina. It is a comprehensive, community-based methodology including research, consultation, and professional training. PECS, or the Picture Exchange Communication System, was developed as an augmentative form of communication that allows those with communication deficits to initiate communication through the exchange of a picture of a desired item and the reciprocal honoring of the request.

[2] Special interest areas (SIAs) are passions that capture the mind, heart, time, and attention of individuals with autism, providing a means through which they view the world (Winter-Messiers, 2007). They have been positively correlated to well-being and self-esteem and are of critical importance to treatment (Winter-Messier). It follows that to encourage growth of self the therapist must embrace the SIA and sensitively coax its expansion toward less rigid expression.

References

American Art Therapy Association. (2009). *Who are art therapists*. Retrieved on January 20, 2011 from http://www.americanarttherapyassociation.org/upload/whoareart therapists2009.pdf

Arguile, F. (1992). Art therapy with children and adolescents. In D. Waller & A. Gilroy (Eds.), *Art therapy: A handbook.* (pp. 140–155). Berkshire, United Kingdom: Open University Press.

Belkofer, C., & Konopka, L. (2008). Conducting art therapy research using quantitative EEG measures. *Art Therapy: Journal of the American Art Therapy Association, 25*(2), 56–63.

Bentivegna, S., Schwartz, L., & Deschner, D. (1983). Case study: The use of art with an autistic child in residential care. *American Journal of Art Therapy, 22*, 51–56.

Betts, D. J. (2001). Special report: The art of art therapy: Drawing individuals out in creative ways. *The Advocate: Magazine of the Autism Society of America, 34*(3), 22–23.

Betts, D. J. (2003). Developing a projective drawing test: Experiences with the Face Stimulus Assessment (FSA). *Art Therapy: Journal of the American Art Therapy Association, 20*(2), 77–82.

Cane, F. (1989/1951). *The artist in each of us.* Washington, DC: Baker-Webster Printing Co.

Craig, J., & Baron-Cohen, S. (1999). Creativity and imagination in autism and Asperger syndrome. *Journal of Autism and Developmental Disorders, 29,* 319–326.

Dewey, J. (1980/1934). *Art as experience.* New York: Perigee Books.

Emery, M. J. (2004). Art therapy as an intervention for autism. *Art Therapy: Journal of the American Art Therapy Association, 21,* 143–147.

Epp, K. (2008). Outcome-based evaluation of a social skills program using art therapy and group therapy for children on the autism spectrum. *Children &Schools, 30*(1), 27–36.

Evans, K. (1998). Shaping experience and sharing meaning: Art therapy for children with autism. *International Journal of Art Therapy, 3*(1), 17–25.

Evans, K., & Dubowski, J. (2001). *Art therapy with children on the autistic spectrum: Beyond words.* London: Jessica Kingsley.

Flaherty, A. W. (2005). Frontotemporal and dopaminergic control of idea generation and creative drive. *Journal of Compartative Neurology, 493,* 147–153.

Ford, T., & Maffeo, N. T. (Producers). (1986). *Babes in toyland.* [DVD]. New York: National Broadcasting Company.

Gabriels, R. (2003). Art therapy with children who have autism and their families. In C. Malchiodi (Ed.), *Handbook of art therapy* (pp. 193–206). New York: The Guilford Press.

Gantt, L., & Tabone, C. (1997). *PPAT rating manual: The Formal Elements Art Therapy Scale (FEATS).* Morgantown, WV: Gargoyle Press.

Gazzaniga, M. (2008). *Learning, arts, and the brain: The Dana Consortium report on arts and cognition.* Washington, DC: Dana Press.

Gilroy, A. (2006). *Art therapy: Research and evidence-based practice.* London: Sage.

Glaaser, J., Goucher, C., Miller, S., & Scheibler, J. (2007, November). *Art therapy and autistic spectrum disorders: Providing creative paths to social-connectedness.* Panel session presented at the 38th annual conference for the American Art Therapy Association, Albuquerque, NM.

Got, I. L. S., & Cheng, S.T. (2008). The effects of art facilitation on the social functioning of people with developmental disability. *Art Therapy: Journal of the American Art Therapy Association, 25*(1), 32–37.

Grandin, T. (1995). *Thinking in pictures.* New York: Doubleday.

Haier, R., J., & Jung, R. E. (2008). Brain imaging studies of intelligence and creativity: What is the picture for education? *Roeper Review, 30*(3), 171–180.

Hornsby, B. (1986). The way it is [Recorded by Bruce Hornsby and the Range]. On *The way it is* [7",12"]. United States: RCA.

Hoy, R. (2007). *Autism and me (film).* London: Jessica Kingsley.

Jung, R. E., Segall, J. M., Bockholt, H. J., Flores, R. A., Smith, S. M., Chavez, R. S., et al. (2010). Neuroanatomy of creativity. *Human Brain Mapping, 31*(3), 398–409.

Kana, R. K., Keller, T. A., Sherkassky, V. L., Minshew, N. J., & Just, M. A. (2006). Sentence comprehension in autism: Thinking in pictures with decreased functional connectivity. *Brain, 129,* 2484–2493.

Kana, R. K., Keller, T. A., Cherkassky, V. L., Minshew, N. J., & Just, M. A. (2008). Atypical frontal-posterior synchronization of Theory of Mind regions in autism during mental state attribution. *Social Neuroscience, 4*(2), 135–152.

Kellman, J. (1999). Drawing with Peter: Autobiography, narrative, and the art of a child with autism. *Studies in Art Education, 40*(3), 258–274.

Lentz, R. (2008). What we talk about when we talk about art therapy: An outsider's guide to identity crisis. *Art Therapy: Journal of the American Art Therapy Association, 25*(1), 13–14.

Lowenfeld, V., & Brittain, W. L. (1987). *Creative and mental growth* (8th ed.). Upper Saddle River, NJ: Prentice Hall Career & Technology.

Malchiodi, C. (Ed.). (2003). *Handbook of art therapy.* New York: The Guilford Press.

Martin, N. (2009). *Art as an early intervention tool for children with autism.* London: Jessica Kingsley.

Minshew, N. (2010, October). *Understanding how the mind and brain think in autism: New advancements in autism diagnosis and intervention.* Conference presentation for Center for Autism and Related Disorders, Kennedy Krieger Institute, Baltimore, MD.

Noble, J. (2001). Art as an instrument for creating social reciprocity: Social skills group for children with autism. In S. Riley (Ed.), *Group process made visible: Group art therapy* (pp. 82–114). Philadelphia: Brunner-Routledge.

Osborne, J. (2003). Art and the child with autism: Therapy or education? *Early Child Development and Care, 173*(4), 411–423.

Parker-Hairston, M. J. (1990). Analyses of responses of mentally retarded autistic and mentally retarded non-autistic children to art therapy and music therapy. *Journal of Music Therapy, 27*(3), 137–150.

Scanlon, K. (1993). Art therapy with autistic children. *Pratt Institute Creative Arts Therapy Review, 14,* 34–43.

Schleien, S., Mustonen, T., & Rynders, J. (1995). Participation of children with autism and nondisabled peers in a cooperatively structured community art program. *Journal of Autism and Developmental Disorders, 25*(4), 397–413.

Seifert, C. (1988). Learning from drawings: An autistic child looks out at us. *American Journal of Art Therapy, 27,* 45–51.

Siegel, D. J. (1999).*The developing mind: How relationships and the brain interact to shape who we are.* New York: The Guilford Press.

Stuss, D. T., Gallup, G. G., & Alexander, M. P. (2001). The frontal lobes are necessary for theory of mind. *Brain, 124,* 279–86.

The Cars. (1984). You might think. On *Heartbeat City*. [7", 12"]. United States: Elektra.

Williams, D. L., Goldstein, G., & Minshew, N. J. (2006). Profile of memory function in children with autism. *Neuropsychology, 20,* 21–29.

Winter-Messiers, M. A. (2007). From tarantulas to toilet brushes: Understanding the special interest areas of children and youth with Asperger syndrome. *Remedial and Special Education, 28*(3), 140–152.

Winnicott, D. W. (1971). *Playing and reality.* London: Tavistock Publications.

Wood, M. (1984). The child and art therapy: a psychodynamic viewpoint. In T. Dalley (Ed.), *Art as therapy* (pp. 50–67). London: Tavistock/Routledge.

CHAPTER 16

Music Therapy Interventions for Social, Communication, and Emotional Development for Children and Adolescents With Autism Spectrum Disorders

DARCY WALWORTH

Introduction

Music therapy is the clinical and evidence-based use of music interventions to accomplish individualized goals within a therapeutic relationship by a credentialed professional who has completed an approved music therapy program (AMTA, 2011a). Music therapists meet with patients and clients to assess the specific need areas for interventions. Once need areas are identified, music therapists will determine individualized goals and objectives for meeting those goals. Documentation is completed after intervention sessions to monitor improvement or attainment of the goals. Termination of services is recommended when all goals are met or when improvement is not seen within the specified time frame for intervention.

Music therapists use a variety of treatment interventions that incorporate preferred music and strategies that best fit the client's interaction and learning style. The highly individualized treatment plans are one of the reasons music therapy can look so different to a person observing several different sessions. Music therapists are adept at assessing client responses in the moment and changing intervention techniques as patients' responses change, always meeting clients where they are to provide the optimal therapeutic interaction between therapist and client.

The idea that music can be therapeutic has a deep history that can be traced back to ancient times as seen in biblical and historical writings in many cultures such as China, India, Greece, and Egypt (Horden, 2000). In America, music therapy began to develop as a therapeutic intervention after World War I and World War II when veterans returned home with physical and emotional traumas. Musicians who visited the hospitals were able to elicit notable change in the emotional and physical responses from the veterans. This ability to change responses resulted in musicians being hired by hospitals to address the various issues their patients faced (AMTA, 2011b). Musicians who were hired realized that training was needed to provide effective interventions for the patients, leading to the formation of college degree programs. Today, colleges in America offer bachelor, master, and PhD levels of degrees in music therapy. The field now encompasses interventions for individuals in medical and psychiatric hospitals, special education in school systems, rehabilitative services, hospice and palliative care, prison inmate programs, physical and substance abuse victims, and private practice services.

Children at risk or diagnosed with autism spectrum disorders (ASD) have shown positive benefits from receiving music therapy interventions. A meta-analysis of music therapy interventions with children and adolescents diagnosed with ASD concluded that all music interventions included in the analysis were effective regardless of the method or purpose of the intervention variable (Whipple, 2004). The dependent variables included in the analysis consisted of social, communication, and cognitive goals such as reducing challenging behaviors, reducing self stimulation behaviors, increasing spontaneous speech and frequency of communicative acts, following instructions during gross motor and computer tasks, identifying pictures, and acquiring a larger vocabulary. This empirical support for inclusion of music therapy as a viable intervention is encouraging as more parents and clinicians look for multidisciplinary team treatment approaches.

Why Music Interventions Work

Music has been shown to contribute to cognitive development, emotion regulation, and social interaction (Juslin & Sloboda, 2001; Trevarthen, 1999) by stimulating neural growth and cortical interconnectivity. Interestingly, individuals with autism spectrum disorders show no deficits in recognizing the emotional content in music (Heaton, Hermelin, & Pring, 1999). Additionally, children with autism spectrum disorders demonstrate superior auditory discrimination skills when compared with neuro-typical children (O'Riordan & Passetti, 2006). These findings suggest that these particular children are amenable to music as part of their therapeutic programming. Neurobiological research into the processing of music suggests that the same area of the brain is activated during auditory processing of music as negative and positive emotions and the visual processing of faces (Koelsch, Fritz, Cramon, Müller, & Friederici, 2006). Children who participate in music therapy interactions will therefore be activating the same brain region to process the music stimuli while they are processing facial inputs of peers in the group and the emotions expressed during the group. Using the intact music-emotion processing to improve the impaired facial and social emotional processing for individuals with ASD may be one reason children show gains in socialization after participating in music therapy sessions. A recent line of neurological research into social connection and connectivity proposes that the human mirror neuron system links music perception, cognition, and emotion through an experiential mechanism (Molnar-Szakacs & Overy, 2006). This system may be the common neural area where combinatorial rules are processed for language, action, and music, which communicate meaning to an individual as well as human affect. Abnormalities of the limbic system such as the amygdala might contribute to an impaired ability to link visual perception of socially and emotionally relevant stimuli with social knowledge and behaviors (Adolphs, Sears, & Piven, 2001). It is theorized that individuals with ASD recruit different neural networks and rely on different strategies when processing facial emotion (Wang, Dapretto, Hariri, Sigman, & Bookheimer, 2004). Taken together, these various research studies provide a promising justification for using music in the treatment of autism spectrum disorders.

Determining Goals to Address Within Music Therapy Sessions

The first step in the treatment process for music therapists is conducting an assessment of a child's strengths and need areas. While some music therapists choose to create a unique assessment for each child, others choose to use an existing standardized assessment tool. There are many different methods of assessments that music therapists report using in school and clinical setting in the course of providing intervention for children with ASD (Layman, Hussey, & Laing, 2002; Wilson & Smith, 2000). One such tool, the Special Education Music Therapy Assessment Process (SEMTAP), sets itself apart as an assessment process rather than an assessment instrument per se. It assesses all of the domain areas for which children can receive music therapy. Many music therapists working in the school setting choose to use the SEMTAP because it conforms to federal education laws and is designed specifically to compliment the IEP for each student

(Brunk & Coleman, 2000, 2002). Another tool being used by music therapists working with children who have communication disorders including ASD is the SCERTS Assessment Model. An analysis of music therapists providing intervention with clients at risk or diagnosed with ASD found the SCERTS tool to be an appropriate assessment option (Walworth, 2007; Walworth, Register, & Engel, 2009). The SCERTS Model assesses strengths and identifies needs for children in the areas of social communication, emotional regulation, and transactional support. The SCERTS is unique in its design in that it not only assesses but also generates specific intervention goals that are measurable and attainable in a 3-month time period.

The skillful application of an established observation procedure can increase the likelihood of capturing an accurate picture of the child (Jellison, 2000). This enables a music therapist to create meaningful and appropriate goals for the music therapy intervention. The establishment of appropriate goals provides the catalyst for the changes a child can experience as a result of participating in music therapy intervention. An experience can be positive for both the client and family without any treatment goals. However, the use of specific goals and objectives provides a framework for progress being made by the child. Additionally, having concrete goals and objectives can open dialogue for collaboration with other treatment team members providing intervention services. Providing comprehensive services to clients allows team members to build on the skills and intervention techniques being addressed in each other's sessions. When children are experiencing strategies to improve similar or related goals across therapeutic environments, the transfer of new skill acquisition is more natural.

How Music Therapy Interventions Meet Goals

Music therapists are able to target music and nonmusic goals when working with ASD children. Some children who have shown a specific interest or talent in playing a musical instrument can benefit from receiving music lessons from a music therapist. A music therapist who is giving music lessons will be able to identify challenges the child faces after conducting the initial assessment. As music lessons progress, a music therapist can use the opportunity of teaching music instrument skills to teach nonmusic skills such as turn taking, following distal points when communicating verbally (pointing away from your body with a finger), regulating when routines change within the session, and using a support system to augment communication during the lesson.

Many music therapists, however, do not provide music lessons but choose to provide interventions solely for the nonmusic goal areas. In this situation, a music therapist will incorporate music into each session as the engagement medium for the acquisition of new skills. It is recommended when interacting with children with ASD that interventions teach functional skills in a conventional, nonthreatening environment with natural reward systems (Lord & McGee, 2001). The natural sequence or flow of a music therapy intervention session will lend itself to opportunities for communication, emotional responses, and socialization. Repair strategies are attempts that a child makes to repair a communication breakdown and will also naturally occur within sessions when a request is unclear or the way to play an instrument being used in the session needs clarification. Instead of forcing an objective into a session plan, music strategies can naturally provide an ideal learning environment for skills a child needs in various settings.

An example of the natural learning environment in music therapy sessions can be seen with children who have difficulty following eye gaze. In this situation, it is helpful for there to be something interesting or intriguing to look at. Music instruments are often colorful and novel and therefore provide a natural interest for following gaze toward an object. Oftentimes, music therapists will use a group setting for children with ASD. There are many benefits to conducting interventions with peers present. Using the same example of eye gaze, there are many natural opportunities for children to follow a therapist's or peer's gaze during songs. When rolling a ball between children and therapist and singing about who has the ball, children will not know to be ready for the ball coming to them unless they are following the ball or the eye gaze of the person passing the ball. A music therapist will structure the activity to set up the child for an opportunity to follow eye gaze instead of the movement of the ball by pausing in the song "I roll the ball to . . . (Pause)." When the child looks at the therapist and sees her eye gaze toward the intended ball receiver, the song then continues ". . . Jesse, he rolls it back to me, rolling, rolling." Music is a natural reinforcer when it is a pleasurable stimulus. Because of this quality, the removal of the stimulus (i.e., interrupting the song) causes a motivation to engage in the desired behavior for the music to continue.

Another common goal area that naturally occurs through music is shared attention. Eye gaze is a skill that is necessary to share attention, so the two skills build on each other. When a music therapist uses Orff xylophones (wooden instruments with removable tone bars) and assigns parts, a natural opportunity is presented to share attention so each child knows when to start and stop playing. This naturally happens within the structure of the song. Each chord or section of the melody will have closure, allowing group participants to shift their attentional focus to the next person playing the continuation of the song. Visual or auditory cues can be used by the music therapist to support children in this task. If nonverbal cues are paired with the musical structure cue, children are given two natural cues for shifting their attention while using an object in a conventional way.

Some children with ASD will immediately spin a drum when they are presented with the instrument and a mallet instead of hitting the drum with the mallet. The natural cue of marching while playing a drum provides an opportunity for children to attend to the action of marching while playing the drum with a mallet.

Improvements in gaze, turn taking, object use, and joint attention for children with ASD have been found when social partners imitate their behavior (Lewy & Dawson, 1992). Songs can naturally incorporate imitation of music behaviors, such as copying rhythm patterns on a drum, or nonmusic behaviors, such as movements and faces. Music therapists can incorporate peer imitation by making group members leaders of the activity that is then copied by the other group members. When children participate in a social group through music, the task of imitating the way an instrument is played requires them to attend to the social partner to pick up the situational cues needed to play the instrument and anticipate the action of the leader.

Music therapists are consulted, contracted, or placed full time into school systems to address barriers to academic learning experienced by some children with ASD. One quality music possesses is the ability to capture attention easily. When children are not attending or engaged in a meaningful way at school, it can be difficult for teachers or peers to reach them verbally. Music, however, provides a new stimulus that often directs attention for shared purposes. When children become dysregulated behaviorally or emotionally, music can soothe and calm based on its predictability and repetition. Establishing a positive association between emotions and music stimuli occurs naturally for many children. Music can also function as a cue. Many people are familiar with the "clean-up" song commonly heard in preschools and day cares. In the same way the clean-up song cues children what task is now at hand, songs can be written by music therapists to cue a child that a certain event is going to occur. For a child who has difficulty transitioning from the classroom to the lunchroom, a song about walking to the door and going to the lunchroom to eat can provide the additional support he needs to make the transition while remaining calm.

Music therapists who provide services in the community clinic or home environments commonly incorporate the parent into the session. This is recommended because children will more readily follow their parent's gaze, will have better affect, and will play with more toys when they are imitating, playing, and involved in communication activities with their parent (Dawson & Galpert, 1990; Rogers, Herbison, Lewis, Pantone, & Reis, 1986; Rogers & Lewis, 1989). Many parents are interested in learning specific techniques for incorporating music into the home environment to help with transition difficulties, behavior outbursts, and responses to their child's attentional focus. While some parents do not think they are "musical" enough to sing with their child at home, the repeated exposure to music during intervention sessions builds their confidence so they are often willing to try singing on their own. By including the parents as members of the treatment team, music therapists are able to find out the greatest needs of the child outside of the clinical intervention setting. Creating meaningful interactions through music for parents and children in between sessions increases the likelihood of a child transferring skills to other settings.

Siblings and friends are also included in music therapy sessions to increase the skills of peers who frequently interact with children with ASD. Peers are able to learn how to initiate positive interactions through songs and music games as well as how to be successful in engaging their sibling or friend into the music activity. Children are wonderful models of appropriate behaviors during music sessions because it is natural to play instruments appropriately versus atypically. The natural imitation and turn taking embedded within many songs creates interactions that do not seem forced for the purpose of learning a new skill.

Successful Applications of Music Therapy Interventions

Playground Case Studies

In an effort to increase social participation and interaction skills on the playground, Kern and Aldridge (2006) investigated four boys aged 3 to 5 years old diagnosed with ASD who were exposed to an outdoor music center added to the playground. The children were recommended for study participation by their teachers and parents. All children exhibited an absence of peer-related interactions on the playground and showed an interest in music. Two peer buddies were chosen from the classmates by the teacher and therapist each day of intervention. The peer buddies displayed an interest in music, typical socialization skills, a positive relationship with the ASD child, and a desire to participate in the intervention.

A covered music hut was constructed on the playground with age-appropriate instruments installed and secured to the structure of the hut. A large variety of instruments was incorporated within the music hut to foster a desire to engage in music play. Each child had a song composed for them by the music therapy researcher that addressed the specific strengths and goals identified by the interdisciplinary team for the study. Teachers were trained in the developmentally appropriate ways of interacting with the children in the sound hut. Additionally, children were familiarized with the songs before interventions in the music hut occurred. Data were collected over a period of 8 months and consisted of a 10-minute sample of the child's playground behaviors for each experimental condition. The number of days observed for each child ranged from 30 to 71 sessions.

Child 1 spent most of his playground time in solitary activities such as riding a tricycle or digging in the sandbox. When he did initiate interactions with other children, it was typically through a negative behavior like taking toys away. This child's peers rarely initiated interactions with him. The highest rate of time spent engaged in peer participation in baseline observations for this child was 18%. With the addition of the music hut without adult assistance, the rate of positive peer interaction ranged from 3 to 40% at the highest level. The addition of the teacher-assisted music hut play increased positive peer interaction to a range of 33 to 68%. The peer-mediated music hut play condition resulted in the most stable levels of positive peer interactions and ranged from 40 to 45%.

Child 2 did not engage in meaningful play of any type on the playground without adult assistance. He most often ran or turned around in circles while singing and signing familiar songs to himself. When not engaging in these aimless wanderings, he often lay on a bench by himself. Both the baseline observations and the music hut with no assistance observations resulted in a maximum rate of 13% of time spent in positive peer interactions. The addition of the teacher mediated interactions in the music hut dramatically raised the amount of time spent engaged in positive peer interactions to 53 to 93%. The peer-mediated condition resulted in this child engaging positively in the range of 43 to 80% of time spent in the music hut.

Child 3 often made his peers afraid to interact with him due to his rough play when he did approach them for interaction. Although he did make some attempts to interact, he most commonly spent his time on the playground by spinning a leaf, wandering aimlessly, or sitting on a bench. He did respond to adult assistance to play meaningfully when prompted. When observed in baseline conditions, this child had a maximum of 15% of his time spent in positive peer interactions. The addition of the music hut to the playground resulted in a range of 0 to 23% of time positively engaged. When a teacher provided assistance in the music hut, it caused a large increase in time spent in positive peer interaction ranging from 33 to 93%. During peer-mediated interventions the amount of time spent in peer interactions ranged from 8 to 33%.

Child 4 would initiate interactions with peers on the playground when he was interested in the object they were playing with. Otherwise, he would run around and chase moving objects such as tricycles around the playground in solitary play. He also would spend time rocking his body back and forth. Baseline observations for this child resulted in a maximum of 5% of time spent engaged in positive peer interactions. There was little change with the addition of the music hut, which resulted in a maximum of 10% of time spent engaged in peer interactions. When teacher-mediated interventions were added, the range of time spent in peer interactions was 28 to 80%. The peer-mediated interventions resulted in 13 to 40% of time spent engaged in positive interactions.

With each child observed, the amount of time spent engaged in unsupported positive peer interaction increased when comparing peer-mediated play with the baseline and the music hut without intervention settings. The most dramatic increases in engagement for each of these children occurred when the teachers assisted with the interactions in the music hut, which is to be expected. The encouraging finding from all of these cases is the rate of interaction increases that was found between peers and the child with autism. These increases occurred without support from teachers or adults in a naturalistic setting. This program is effective over time and increases communicative attempts between children on the playground.

Self-Contained Classroom Case Studies

Brownell (2002) conducted a series of four case studies with male children aged 6–9 years old who exhibited problem behaviors in the school setting in a self-contained classroom. The children were individually referred for music therapy intervention by their teacher and were all verbal with at least prereading skills. Target behaviors for the four children were talking less about television, listening to directions and following them, and using a quiet voice, for two of the case study subjects. The interventions used in the treatment conditions were social stories written specifically about the child's desired behavior change that were either sung or read verbally. The three treatment conditions each child received were baseline (A), reading the social story (B), and singing the story (C) presented in ABAC/ACAB order. Baseline frequencies of each targeted behavior were tallied during 1-hour segments prior to the social story intervention beginning and again between types of treatment conditions. One-hour observations of behaviors immediately following the interventions were conducted in the classroom at the same time of day as baseline observations.

The first child in the case studies was causing disruptive behavior in the classroom when making repetitive statements from movies or television. This child's teacher referred him for the music therapy intervention with the goal of reducing the amount of TV talk in the classroom. The intervention treatments were scheduled during the time of day the teacher identified as the most problematic for the child, when he consistently made the greatest frequency of TV talk statements. When comparing the frequencies of TV talk between treatment conditions, there were significantly fewer echolalia television statements made by the child following the social story reading and singing conditions ($p < .05$). The lowest levels of TV talk were made after the music therapy interventions when the social story was sung.

The second child in the case studies was referred by his teacher for lack of responsiveness accompanied by flat affect when verbal directions were given to the child. This behavior was persistent in all settings and throughout the entire day. Comparison of treatment conditions found significant differences between baseline and treatment conditions ($p < .05$) for the number of times a direction was repeated before the child responded. Both the singing and reading of the social story resulted in decreased numbers of directives stated by the teacher. Interestingly, the observation of baseline behaviors in the middle of the treatment conditions also showed an improvement in behavior, suggesting the child transferred the knowledge gained about following directions to the classroom without having the intervention that day.

The third and fourth children were both referred by their teachers for interventions addressing decreasing their vocal volume when speaking in the classroom. The third child often scared other students in the classroom when using his loud shouting voice, resulting in behavior disturbances from his peers. The behaviors occurred throughout the day, so the intervention session was selected to occur in the morning. The baseline measurement consisted of the number of times the teacher verbally cued the child to use his quiet voice or shushed him. A significant reduction in the number of time the teacher cued him to use his quiet voice was found after both the reading and the singing treatment interventions.

The fourth child in the case studies also displayed a loud shouting voice and commonly made loud nonsense noises, leading to classroom behavior disturbances. Many times, this child was removed from the classroom to allow other students the ability to stay regulated and be able to participate in the classroom instruction time. The baseline measurement consisted of the number of times the teacher verbally cued the child to use his quiet voice or shushed him. Since his behaviors occurred throughout the day, the afternoon was chosen to implement the intervention sessions. The number of times the teacher cued him to use his quiet voice or shushed him was significantly lower after both of the intervention sessions.

When looking at the data for all four case studies, it is apparent that the negative behaviors occurred with the lowest total frequency after the music assisted social story conditions (Brownell, 2002). While there were not overall significant differences found between the reading and singing social story interventions, the trends toward music being very effective at reducing problem behaviors in the classroom is promising and warrants further investigation. It is possible that with more than two intervention sessions the behaviors could have a more lasting change for children with ASD.

Preschool Case Studies

Kern, Wolery, and Aldridge (2007) conducted two case studies with 3-year-old children in a preschool setting. Both children had a very difficult time transitioning into the classroom each morning to begin the day at preschool. Parents, teachers, and therapists recommended that both children receive assistance from the music therapist to address this issue. The music therapist consulted with teachers to incorporate a song into the morning transition time from home into the classroom for the two children. Before the study began, common behaviors for the first child in the case studies were lying on the floor outside of the room, screaming, and refusing to enter the room. Common behaviors for the second child consisted of entering the room but refusing to let go of his caregiver and crying.

Both boys had limited speech and used the Picture Exchange Communication System (PECS) to augment their communication with others (Frost & Bondy, 2002). The PECS system uses small picture cards of images paired with words to augment the communication ability for children at risk or diagnosed with communication disorders. These children were used to seeing a PECS symbol of a stick figure waving with the word *hello* when they entered the classroom. This symbol was incorporated into the music therapy routine created to help their morning transition go more smoothly. The music therapist providing intervention composed unique songs that addressed the five desired morning routine steps to disengage from the caregiver and integrate into the classroom. Staff and caregivers were given a CD to practice the songs and learn them for incorporating into the morning transition time. A multiple baseline design was used to compare behavioral responses with the interventions for each child. The baseline condition incorporated a five-step transition sequence that was followed verbally by staff and caregivers. The music therapy intervention condition used the same five-step routine, with the alteration of singing the steps instead of verbally stating them. The music therapist composed each song based on the child's personality and music preferences.

The first child reported in this case study had very positive responses to the music intervention compared with the verbal statements for each morning routine step. The number of steps completed independently never rose above two with the verbal statements condition. After music intervention was initiated this child's independent behaviors showed a steady increase and stabilized at four positive behaviors of the desired five steps during morning transition time. Returning to the baseline verbal condition resulted in the number of independent behaviors immediately dropping back to two independent responses. The initiation of the music condition caused an increase in independent responses that stabilized again at the four-responses rate.

The second child in the case studies also had positive results with the music intervention once it was modified to not include saying good-bye in the classroom but saying good-bye to his caregiver at the door. Similarly, both baseline verbal condition responses were low and were primarily in the two- to three-responses range. During the two modified music intervention conditions, responses were consistently three independent responses and four independent responses of the five-step transition routine. Peers within the classroom responded positively to the music routine by coming up to this child independently and engaging in a social exchange.

The results from Kern et al. (2007) provide another documented intervention that can be implemented by teachers, families, and music therapists. The addition of singing to instructions that are typically stated verbally is a simple modification to make for transition times. Children are able to participate in the sung instructions by singing the lyrics themselves or humming along in their head. When a statement is made verbally to a child there is no joint involvement required from the child during the statement. The simple fact that singing is naturally a multiple person activity may be the reason the children in these case studies had more positive responses during the singing condition. For teachers or parents who do not consider themselves musically talented enough to sing, it is important to remember that a performance is not required for this intervention. When targeted singing is occurring with a child, the quality of the singing is not as important as the engagement of child with the singer. To make the experience more comfortable for parents and teachers, familiar melodies can be used with words changed to incorporate the intervention goals. In this situation, it may be more effective to use a song melody that is not already familiar for the child with autism so there is no confusion about which lyrics are recalled in the moment of the intervention.

Guidelines for Using Music Therapy

Music therapists can be consulted to target specific communication and behavioral needs of children with autism in the school setting or the home setting or to cotreat with therapists using different treatment modalities. The role of the music therapist as an observer within a naturalistic setting is a valuable asset when trying to determine the most effective time and mode for implementing intervention services. Music therapists have specific training to assess antecedents to problem behaviors and to determine meaningful motivators for each child or client. Anytime music therapy is used to address outcomes for children with ASD, an assessment is first completed. Therapist-generated assessments as well as standardized assessments can be conducted. Only after the assessment is complete will a music therapist know which target areas to address therapeutically in sessions. At this point, a session treatment plan is created to allow documentation of goals that are met over time. Without an assessment, the intent of the therapeutic process is unclear and not as purposeful.

The existing published literature in peer-reviewed journals using experimental control conditions for music therapy interventions with children with autism has demonstrated positive outcomes for problem behaviors (Brownell, 2002), communication (Buday, 1995; Edgerton, 1994; Kern et al., 2007; Wimpory, Chadwick, & Nash, 1995), emotional regulation (Katagiri, 2009; Kim, Wigram, & Gold, 2009), and social interaction (Kern & Aldridge, 2006; Kern et al., 2007, Kim, Wigram, & Gold, 2008; Kim et al., 2009; Pasiali, 2004; Wimpory, Chadwick, & Nash, 1995).

Both behavioral and improvisational styles of interaction have shown positive outcomes for children with autism. The common thread between both styles of intervention is the assessment of the current state of the child with autism and responding with a music stimulus. Using live music gives the child and therapist the ability to communicate through the music instead of through verbalizations. Musical attunement can be used to facilitate joint attention and nonverbal socialization (Kim et al., 2008). Musical attunement is a specialized technique of improvisational music therapy and one that is commonly used by therapists providing improvisational methods of treatment. The music therapist very carefully matches children's musical and nonmusical expressions with the live music they are providing. This allows the children to connect their current state with therapist responses.

Behavioral interventions typically choose the goals to address after the assessment process is completed. According to Lord and McGee (2001), language and communication goals should be met within a 2- to 3-month time frame. If the ongoing assessment process shows that no gains are being made by the client it is recommended that the treatment strategy be changed. The importance of having behaviors to track is paramount within this framework. Once the targeted behaviors are identified, the process of observing and recording those behaviors over time begins. It is often clear early in the treatment process which behaviors are showing improvement in response to the music interventions.

The selection of how music will function within the session is the next step in the treatment process. Music has the ability to act as a reinforcer for desired behaviors, structure for the entire session, motivator to communicate, means of expressing emotions, catalyst for dramatic/imaginative play, engagement for focusing attention, and facilitator of social experiences. Choosing which function music will serve in the session is based on the culmination of a music therapist's training. As the session progresses, a music therapist continually assesses client responses and chooses the next function music will serve. With each selection of music function, the client's needs are being met and skills are being built upon. Documenting that acquisition of skills has occurred is seen when progress notes are reviewed. Without the assessment and documentation steps of the treatment process, a music therapist is able to tell only anecdotally what progress the client is making.

Music therapy is a promising intervention for children with ASD. As more findings are reported in peer-reviewed sources it will become clear which treatment interventions have high success rates. The movement of autism research to random assignment large group designs requires music therapists to participate in multisite studies and to use a protocol for treatment intervention. Although the music therapy process is highly individualized for each child, it is possible to employ similar strategies to determine if common responses can be found. The studies reviewed in this chapter highlight the successful application of specific strategies that could be replicated in the future for other music therapists with similar clients. Music serves multiple functions for children with autism and is able to shape behaviors, emotions, and communication.

References

American Music Therapy Association. (2011a). *What is music therapy?* Retrieved from http://www.musictherapy.org/faqs.html

American Music Therapy Association. (2011b). *What is the history of music therapy as a health care profession?* Retrieved from http://www.musictherapy.org/faqs.html

Adolphs, R., Sears, L., & Piven, J. (2001). Abnormal processing of social information from faces in autism. *Journal of Cognitive Neuroscience, 13,* 232–240.

Brownell, M. D. (2002). Musically adapted social stories to modify behaviors in students with autism: Four case studies. *Journal of Music Therapy, 39,* 117–144.

Brunk, B. K., & Coleman, K. A. (2000). Development of a special education music therapy assessment process. *Perspectives, 18,* 59–68.

Brunk, B. K., & Coleman, K. A. (2002). A special education music therapy assessment process. In B. Wilson (Ed.), *Models of music therapy interventions in school settings* (2nd ed., pp. 69–82). Silver Spring, MD: American Music Therapy Association.

Buday, E, M. (1995). The effects of signed and spoken words taught with music on sign and speech imitation by children with autism. *Journal of Music Therapy, 32,* 189–202.

Dawson, G., & Galpert, L. (1990). Mother's use of imitative play for facilitating social responsiveness and toy play in young autistic children. *Development and Psychopathology, 2,* 151–162.

Edgerton, C. L. (1994). The effect of improvisational music therapy on the communicative behaviors of autistic children. *Journal of Music Therapy, 31,* 31–62.

Frost, L., & Bondy, A. (2002). *PECS: The Picture Exchange System Training Manual* (2nd ed.). Newark, DE: Pyramid Educational Consultants, Inc.

Heaton, P., Hermelin, B., & Pring, L. (1999). Can children with autistic spectrum disorders perceive affect in music? An experimental investigation. *Psychology of Medicine, 29,* 1405–1410.

Horden, P. (Ed.). (2000). *Music as medicine: The history of music therapy since antiquity.* Aldershot: Ashgate.

Jellison, J. A. (2000). A content analysis of music research with disabled children and youth (1975–1999): Application in special education. In: *Effectiveness of music therapy procedures: Documentation of research and clinical practice* (3rd ed., pp. 199-264). Silver Springs, MD: American Music Therapy Association.

Juslin, P., & Sloboda, J. A. (Eds.). (2001). *Music and emotion: Theory and research.* Oxford: Oxford University Press.

Katagiri, J. (2009). The effect of background music and song texts on the emotional understanding of children with autism. *Journal of Music Therapy, 46,* 15–31.

Kern, P., & Aldridge, D. (2006). Using embedded music therapy interventions to support outdoor play of young children with autism in an inclusive community-based child care program. *Journal of Music Therapy, 43,* 270–294.

Kern, P., Wolery, M., & Aldridge, D. (2007). Use of songs to promote independence in morning greeting routines for young children with autism. *Journal of Autism and Developmental Disorders, 37,* 1264–1271.

Kim, J., Wigram, T., & Gold, C. (2008). The effects of improvisational music therapy on joint attention behaviours in autistic children: A randomized controlled study. *Journal of Autism and Developmental Disorders, 38,* 1758–1766.

Kim, J., Wigram, T., & Gold, C. (2009). Emotional, motivational and interpersonal responsiveness of children with autism in improvisational music therapy. *Autism, 13,* 389–409.

Koelsch, S., Fritz, T., Cramon, Y., Müller, K., & Friederici, A. D. (2006). Investigating emotion with music: An fMRI study. *Human Brain Mapping, 27,* 239–250.

Layman, D. L., Hussey, D. L., & Laing, S. J. (2002). Music therapy assessment for severely emotionally disturbed children: A pilot study. *Journal of Music Therapy, 39,* 164–187.

Lewy, A. L., & Dawson, G. (1992). Social stimulation and joint attention in young autistic children. *Journal of Abnormal Child Psychology 20*(6), 555–566.

Lord, C., & McGee, J. P. (Eds.). (2001). *Educating children with autism.* Washington, DC: National Academy Press.

Molnar-Szakacs, I., & Overy, K. (2006). Music and mirror neurons: From motion to "e"motion. *SCAN, 1,* 235–241.

O'Riordan, M., & Passetti, F. (2006). Discrimination in autism within different sensory modalities. *Journal of Autism and Developmental Disorders, 36,* 665–675.

Pasiali, V. (2004). The use of prescriptive therapeutic songs in a home-based environment to promote social skills acquisition by children with autism: Three case studies. *Music Therapy Perspectives, 20,* 11–20.

Rogers, S. J., Herbison, J., Lewis, H., Pantone, J., & Reis, K. (1986). An approach for enhancing symbolic, communicative, and interpersonal functioning of young children with autism and severe emotional handicaps. *Journal of the Division of Early Childhood, 10,* 135–148.

Rogers, S. J., & Lewis, H. (1989). An effective day treatment model for young children with pervasive developmental disorders. *Journal of the American Academy of Child and Adolescent Psychiatry, 28,* 207–214.

Trevarthen, C. (1999). Musicality and the intrinsic motive pulse: Evidence from human psychobiology and infant communication. In *"Rhythms, music narrative, and the origins of human communication"*. *Musicae Scientiae, Special Issue, 1999-2000*, 157–213. Liége: European Society for the Cognitive Sciences in Music.

Walworth, D. D. (2007). The use of music therapy within the SCERTS Model for children with autism spectrum disorder. *Journal of Music Therapy, 44*, 2–22.

Walworth, D. D., Register, D., & Engel, J. (2009). Using the SCERTS model assessment tool to identify music therapy goals for clients with autism spectrum disorder. *Journal of Music Therapy, 46*(3), 204–16.

Wang, A. T., Dapretto, M., Hariri, A. R., Sigman, M., & Bookheimer, S. Y. (2004). Neural correlates of facial affect processing in children and adolescents with autism spectrum disorder. *Journal of the American Academy of Child & Adolescent Psychiatry, 43*(4), 481–490.

Whipple, J. (2004). Music in intervention for children and adolescents with autism: A meta-analysis. *Journal of Music Therapy, 41*, 90–106.

Wilson, D. L., & Smith, D. S. (2000). Music therapy assessment in school settings: A preliminary investigation. *Journal of Music Therapy, 37*, 95–117.

Wimpory, D., Chadwick, P., & Nash, S. (1995). Brief report: Musical interaction therapy for children with autism: An evaluative case study with two-year follow-up. *Journal of Autism and Developmental Disorders, 25*, 541–552.

CHAPTER 17

Moving Into Relationships

Dance/Movement Therapy With Children With Autism

CHRISTINA DEVEREAUX

Autism spectrum disorders (ASD) are characterized by widespread abnormalities of social interactions and communication as well as restricted interests and repetitive behavior (APA, 2000). As of 2010, 1 in 110 individuals was diagnosed with autism spectrum disorders. These statistics, according to Autism Speaks (2010), are more common than pediatric cancer, diabetes, and AIDS combined. Furthermore, autism reportedly occurs four times more often in boys than in girls and occurs in all racial, ethnic, and social groups (NINDS, 2008). Early warning signs and subsequent diagnosis of the disorder are first suspect when developmental milestones appear to not be met.

Currently, there is no cure for autism; however, therapies and behavioral interventions designed to remedy specific symptoms can bring about substantial improvement (Koegel, Koegel, Fredeen, & Gengoux, 2008; Ortega, 2010; Rogers & Vismara, 2008). Such intervention may help to lessen disruptive behaviors and to develop coping skills that allow for greater independence. However, just as there is no one symptom or behavior that identifies individuals with ASD, there is no single treatment that will be effective for all children on the spectrum. Treatment must be tailored to children's unique strengths, challenges, and need level.

Effective treatment plans focus on therapies and interventions that target the core symptoms (i.e., impaired social interaction, problems with verbal and nonverbal communication, and obsessive or repetitive routines and interests); early intervention is critically important. A highly recognized treatment called applied behavior analysis (ABA), a systematic method using behavioral trials to improve social behavior, has received a lot of attention in bringing about behavioral changes with children with ASD (Jensen & Sinclair, 2002; Ortega, 2010; Schreibman, 2000; Smith, Mozingo, Mruzek, & Zarcone, 2007). However, other treatment approaches may play an important role in improving verbal and nonverbal communications skills and reducing other associated symptoms in social engagement (Levy, Mandell, Merhar, Ittenbach, & Pinto-Martin, 2003; Merna, 2010; Smith, 1999, 2008). Among these complementary approaches is the discipline of dance/movement therapy (DMT), which may be conducted in individual, group, or family formats and can be integrated into other therapeutic programs.

This chapter discusses the use of dance/movement therapy and how the therapeutic process can serve both as a bridge for contact and a vehicle for expressive communication for individuals with autism (ADTA, 2011). Particular emphasis is placed on DMT's unique facility for understanding, reflecting, and expanding nonverbal expression and how this can help those with autism to improve socialization and communication and to build body awareness and can enhance relational engagement. Supportive literature addressing concepts in neuroscience, social engagement theories, attachment, and infant research complements the discussion. Case illustrations are highlighted to provide concrete examples of these theoretical concepts.

Dance/Movement Therapy: Assumptions and Principles

According to the American Dance Therapy Association (ADTA, n.d.), DMT is known as "the psychotherapeutic use of movement to promote emotional, cognitive, physical, and social integration of individuals." DMT is practiced in a wide variety of settings supporting a range of populations and can be used with people of all cultural, racial, and ethnic groups.

Dance/movement therapists view movement of the body as both expressive and communicative and use it both as a method of assessing individuals and the mode for clinical intervention. It is based on the belief that there is a fundamental interconnection between the mind and body, underscoring the assumption that whatever is impacting the body will reciprocally impact the mind. Therefore, a core principle in DMT stresses that healthy overall functioning relies on the integration of both the mind and body (Levy, 2005). When there is a lack of mind–body integration, individuals may suffer from a variety of psychological disorders. Similarly, there is a foundational belief that examining one's movement vocabulary or range "opens a door to the study of patterns of early development, coping strategies, and personality configurations" (Kestenberg, Loman, Lewis, & Sossin, 1999, p. 2). An increased integration of one's body parts and awareness of others expands individuals' movement vocabulary, thus increasing their ability to communicate their needs and desires.

DMT focuses directly on movement behavior as it emerges out of the developed therapeutic relationship. Dance/movement therapy pioneer Marian Chace emphasized that "the therapeutic relationship is core to the meaning of movement structures that evolve between the dance therapist and those with whom he/she works and it is the interactive process that enables change" (cited in Fischer & Chaiklin, 1993, p. 138). Furthermore, because "movement is a universal means of communication" (Erfer, 1995, p. 196), it is an especially useful therapeutic approach with individuals with autism that can provide both a direct link to feelings and bridge a connection or relationship with others. Dance/movement therapists "have a unique facility for understanding, reflecting, and expanding nonverbal expressions that can help those with autism to improve socialization and communication, build body awareness, and can directly affect motor deficits" (ADTA, n.d). Further, because many children with autism spectrum disorders either have limited speech or remain nonverbal most of their life (Luyster, Kadlec, Carter, & Tager-Flusberg, 2008), movement can serve as the common language for building communication.

Dance/Movement Therapy and Autism Spectrum Disorders

There is much published literature dating back to the 1960s exploring the powerful therapeutic connections that have occurred between individuals with autism spectrum disorders through the process of dance/movement therapy (e.g., Adler, 1968; Cole, 1982; Erfer, 1995; Kalish, 1968; Loman, 1995; Siegel, 1973). Despite these long-standing discussions about DMT's positive therapeutic outcomes with the treatment of autism, few empirically based studies address the treatment of DMT within the context of broader evidenced-based practice. Much of the published and nonpublished literature in DMT and ASD is qualitative in nature (case studies) and occurred between a short- to midterm duration of treatment interval, making it difficult to examine long-term treatment outcomes (Merna, 2010). Yet in Merna's conceptual content analysis study examining this existing DMT and autism literature, results reported 1,084 treatment outcomes in the areas of social relatedness, communication, and restrictive, repetitive behaviors strongly suggesting that DMT can addresses the core deficits and clinical issues associated with an ASD diagnosis as defined by the American Psychiatric Association (2000). Merna indicates, "This result alone shows evidence that DMT has the ability to produce positive outcomes for nonverbal and preverbal children with ASD" (p. 176) and "provide a window into DMT's possible potential to become an evidence-based practice" (p. 174).

Current trends in neuroscience, social engagement theories, and infant research are also highlighting the importance of the inclusion of the body in therapy (Ogden, Minton, & Pain, 2006; Rothschild, 1999), underscoring the importance of treatment approaches that address relational interaction (Greenspan & Wieder, 1997, 1999; Schore, 2003). Both relational interaction and body integration are concepts that DMT has been practicing with children with autism spectrum disorders for decades (Adler, 1968; Baudino, 2010; Erfer, 1995, Kalish, 1968; Levy, 1988; Loman, 1995; Tortora, 2006).

Much of the dance/movement therapy treatment with autism takes a developmental and relational, rather than a behavioral, approach where the focus is on assisting the individual with ASD in rechoreographing developmental stages by "go[ing] back completely to the infantile developmental stages, working through them as the child is ready and capable of doing so" (Chace, 1993, p. 353). According to Loman (1995), "Even normal children in any phase of development may regress at times in order to sense the mastery in the previous phase" (p. 216). However, dance/movement therapy provides children with autism spectrum disorders "the opportunity to experience a "second chance" at development and, with the support and assistance from the dance/movement therapist, establish the developmental foundation for further social, emotional and cognitive growth" (Merna, 2010, p. 117).

Theoretical Foundation: Attunement, Mutual Regulation, and Expanding the Window of Tolerance

Kanner stated that children with autism "[shut] out anything that comes to [them] from the outside" (as cited in Erfer, 1995, p. 192). This makes communication extremely difficult, establishing the importance of incorporating movement as a method of communication. Beginning this communication involves the careful use of attunement to establish empathy and adjustment to develop trust (Kestenberg, as cited in Loman, 1995, p. 222), which facilitates the transition from inner to outer (environmental) stimuli.

Mirroring, Attunement, and Empathy

Through the use of a traditional dance/movement therapy technique called *mirroring* or *empathic reflection* (Chaiklin & Schmais, 1993), the therapist reflects individuals' body rhythms, movement patterns, or vocalizations to begin the process of relationship formation. The goal is to attune to clients where they are both physically and emotionally and to establish a trusting therapeutic movement relationship-building awareness of the self and other. This is particularly important for individuals with autism where there are core challenges in social interaction, imitation, and reciprocal relational engagement. Hadjikhani (2007) describes the importance of treatment approaches for autism "consisting in a training of imitative skill may be a valid way to develop not only imitation per se, but also socio-cognitive aspects in autism" (p. 160). However, according to Chaiklin and Schmais:

> There is a fine line between empathy on a movement level and mimicry. Mimicry involves duplicating the external shape of the movement without the emotional content that exists in the dynamics and in the subtle organization of the movement. . . . Empathy meant sharing the essence of all nonverbal expression resulting in . . . direct communication. (p. 86)

Therapeutic interactions that are not only imitating or reflecting back the movement action but are also attuning to children's emotional state meets them where they are and also sends the nonverbal message, "I hear you, I understand you, and it's okay." As more awareness of the self develops, those with autism can develop increased awareness of others and their surroundings. Recognizing and responding to another person, increasing eye contact, participating in shared experiences and engaging in shared focus, breaking through isolation, decreasing the interpersonal distance that is part of the social isolation, and developing trust are all treatment goals in dance/movement therapy with individuals with autism.

The process of moving with someone through the art of dance empathically connects the therapist with the individual with autism so that the experience of attunement can begin. This attunement is "a kinesthetic and emotional sensing of others" (Erskine, 1998, p. 236). By "knowing [the child's] rhythm, affect, and experience by metaphorically being in its skin . . . it goes beyond empathy to create a two-person experience of connectedness by providing a reciprocal affect and/or resonating response" (Erskine, p. 236). In dance/movement therapy, attunement is communicated not just by what is said but also by facial or body movements, signaling to children that their affect and needs are perceived, are significant, and make an impact on another (Devereaux, 2008).

To enter into this communication, Schore (2003) asserts that one must be psychobiologically attuned not so much to children's overt behavior as to the reflections of the rhythms of his internal state. According to Schore (2001), these affective attunements, both spontaneously and nonverbally, are "the moment-to-moment expressions of [one's] regulatory functions occur[ing] at levels beneath awareness" (p. 14).

Schore (2003) also stresses that attunement involves all of the senses and much also depends on sensitive attunement to sound, tone of voice, and the rhythms of speech. In addition, he also asserts the essential role of the occurrence of playful interactions between a dyad, where there is an amplification of excitement that occurs between both parties during the interactive play and then a capacity for each participant in the interaction to become centered again and self-contained in the presence of each other.

Because many of these attuned interactions occur on a nonverbal level, dance/movement therapy can be an ideal treatment intervention in supporting the development of empathy an experience that individuals with autism are lacking (Lombardo, Barnes, Wheelwright, & Baron-Cohen, 2007). This is done through relational dances and movement interactions such as trying on various body shapes, exaggerating or exploring various movement dynamics, and engaging in heightened moments of rhythmic synchrony. In essence, it is the interactive movement relationship that is essential in the dance/movement therapy treatment process. Later in this chapter, case illustrations highlight these important distinctions.

Self- and Mutual Regulation: Mutual Influences

The importance of an interactive cycle between two individuals continues to be highly explored in parent–infant research focusing on mutual/interactive regulation (e.g., Beebe & Lachmann, 1998; Brazelton, 1982; Stern, 1985; Tronick, 1980, 1998, 2003). During interactive moments poignant with affect, mother and baby help regulate and transform each other's internal and external worlds (Stern, Hofer, Haft, & Dore, 1985). The baby feels these experiences. At the same time the baby feels, the baby senses the feeling of the other. It is the sharing and *interactive/mutual regulation* during these times of shared moments where mother and child are attuned in a synchronistic nonverbal exchange (Stern, 1985). These shared experiences enhance the initial bond developed by the child and the mother. According to Beebe and Lachmann (1998), during these shared experiences "contingencies flow in both directions between partners. That is, the behavior of each partner is contingent upon (influenced by) that of the other" (p. 485).

This infant mental health literature is significant to understanding the mutuality and importance of the interactive movement relationship between the dance/movement therapist and the individual with autism. Fischer and Chaiklin (1993) discuss:

> The dance therapist in the role of participant observer must have a clear realization and responsibility for his or her own dance in relation to the other individual. Just as the tension of any existing anxiety present in the mother induces anxiety within the infant, such tension in the therapist will affect the interaction. The meeting in movement of the therapist and the client assumes that both are part

of the dialogue, even though one is identified as helper and the other as needing help (p. 139).

To illustrate this, I describe a personal experience as a dance/movement therapist in interaction with a child and its influence on me.

As I began to expand my practice into working with children who had been diagnosed on the autism spectrum, I found myself seeking moments of relational contact that I was so used to during times of interactive engagement through the dance/movement process with non-ASD clients. However, in working with my clients on the autism spectrum, I often found that these moments were fleeting. I discovered that reciprocal moments of engagement through eye contact or spontaneous initiated gestures became critical.

I vividly remember a particular time during a dance/movement therapy group of children with autism spectrum disorders in a public school. All of these children had limited verbal language and were fairly lower functioning. Often times, there was very limited eye contact, and the focus of the session was to connect the children to their bodies, to build body awareness, and to support them in building relational connections with others. As we were engaging in a movement warm-up, stretching and expanding our limbs out into the space, carving out space around us, tapping and defining our body parts, I simultaneously labeled the names of our body parts. As I identified "head, ears, toes, knees, elbows, fingers" the children began to discover their own body part connections. Erfer (1995) asserts "naming body parts as they are touched and moved provides a cognitive link to the physical actions" (p. 201). As this occurred, we began to spontaneously twist our bodies from side to side. I mirrored this movement development and encouraged the group to expand the twist. As we did this, I noticed the child to my left, one who often was engaged in self-stimulatory, repetitive, restrictive, behavior such as flapping her hands or jumping up and down. She was typically relationally disconnected and minimally communicative. I caught her eye as we were twisting side to side moving in opposite directions. We would twist away from each other, then toward each other, and then back again. The moments of twisting toward each other appeared to enliven her. It was clear that she was actually "seeing" me. We were engaging in a dyadic dance. At that moment, I reached my hands out as if to signal some direct physical contact with her (like a "high five") action, and she took me up on this offer, meeting my hand with hers in a spontaneous high five but still fixated on my gaze and smiling from ear to ear. I then guided the group in expanding this movement and invited the group to "say hello to the person next to you," at which point she twisted away from me and then back to me again, raising her hand in the high-five gesture, meeting my hand with hers in physical contact and then uttering the word "Hi."

It was during this interactional exchange that I was reminded not only of the power of movement but also of my own embodied sense of the impact of mutual engagement with these children.

When emotional energy is exchanged between two people, their internal worlds resonate with each other. Lewis, Amini, and Lannon (2000) refer to this phenomenon as *limbic resonance*. Limbic resonance allows two people to tune into another's inner world. In the most growth-enhancing environments, good responses get mirrored and the child replies by creating a similar response. During this dyadic dance, the child and the therapist are together in a state of coregulation of affect. As it gets more complex, children are less dependent on the therapist and further are able to develop the ability to self-regulate. Lewis et al. (2000) refer to this synchronistic exchange as limbic regulation where as the limbic brains in dyadic connections are jointly or coregulating each other.

In dance/movement therapy, the therapist serves as "a catalyst, gradually assisting in the expansion and elaboration of the patient's movements until they reach full expressivity—yet always watching the patient's emotional and kinesthetic reactions to this change and adjusting their empathic movements accordingly" (Merna, 2010, p. 111).

The previous discussion highlighting interactive components of the therapeutic process is a clear reminder that healthy development is an interactive cycle that *requires* relationship with the other and relationship with the self. Both are essential. Therefore, we can assume that not only does the child with ASD impact the therapist, who then can make careful movement adjustments to amplify and expand the expressive communicative gestures, but also the therapist can then assist the child in modulating states of hyper- or hypo-arousal by attending to each client's "Window of Tolerance." This is discussed in the next section.

Window of Tolerance

Ogden et al. (2006) identify a theory of modulating arousal in clients who are experiencing trauma referred to as the window of tolerance (p. 26). Ogden et al. see significant application of this work with children with autism spectrum disorders. They discuss that we all have an "optimal arousal zone" where our nervous system is neither overactivated (hyper-aroused) or underactivated (hypo-aroused). We help our clients by working within the optimal arousal zone:

> When hyper-aroused, clients experience too much arousal to process information effectively ... and can be tormented by body sensations. But when hypo-aroused, clients suffer another kind of torment stemming from a dearth of emotion and sensation.... (p. 26)

Dance/movement therapists work to assist children with autism to regulate their nervous system from falling between the two extremes of arousal called the window of tolerance (p. 27) through interactive regulation and by channeling stimulatory behavior into expressive communication:

> When clients are working within a window of tolerance, information received from both internal and external environments can be integrated. They can continually process the ongoing barrage of sensory information while assimilating prior input. (Ogden et al., 2006, p. 27)

An important distinction in the dance/movement therapy approach is that DMTs observe movement gestures from children with autism, including repetitive, restrictive, or self-stimulatory behaviors, as communicative expressions. Therefore, through the use of mirroring and empathic reflection, rather than encouraging the disengagement of a particular stereotyped pattern (trying to stop it), the dance/movement therapist may initially begin to kinesthetically attune to these gestures and then work to channel these movements into healthier interactively regulated movement sequences. Chace (1993) discusses that "you work with the autistic person's natural movement, enlarging them, broadening them- yet taking the leadership in movement from the patient" (p. 353).

Because it is characteristic that individuals with autism engage in ritualistic, repetitive, and stereotypical movements including restricted patterns in space (e.g., pacing in a circle), rocking, and perseveration on one body part (e.g., flapping arms or wiggling fingers in front of the eyes) (Torrance, 2003; Tortora, 2006), examining these actions as communication signals reflecting the perspective of the three zones of arousal is a valuable tool for dance/movement therapy intervention. Restrictive, repetitive, or self-stimulatory movements act like a barrier for these children from engaging with others within the external environment by either keeping them stuck in their own self-stimulation or used to avoid contact with others (Duggan, 1978; Parteli, 1995). Parteli suggests that these stereotyped movements are forms of expressive communication, and thus it is possible to use these movements to build a connection with children and assist them in slowly breaking down the aforementioned barrier. DMTs focus on increasing children's movement repertoire by expanding the repetitive, restricted movement patterns into expressive dances in turn provides a broader range of responses that children can use to communicate and cope within their environment. As this happens the children can slowly begin to expand away from their private worlds into the outside environment to allow a relationship to form.

An example of this is described in the case of Jack, an 8-year-old child diagnosed with ASD who worked with me in once-a-week, 45-minute dance/movement therapy sessions. He could often become overstimulated by environmental stimuli and responded to this activation in his nervous system through hyper-arousal. His body communicated this hyper-arousal through self-stimulatory, repetitive movements and gestures, typically via jumping up and down quickly, clapping his hands, and making audible "ahhhh" sounds. This quickly escalated by jumping around the space and physically crashing into others or objects in the room that on many occasions became dangerous, not only to Jack's own physical safety but also to the other children and adults.

These movement presentations were signals that Jack had moved beyond his window of tolerance, out of his optimal arousal zone, and was moving into a hyper-aroused state. I used his movements first to attune with his body state and coregulated his experience through slowing down my own body so that a collaboratively improvised dance developed through the dyadic non-verbal exchanges in the movement process. This dance assisted Jack in modulating his repetitive movement patterns and empowered him to activate his own regulatory capacities. As I engaged Jack in an attuned movement communicative dialogue, the once self-stimulatory movement developed into a dance of stop and go, allowing Jack to initiate the verbal command of stop and go and thus to take full mastery over his own movement impulses. Most importantly, the initial self-stimulatory, hyper-aroused, repetitive movement sequences that kept him from engaging with others instead became the direct route for connective and expressive social communication.

Dance/Movement Therapy in Group Treatment

Dance/movement therapist Greer-Paglia's (2006) Harvard University study compared data collected on students with autism participating in creative dance and "circle time," a typical classroom activity with similar social objectives, to explore social competence. The results of her study not only suggested that creative dance was beneficial as a social intervention for children with autism but also discovered that in a relatively brief amount of time (12 weeks) the performance gap in social competence between verbal and nonverbal students with ASD was smaller in the creative dance condition than in the circle time condition. Greer-Paglia's findings provide a strong supportive framework for the distinct differences that the dance/movement therapy group approach provides children with ASD, especially within an educational system.

Group dance/movement therapy sessions typically begin with a warm-up. This is an opportunity not only for physical warming of the body but also for the therapist to assess the emotional needs of the clients, to establish direct communication, and to build a sense of group unity and trust. Marian Chace described the warm-up phase as the "testing period" (Levy, 2005, p. 25) where comfort between clients could be explored. Groups often begin through facilitation in a circle formation so that group communication can occur easily and a therapeutic container or "holding environment" (Winnicott, 1971) is developed. Next, a period of broadening, expanding, and clarifying movement actions continues during a period of theme development. For children with autism spectrum disorders this is a time for "working on concepts, developing themes...practicing motor skills, and developing socialization" (Erfer, 1995, p. 201). During this portion of the group process, a strong emphasis is placed on movements that assist the group in joining together and building connections on a movement level (moving closer together, reaching toward each other) and engaging in synchronistic rhythmic action. Group rhythmic action provides a sense of organization to the group (Levy, 2005). With children on the autism spectrum, repetition and predictable movement sequences can assist with the establishment of trust, can gain mastery over movement, and can build movement repertoire. During the closure portion of the session, the primary goal is to regulate the body, to integrate their movement experiences, and to assist them in staying within their optimal arousal zone. The dance/movement therapist incorporates and models ways to allow the body to become relaxed and settle after expansive movement. Chace described this stage as "a supportive closure that allow[s] patients to leave with some sense of satisfaction and resolve" (Levy, 2005, p. 26).

The next section describes a group dance/movement therapy session that occurred with children with ASD in a special education setting. The example explores a typical group that occurred with approximately 5–6 children all diagnosed with ASD. This session occurred after several months of weekly treatment and already established therapeutic relationships with the group facilitator. Classroom teachers and classroom aides also participated fully in the group process. Their participation not only assisted in providing additional behavioral and adult support but also served as a simultaneous opportunity for the children and the teachers to build healthy social relationships. Specific interventions are identified where dance/movement therapy supported the children in enhancing body awareness, expanding emotional expressiveness, and building greater relational connections with others.

The Dance/Movement Therapy Group: A Case Example

As I open the door of the room, I am immediately greeted with smiles, "hellos," and some hugs. This indicates to me that the children are establishing a relationship, as they are now relationally greeting me, and initiating contact. As I set up my music, the children are moving with excitement that it is time for dance therapy. They slip their shoes off and meet me in the center of the room where there is space large enough for dancing and expression. I greet them all with smiles and assess if we should begin on the floor (to help ground them) or if they are ready to begin standing. I examine their movement energy, their engagement in reciprocal eye contact, and any verbalization that is present. I decide to invite them to begin standing, and we make a circle formation. I place spot markers on the floor that define their personal space within the circle and provide a visual tool to build spatial awareness.

I assist the children through a movement warm-up by supporting them in reconnecting to their bodies and helping them identify how their bodies can move and are connected. We greet our toes, fingers, knees, elbows, and other parts of ourselves and experiment with how we want to move. I scan the room and acknowledge any differences in how each child is exploring different body parts, sending the message that individual movement expression is invited and encouraged. All of this is done with the support of rhythmic music to help in organizing the group and provide some unity. It is this moment where I sense that the group has begun to attune to each other. I suggest that we begin to greet each other by encouraging eye contact around the circle and simple "hello" waving gestures. I notice that they are doing this greeting gesture in their own expressive way. I take this as a cue for each of them to have their own moment of individual expression and to further assess each individual child's particular need level. The children are encouraged to do a solo dance in the center of the circle as their classmates and teachers cheer them on. One by one, each of the children goes into the middle of the circle while the rest of the group either follows how the solo dancer is moving or we add an accompanied rhythmic sound (such as a clap or a knee tap) to keep the group connected. We chant together, "Johnny can move however he wants," acknowledging by name the person dancing in the center. In this group, it appears to be a liberating experience that the children have choices, expressivity, and creativity and can decide how they want to greet each other and how their body wants to move for that particular day. Occasionally, I notice that the open expressive time can be too much for some children, so I attend to this by regulating any hyper-aroused state by lowering my voice, bringing my body to a lower level, or adding a strong downbeat as an organizing tool. I am careful to attend not just to the children's individual movements but to the group's energy as a whole. During extensive periods of exertion of high intensity and energetic bursts, I am conscious to follow this with modulated movements that are grounding and containing (e.g., tapping body parts, holding hands in a circle and moving it in and out, or bringing the movement to the ground to explore the low level).

With children who have difficulties being in relationship with others, such as those with autism spectrum disorders, initiating can be difficult. Modeling different ways to move, expanding their repertoire, and encouraging creativity has allowed the children to discover that they have choices too. I've noticed over time that their expression has expanded; they are more creative, spontaneous, and joyful as they engage in their solo dances and observe how different each other is in their movement repertoire. Today I am surprised as Matthew spontaneously wiggles his hips from side to side during his solo dance rather than engaging in his typical stereotyped movement of running around in the circle. I comment on this, recognizing that we have seen a different part of him. He responds to my acknowledgment by expanding his hip movement into a spin around on one leg. It is clear that his broadening range of movement is a reflection of increased awareness of his body. His expansive movement repertoire is also giving him more possibilities of being in the environment rather than staying within restrictive, repetitive patterns.

The session continues as we engage further in moving together as one group in synchrony, a powerful experience that bonds us. As we are moving together in the same rhythm to the percussive music, we can't help but feel connected, relational, and together. We are swept up with the experience of joining in a synchronistic dance together. Erfer (1995) notes that "rhythm is a meaningful organizer of impulses" (p. 201). Depending on the need level of the children in the moment, I vary what happens next from session to session. At times I might support them in taking on extended leadership, exploring and moving out into the space around us, or become engaged in some imagery that will only deepen our connection to each other and to their body. We may work with defining our personal space around us or on building impulse and body control with an expressive game of "freeze dance." We may connect our movements to verbalizations, feelings, or images. However, today, I invite the group to change the circle formation into a line to create a human train. I am sensing that the group is unified today, yet there is need for individual expression. I encourage David to start as our leader, guiding the group around the room wherever he wants to go. I specifically choose David to begin, as I noticed during the solo dances that he appeared to be struggling with maintaining focus when another child was in the middle and wandered away from the circle several times. He is thrilled with this opportunity and meanders throughout the space, first staying within the circular pathway but, with encouragement, breaking out of the circle formation into the space. He is experimenting with how his own movement choices impact the group. Spontaneously, David speeds up the tempo of his leadership and visibly looks behind him to see how the group responds to this conscious change. The group responds to this intervention by mirroring and following this change in pace. It is an incredible moment where David has mastery over his own impulses and they become channeled into expressive communicative movements toward the entire group.

Oftentimes, the teachers will tell me during consultations about a particular theme that they are working on in the classroom, such as "opposites" or "directions" or "animal imagery." Moving with these themes is a wonderful opportunity for the children to embody their learning: to deepen their cognitive understanding of the concept on a body level and to experientially explore it. We'll move "opposites" of big/small, slow/fast, up/down, in/out, forward/backward. All this time, they are learning, however, most of all they are enhancing their expression and channeling their feelings.

As the session comes to an end, I bring out a large tactile stretch band in a circular shape to bring them back to the circle formation help the children reconnect to their own sensory experiences. The use of props (stretch fabrics, scarves, balls, and music) during sessions serves as a connective tool—as a less threatening way to bridge connection in the group, from client to client, therapist to client, client to therapist, or client to imagination and exploration. These tools can also assist in providing a means of contact between therapist and client and also as a way "to express feelings and thoughts, which create an outlet for imagination and exploration" (Baudino, 2010, p. 126). Connective tools also serve as useful assessment tools: they evoke interest in the children, induce movement, and divert attention away from the internal stimuli (Mendelsohn, 1999).

During the closure portion of the session, I change the tone of the environment by putting on slower, soothing music. I incorporate and model ways to allow the body to become relaxed and settle after expansive movement. The tactile circular stretch band aids in defining the emotional holding environment that was established and allows the children to push against the boundaries of space within a safe container. The children explore the edges of the space around them and take some risks and venture out beyond the space in the circle to press their body against the fabric in another location within the circle. This exploration time is encouraged. I am assisting them in feeling the flexibility of the therapeutic container while they are engaged in sensory experiences. Staying within the contained tactile space, I encourage the children to find their way down to the ground, as a literal experience of landing at the end of the session. Together, we lean backward with the support of the fabric and feel ourselves held by the group. It is at this point of the session that I'm in awe. The children seem settled and connected to themselves and each other and have allowed themselves to become passive and relaxed (an experience the teachers tell me doesn't happen often in the classroom). At the end of the session, a teacher's aide says to me, after witnessing the transformation from the beginning to the end of the session, "It is as if they have become alive." As I gather my music and props, I am then reminded that I too am mutually influenced and swept up by the connective energy.

Discussion

After a year of weekly DMT sessions, teachers commented on the children's ability to have more awareness of themselves and others through increased eye contact, increased verbalization, and enhanced identification and awareness of specific body parts. In addition, gross motor coordination expanded and was reflected in movements such as crawling, jumping, swinging, pushing, rocking, and reaching. Furthermore, the sessions assisted directly in regulating classroom behavior, channeling and containing outbursts, and decreasing acting out and anxiety. For example, one student who could initially become highly hyper-aroused following any kind of contact (e.g., eye contact, holding hands, verbal prompting) now is fully initiating "partner dances" during sessions, moving together with an adult with the connection with a dancing scarf, and initiating contact with verbal greetings and gesturing toward others to hold hands. This was an example that the children appeared to have an increased ability to tolerate physical and relational contact with adult and peers for an expanded period of time.

The children began to demonstrate an expansion of body control and enhanced focus and attention. For example, during a "freeze dancing" exploration, the children more easily followed internal cues to stop and freeze their body into creative shapes rather than having limited awareness of external cues such as music, drumbeats, or verbal prompting.

In addition to the increased body and relational awareness, the sessions also assisted the integration of their cognitive learning, as the movement process was also used to expand and enhance their academic skills. (i.e., abstract concepts of "in/out" "above/below" "over/under" were explored through the movement process so the children could embody these concepts, verbalize them, and then translate them further in other subjects). Some children explored more direct connections between body parts and their functionality and experientially explored this relationship—for example, identifying internal organs such as heart and lungs during the closure of the session so they could attend to their own body's natural built-in coping skills to modulate arousal. For the higher-functioning children, more abstract concepts were explored such as identification and exploration of specific feeling states and differentiation between their own feeling state and that of their peers'. The children's reflections back and mirroring of embodied feeling states of their peers revealed many students' increased capacity for empathy; something that is a significant gain within the autism population.

Conclusion

In summary, dance/movement therapy provides a vehicle for the therapist and client to engage in a movement dialogue through the body. During this process, the client's movement presentations are viewed as communicative expressions that are then reflected, amplified, and channeled into relational dances. Current research in neuroscience and infant research supports the inclusion of the body and relational experience for the development of a child's brain. Attuned communication leads to mutually regulated movement dances that assist clients in expanding their window of tolerance and staying within the present moment without engaging in self-stimulatory behavior. This can be done in both a group and individual context.

As discussed in the case illustrations, dance/movement therapy's embodied exploration of interactive engagement within the sessions helps children with autism spectrum disorders to increase their capacity for empathy and social connections. Through the establishment of a trusting therapeutic relationship, the children had an increased ability to develop more awareness of themselves and others, increased eye contact, increased verbalization, and enhanced identification and awareness of specific body parts emerged through expressive movement experiences through attuned experiences.

References

Adler, J. (1968). The study of an autistic child. In the *Annual proceedings of the American Dance Therapy third annual conference* (pp. 43–48). Columbia, MD: ADTA.

American Dance Therapy Association. (ADTA). (2011). *What is dance/movement therapy*. Retrieved on April 26, 2011 from http://www.adta.org/Default.aspx?pageId=378213

American Dance Therapy Association. (ADTA). (n.d.) *Dance/Movement therapy & autism*. Retrieved on April 26, 2011 from http://www.adta.org/Default.aspx?pageId=378243

American Psychiatric Association. (APA). (2000). *Diagnostic and statistical manual of mental disorders* (4th ed., text rev.). Washington, DC: Author.

Autism Speaks. (2010). Autism: What is it? Retrieved August 21, 2010 from http://www.autismspeaks.org/whatisit/index.php

Baudino, L. (2010). Autism spectrum disorder: A case of misdiagnosis. *American Journal of Dance Therapy, 32,* 113–129.

Beebe, B., & Lachmann, F. M. (1998). Co-constructing inner and relational processes. Self and mutual regulation in infant research and adult treatment. *Psychoanalytic Psychology, 15*(4), 480–516.

Brazelton, T. B. (1982). Joint regulation of neonate-parent behavior. In E. Tronick (Ed.), *Social interchanges in infancy: Effect, cognition, and communication* (pp. 7–22). Baltimore, MD: University Park Press.

Chace, M. (1993). Audio taped discussion: Body image. In S. Sandel, S. Chaiklin, & A. Lohn (Eds.), *Foundations of dance/movement therapy: The life and work of Marian Chace* (pp. 352–364). Columbia, MD: The Marian Chace Memorial Fund of the American Dance Therapy Association.

Chaiklin, S., & Schmais, C. (1993). The Chace approach to dance therapy. In S. Sandel, S. Chaiklin, & A. Lohn (Eds.), *Foundations of dance/movement therapy: The life and work of Marian Chace* (pp. 75–97). Columbia, MD: The Marian Chace Memorial Fund of the American Dance Therapy Association.

Cole, I. (1982). Movement negotiations with an autistic child. *Arts in Psychotherapy, 9*(1), 49–53.

Devereaux, C. (2008). Untying the knots: Dance/movement therapy with a family exposed to domestic violence. *American Journal of Dance Therapy, 30*(2), 58–70.

Duggan, D. (1978). Goals and methods in dance therapy with severely multiply handicapped children. *American Journal of Dance Therapy, 2*(1), 31–34.

Erfer, T. (1995). Treating autism in public schools. In F. Levy (Ed.), *Dance and other expressive therapies when words are not enough* (pp. 191–211). New York: Routledge.

Erskine, R. (1998). Attunement and involvement: Therapeutic responses to relational needs. *International Journal of Psychotherapy, 3*(3), 235–244.

Fischer, J., & Chaiklin, S. (1993). Meeting in movement: The work of therapist and client. In S. Sandel, S. Chaiklin, & A. Lohn (Eds.), *Foundations of dance/movement therapy: The life and work of Marian Chace* (pp. 136–153). Columbia, MD: The Marian Chace Memorial Fund of the American Dance Therapy Association.

Greenspan, S., & Wieder, S. (1997). Developmental patterns and outcomes in infants and children with disorders in relating and communicating: A chart review of 200 cases of children with Autistic Spectrum Diagnoses. *Journal of Developmental and Learning Disorders, 1*(1), 87–141.

Greenspan, S., & Wieder, S. (1999). A functional developmental approach to autism spectrum disorders. *Journal of the Association for Persons with Severe Handicaps, 24*(3), 147–161.

Greer-Paglia, K. (2006). *Examining the effects of creative dance on social competence in children with autism: A hierarchical linear growth modeling approach.* Unpublished doctoral dissertation, Harvard University, Cambridge, MA.

Hadjikhani, N. (2007). Mirror neuron system and autism. In P. Carlisle (Ed.), *Progress in autism research* (pp. 151–166). New York: Nova Science Publishers.

Jensen, V. K., & Sinclair, L. (2002). Treatment of autism in young children: Behavioral intervention and applied behavior analysis. *Infants & Young Children, 14*(4), 42–52.

Kalish, B. (1968). Body movement therapy for autistic children: A description and discussion of basic concepts. *Proceedings of the American Dance Therapy Association Third Annual Conference*, 49–59.

Kestenberg, J. A., Loman, S., Lewis, P., & Sossin, K. (1999). *The meaning of movement.* Netherlands: Gordon and Breach Publishers.

Koegel, L., Koegel, R., Fredeen, R., & Gengoux, G. (2008). Naturalistic behavioral approaches to treatment. In K. Chawarska, A. Klin, & F. Volkmar (Eds.), *Autism spectrum disorders in infants and toddlers* (pp. 207–242). New York: Guilford Press.

Levy, F. (1988). *Dance movement therapy: A healing art.* Reston, VA: American Alliance for Health, Physical Education, Recreation, and Dance.

Levy, F. (2005). *Dance movement therapy: A healing art* (rev. ed.). Reston, VA: American Alliance for Health, Physical Education, Recreation, and Dance.

Levy, S., Mandell, D., Merhar, S., Ittenbach, R., & Pinto-Martin, J. (2003). Use of complementary and alternative medicine among children recently diagnosed with autism spectrum disorder. *Developmental and Behavior Pediatrics, 24*(6), 418–423.

Lewis T., Amini, F., & Lannon, R. (2000). *The general theory of love.* New York: Random House.

Loman, S. (1995). The case of Warren: A KMP approach to autism. In F. Levy, J. Fried, & F. Leventhal (Eds.), *Dance and other expressive art therapies: When words are not enough* (pp. 213–223). New York: Routledge.

Lombardo, M. V., Barnes, J. L., Wheelwright, S. J., & Baron-Cohen, S. (2007). Self-referential cognition and empathy in autism. *PLoS ONE, 2*(9), e883. doi:10.1371/journal.pone.0000883

Luyster, R., Kadlec, M., Carter, A., & Tager-Flusberg, H. (2008). Language assessment and development in toddlers with autism spectrum disorders. *Journal of Autism and Developmental Disorders, 38,* 1426–1438.

Mendelsohn, J. (1999). Dance/movement therapy with hospitalized children. *American Journal of Dance Therapy, 21*(1), 65–80.

Merna, M. (2010). Compiling the evidence for dance/movement therapy with children with autism spectrum disorders: A systematic literature review. Unpublished master's thesis, Drexel University, Philadelphia.

National Institute of Neurological Disorders and Stroke. (NINDS). (2008). Retrieved January 30, 2008 from http://www.ninds.nih.gov/

Ogden, P., Minton, K., & Pain, C. (2006). Window of tolerance: The capacity for modulating arousal. In P. Ogden & K. Pain (Eds.), *Trauma and the body* (pp. 26–40). New York: Norton.

Ortega, J. (2010). Applied behavior analytic intervention for autism in early childhood: Meta-analysis, meta-regression and dose-response meta-analysis of multiple outcomes. *Clinical Psychology Review, 30,* 387–399.

Parteli, L. (1995). Aesthetic listening: Contributions of dance/movement therapy to the psychic understanding of motor stereotypes and distortions in autism and psychosis in childhood and adolescence. *Arts in Psychotherapy, 22*(3), 241–247.

Rothschild, B. (1999). *The body remembers: The psychophysiology of trauma and trauma treatment.* New York: Norton.

Rogers, S., & Vismara, L. (2008). Evidence-based comprehensive treatments for early autism. *Journal of Clinical Child and Adolescent Psychology, 37*(1), 8–38.

Schore, A. N. (2001). Effects of a secure attachment relationship on right brain development, affect regulation, and infant mental health. *Infant Mental Health Journal, 22,* 7–66.

Schore, A. N. (2003). *Affect regulation and the repair of the self.* New York: Norton.

Schreibman, L. (2000). Intensive behavioral/psychoeducational treatments for autism: Research needs and future directions. *Journal of Autism and Developmental Disorders, 30*(5), 373–378.

Siegel, E. (1973). Movement therapy with autistic children. *Psychoanalytic Review, 60*(1), 141–149.

Smith, T. (2008). Empirically supported and unsupported treatments for autism spectrum disorders. *Scientific Review of Mental Health Practice, 6*(1), 3–10.

Smith, T. (1999). Outcome of early intervention for children with autism. *Clinical Psychology: Science and Practice, 6,* 33–49.

Smith, T., Mozingo, D., Mruzek, D., & Zarcone, J. (2007). Applied behavior analysis in the treatment of autism. In E. Hollander & E. Anagnostou (Eds.), *Clinical manual for the treatment of autism* (pp. 153–177). Washington, DC: American Psychiatric Publishing.

Stern, D. (1985). *Interpersonal world of the infant.* New York: Basic Books, Inc.

Stern, D., Hofer, L., Haft, W., & Dore, J. (1985). Affect attunement: The sharing of feeling states between mother and infant by means of inter-modal fluency. In T. Field & N. Fox (Eds.), *Social perception in infants* (pp. 249–268). New York: Ablex Publishing.

Torrance, J. (2003). Autism, aggression and developing a therapeutic contract. *American Journal of Dance Therapy, 25*(2), 97–109.

Tortora, S. (2006). *The dancing dialogue.* Baltimore, MD: Paul H. Brookes Publishing.

Tronick, E. (1980). On the primacy of social skills. In D. B. Sawin, L. O. Walker, & J. H. Penticuff (Eds.), *The exceptional infant: Vol. 4. Psychosocial risks in infant-environmental transactions* (pp. 144–158). New York: Brunner/Mazel.

Tronick, E. (1998). Dyadically expanded states of consciousness and the process of therapeutic change. *Infant Mental Health Journal, 19,* 290–299.

Tronick, E. Z. (2003). Things still to be done on the still-face effect. *Infancy, 4*(4), 475–482.

Winnicott, D. W. (1971). *Playing and reality.* London: Tavistock/Routledge.

Index